IMMUNOBIOLOGY OF PROTEINS AND PEPTIDES IV

T-CELL RECOGNITION AND ANTIGEN PRESENTATION

ADVANCES IN EXPERIMENTAL MEDICINE AND BIOLOGY

Recent Volumes in this Series

Volume 218
CORONAVIRUSES
Edited by Michael M. C. Lai and Stephen A. Stohlman

Volume 219
REGULATION OF OVARIAN AND TESTICULAR FUNCTION
Edite by Virendra B. Mahesh, Dharam S. Dhindsa, Everett Anderson, and Satya P. Kalra

Volume 220
CONTINUOUS TRANSCUTANEOUS MONITORING
Edited by Albert Huch, Renate Huch, and Gosta Rooth

Volume 221
MOLECULAR MECHANISMS OF NEURONAL RESPONSIVENESS
Edited by Yigal H. Ehrlich, Robert H. Lenox, Elizabeth Kornecki, and William O. Berry

Volume 222
OXYGEN TRANSPORT TO TISSUE X
Edited by Masaji Mochizuki, Carl R. Honig, Tomiyasu Koyama, Thomas K. Goldstick, and Duane F. Bruley

Volume 223
UREMIC TOXINS
Edited by Severin Ringoir, Raymond Vanholder, and Shaul G. Massry

Volume 224
UROGENITAL INFECTIONS
Edited by Amedeo Bondi, Donald D. Stieritz, John M. Campos, and Linda Ann Miller

Volume 225
IMMUNOBIOLOGY OF PROTEINS AND PEPTIDES IV: T-CELL RECOGNITION AND ANTIGEN PRESENTATION
Edited by M. Zouhair Atassi

A Continuation Order Plan is available for this series. A continuation order will bring delivery of each new volume immediately upon publication. Volumes are billed only upon actual shipment. For further information please contact the publisher.

IMMUNOBIOLOGY OF PROTEINS AND PEPTIDES IV

T-CELL RECOGNITION AND ANTIGEN PRESENTATION

Edited by

M. Zouhair Atassi

Baylor College of Medicine
Houston, Texas

PLENUM PRESS • NEW YORK AND LONDON

Library of Congress Cataloging in Publication Data

International Symposium on the Immunobiology of Proteins and Peptides (4th: 1986: Las Vegas, Nev.)
Immunobiology of proteins and peptides IV: T-cell recognition and antigen presentation / edited by M. Zouhair Atassi.
p. cm. (Advances in experimental medicine and biology, v. 225)
"Proceedings of the Fourth International Symposium on the Immunology of Proteins and Peptides, held November 30–December 4, 1986, in Las Vegas, Nevada"—T.p. verso.
"Sponsors of the symposium, Abbott Laboratories... [et al.]"—T.p. verso.
Includes bibliographies and index.
ISBN-13: 978-1-4684-5444-4 e-ISBN-13: 978-1-4684-5442-0
DOI: 10.1007/978-1-4684-5442-0
1. T cells—Congresses. 2. T cells—Receptors—Congresses. 3. Antigen presenting cells—Congresses. 4. Antigens—Congresses. I. Atassi, M. Z. II. Abbott Laboratories. III. Title. IV. Title: T-cell recognition and antigen presentation V. Series. [DNLM: 1. Antigen-Presenting Cells—immunology—congresses. 2. Antigens, Immune Response—immunology—congresses. 3. Lymphocytes—immunology—congresses. W1 AD559 v.225 (p) / QW 568 I613 1986i]
QR185.8.T2I58 1986 87-29231
612'.118222—dc19 CIP

Proceedings of the Fourth International Symposium on the Immunobiology of Proteins and Peptides, held November 30–December 4, 1986, in Las Vegas, Nevada

Scientific Council of the Symposium

M. Z. Atassi, Chairman
H. L. Bachrach
E. Benjamini
D. Morrison
G. S. Bixler, Jr., Meeting Secretary
N. J. Calvanico, General Secretary

Major sponsors of the Symposium

Abbott Laboratories
Amgen
Merck Sharp and Dohme Research Laboratories
National Aeronautics and Space Administration
Office of Naval Research
United States Army Medical Research and Development Command

The following organizations also contributed to the Symposium:

Smith Kline and French Laboratories
Pharmacia
Fisher Scientific Company
Upjohn

Softcover reprint of the hardcover 1st edition 1987
A Division of Plenum Publishing Corporation
233 Spring Street, New York, N.Y. 10013

SCIENTIFIC COUNCIL OF THE SYMPOSIUM

M.Z. Atassi, Chairman
H.L. Bachrach
E. Benjamini
D. Morrison
G.S. Bixler, Jr., Meeting Secretary
N.J. Calvanico, General Secretary

THE FOLLOWING ORGANIZATIONS WERE THE MAJOR SPONSORS OF THE SYMPOSIUM

Abbott Laboratories
Amgen
Merck Sharp and Dohme Research Laboratories
National Aeronautics and Space Administration
Office of Naval Research
United States Army Medical Research and Development Command

THE FOLLOWING ORGANIZATION ALSO CONTRIBUTED TO THE SYMPOSIUM

Smith Kline and French Laboratories
Pharmacia
Fisher Scientific Company
Upjohn

PREFACE

This symposium was established in 1976 for the purpose of bringing together once every two or three years, active investigators in the forefront of contemporary immunology, to present their findings and to discuss their significance in the light of current concepts and to identify important new directions of investigation. The founding of the symposium was stimulated by the achievement of major breakthroughs in the understanding of the immune recognition of proteins and peptides. We believed that these breakthroughs will lead to the creation of a new generation of peptides which should have enormous potential in biological, therapeutic and basic applications. This anticipated explosion has finally occurred and many applications of these peptides are now being realized.

The main symposia topics of the fourth symposium were: T-cell recognition of proteins, structure and function of the T-cell receptor, presentation of protein antigens, recycling and activation of membrane receptor molecules, Ir-gene control of T-cell responses and methods of cell separation. The molecular features recognized by antibodies on proteins were the first immune recognition sites to be localized and confirmed by synthetic peptides. The complete antigenic structures of several proteins have been defined, and individual antigenic sites have been described on many more proteins. More recently, major breakthroughs have been reported in the immune recognition of proteins by T cells. Now, the complete T-cell recognition profiles of several proteins and a few more individual T sites on some proteins have been localized. Many of these molecules are discussed in this volume.

The diversity of antibody specificity occupied center stage in immunology for over three decades. The diversity in T-cell specificity and its understanding in molecular terms had to await the advent of the recent powerful tools of molecular biology. In this volume, the structure of the T-cell receptor and its relationship to immune recognition by T cells are discussed.

Having acquired a great deal of knowledge about protein molecular features that are recognized by antibodies and by T-cells, it has become feasible, using precise molecular tools to investigate the first phases of recognition by the immune system. For a long time, it has been believed, and many experiments were so designed to show, that the first critical steps of immune recognition involved internalization and degredation of the protein by the antigen-presenting cells and then the reappearance of protein fragments on the surface of the antigen-presenting cells which then present these fragments to the T-cells. Thus, the fragments constitute the target of recognition. However, in the last 5-6 years, a small, greatly outnumbered group of investigators have reported studies that would suggest that the accessory cells present protein antigen in intact form to the T-cell. In other words presentation is independent of processing. In this volume, proponents of both schools of thought present some of their findings and viewpoints. It has also been suggested recently that antigen presentation may not be entirely unrelated to other membrane-mediated cellular activation phenomena. The resemlance, if any, of these systems to immune recognition is, therefore, examined, and the latest concepts of recycling and activation of membrane receptor molecules are discussed in this volume.

The interaction of cells and molecules which generate an immune response are controlled and regulated at various steps in the pathway. Manipulation and therapeutic exploitation of the immune system cannot be obtained without detailed understanding of these intricate networks of recognition and regulation. Some of the molecules that control and regulate the immune system are discussed in this volume.

Cellular studies in immunology are highly dependent on the ability to isolate the appropriate cell lines and clones. The procedures presently employed have been quite effective. But yet new and promising technologies are emerging. The ability to preform cell separations in microgravity may prove to be one of the most important biologically-related fringe benefits of the space program. The current status of these invesitgations is reviewed.

M.Z. Atassi

CONTENTS

THE MAJOR HISTOCOMPATIBILITY COMPLEX AND PROTEIN RECOGNITION

BY T LYMPHOCYTES

Jan Klein

Max-Planck-Institut für Biologie
Abteilung Immungenetik
Tübingen, Federal Republic of Germany

Twosome and Threesome Relations

In biochemistry all good things come in twos -- as pairs of receptors and their ligands (Fig. 1). An enzyme interacts with its substrate and thus initiates or accelerates a chemical reaction. A hormone binds to its receptor and thus regulates a physiological process. A regulatory protein attaches to a promoter region of DNA and thus activates a gene. And so on. In immunology, on the other hand, the best things come in threes. Here, the T-cell receptor (Tcr) curiously enough does not react with one but with two ligands simultaneously: with an antigen and with major histocompatibility complex (Mhc) molecules (Fig. 2). The immune system, to be sure, has not completely abandoned the old-fashioned twosome relationship (antibodies react with antigens and antigens only), but the most profound event in the immune response, the initial distinction between self and nonself, is a threesome affair.

So strange is the notion of a single receptor recognizing two ligands simultaneously that some immunologists have tried to argue around it. They came up with the idea that in reality the Mhc molecule (self) is the receptor for the antigen (nonself) and the Tcr is the receptor for the modified self -- for the Mhc molecule altered by the interaction with the antigen (Zinkernagel and Doherty, 1974; Ohno et al., 1981; Sherman, 1982). It is a strange idea because it presupposes that a single "receptor" (the Mhc

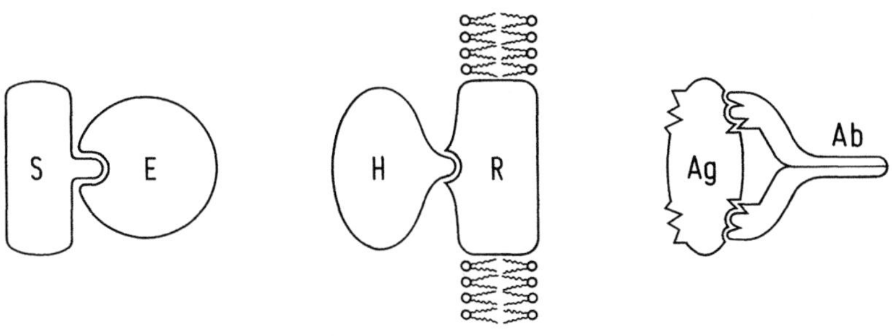

Fig. 1. Twosome interactions in biochemistry and immunology.

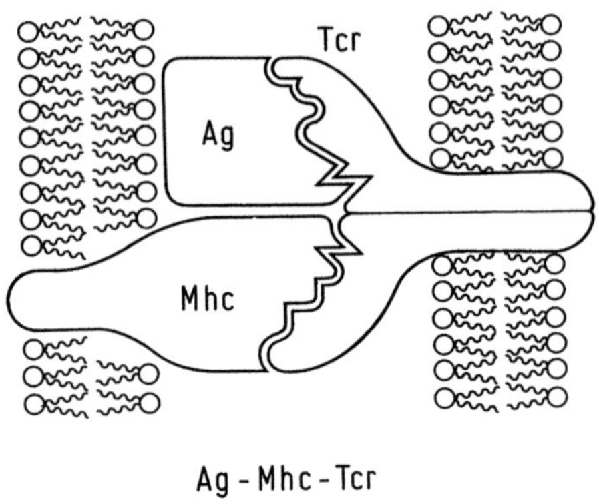

Fig. 2. The threesome interaction of antigen (Ag), major histocompatibility complex (Mhc) molecule, and the T-cell receptor (Tcr).

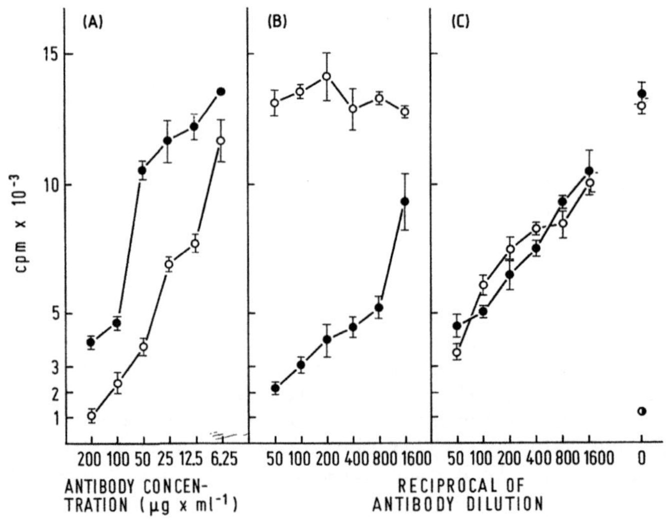

Fig. 3. Antibody blocking of T cell responses to liposome-bound antigens. IL-2 production by the pigeon cytochrome c (PCC)+E^k specific hybridoma in response to liposomes carrying PCC and E^k molecules (●) and liposomes carrying PCC alone (O) was tested in the absence of APC. Antibodies added to the culture were (A) C13, IE5 (PCC specific), (B) 13/18 (E^k specific) and (C) GK 1.5 (L3T4 specific). The semi-closed circle represents the medium control. Each point represents the arithmetic mean ± SD (vertical bars) of triplicate cultures. E^k = class II molecule controlled by the mouse Mhc. (From Walden et al., 1986a).

molecule) can specifically recognize a very large number of ligands (different antigens) and that each of these ligands can alter the Mhc molecule in a specific way. Yet, until recently there has been no convincing experimental evidence to disprove the altered-self hypothesis. Only now can the hypothesis safely be discarded. Walden and his colleagues (1986a) have demonstrated that T cells stimulated by an antigen (pigeon cytochrome c) together with self class II Mhc molecules can be restimulated with the antigen alone, in the absence of any Mhc molecules (Fig. 3). To achieve this, they conjugated the antigen to the lipids of a liposome which they then added instead of antigen presenting cells (APC), to the primed T cells. The lymphocytes responded to the antigen by increased incorporation of tritiated thymidine, proliferation, and, in other experiments, also by the production of interleukin-2 (IL-2) -- a sure sign of their activation. Similar activation could also be achieved with other antigens (e.g., lactate dehydrogenase B or keyhole-limpet hemocyanin). The T-cell proliferation could be blocked by the addition to the culture of antibodies specific for the antigen, but not by antibodies specific for class II molecules, thus confirming that these molecules, which normally provide the context for antigen recognition, were not involved in the T lymphocyte activation in this particular experiment. The T cells could be restimulated only with the same antigen that was used for their priming; unrelated antigens failed to elicit any significant response, indicating that the response was as specific as that occurring in the context of Mhc molecules.

Clusters, Grids, and Affinities

An analysis of the conditions under which antigen alone, without Mhc molecules, could restimulate T cells revealed that a relative rigidity of the liposome bilayer and a relative high density of the antigenic molecules conjugated to the lipids was required. This observation suggests, in turn, that clustering of Tcr may be necessary for lymphocyte activation and that the affinity of receptor-ligand interaction is, not surprisingly, critical for the initiation of the response. These two requirements may be interrelated. It is possible that under physiological conditions, the Mhc molecules are responsible for clustering the receptors, either because they are present at high density on the APC or because they themselves occur in patches in the plasma membrane. In the rigid liposome, the antigen molecules form a relatively immobile, dense grid which favors clustering of receptors interacting with the individual antigenic determinants. This interpretation is supported by the observation that multivalent antigens, such as those generated by the conjugation of multiple haptenic groups to a carrier molecule, can also function without Mhc molecules when they interact with Tcr (Carel et al., 1983; Rao et al., 1984a,b; Siliciano et al., 1985a,b, 1986).

The ease with which T-cell proliferation can be blocked with antigen-specific antibodies when the antigen is presented on liposomes contrasts with the difficulties other investigators have had attempting to block presentation by APC. The reason for this difference may again lie in the affinity and the geometry of interactions between the Tcr, the antigen, and the Mhc molecules. One can imagine that in a physiological situation, the initial interaction of the Tcr is with the Mhc molecules of the APC. Such an interaction may occur all the time but its affinity is so weak that it does not lead to activation of the T lymphocyte. The weak bonds between the Tcr and the Mhc molecules may constantly form and break without any consequence to the cells involved. When Mhc-specific antibodies are present they may bind to the Mhc molecules with high affinity and thus block the Tcr-Mhc molecule interaction and hence also antigen presentation. Blocking of antigen presentation by Mhc-specific monoclonal antibodies has been demonstrated repeatedly in a number of laboratories (e.g., Baxevanis et al., 1980; Lerner et al., 1980). If Mhc-specific antibody is not present, the Tcr-Mhc molecule interaction is stabilized by the interaction with antigen.

The density of the antigen on the APC and its affinity for the Tcr are too low to even initiate the T-cell:APC interaction. It is only when the Tcr, weakly interacting with Mhc molecules on the APC, encounters the antigen that a strong bond between the two cells snaps in. The affinity interaction in the threesome complex is now so high that the antigen-specific antibody cannot compete successfully with it. Since the antibody also does not interfere with the initial recognition of the Mhc molecules by the Tcr, it often does not block antigen presentation, particularly when it is specific for a different determinant on the antigen molecule than the Tcr is, which happens most of the time. Only when conditions are favorable for the antibody, can it block antigen presentation. Only on the liposomes, where the Tcr is forced to initiate the recognition via the antigen rather than via the Mhc molecules, and the affinity of the recognition remains relatively low for the individual Tcr-Mhc molecule pairs (but the avidity of all the interactions is high), does the antibody compete successfully with the Tcr and blocks T-cell activation. In experiments in which antigen presentation by APC could be blocked (Corradin and Engers, 1984; Lamb et al., 1984), it may have been the nature of the antigen or even other factors that brought the experiment to a successful conclusion.

The Form of the Presented Antigen

The antigen used for the experiment depicted in Figure 3 was a whole protein, which was covalently coupled to the liposome. The only cell in this system was the T lymphocyte with receptors specific for this antigen. There was thus no cell available that could "process" the protein by degrading it into peptides. Walden and his colleagues (1985, 1986a,b) tested several other antigens for their ability to be presented by liposomes (i.e., cytochrome c, insulin, lactate dehydrogenase B, lysozyme, ovalbumin, and keyhole limpet hemocyanin) and obtained in all instances the same result: a whole protein molecule attached to a lipid bilayer can be recognized specifically by the Tcr of activated T lymphocytes.

This observation opposes the current dogma according to which large proteins are taken up by the APC, sequestered into the lysosomal compartment, degraded into peptides, and the peptides returned to the cell surface where they associate with Mhc molecules (Grey and Chesnut, 1985). Only if so processed can the antigens be recognized by the T cells. We have discussed the merits of the antigen processing hypothesis elsewhere (Klein et al., 1985; Klein and Walden, 1986) and I will therefore not repeat the arguments here. Suffice to say that now even the proponents of the hypothesis admit that at least some quite large protein molecules, such as fibrinogen, need not be processed at all to be recognized by T cells (Allen et al., these proceedings). They admit further that for other antigens the processing may constitute the mere unfolding of a globular protein and that this event can take place on the cell surface rather than inside the cell (Streicher et al., 1984; Kovač and Schwartz, 1985). These conclusions may be paving the way for a reconciliation of the two originally so diametrically opposite views of antigen presentation. It is clear, however, that whatever compromise is reached in the end, the original hypothesis of antigen processing encompassing all the large proteins is no longer valid and that whatever happens to the presented antigen can happen at the cell surface without the protein having to actually enter the cell.

Consequences of Mhc Polymorphism

The fact that the Tcr recognize not one but two ligands simultaneously is strange. But perhaps even more curious is the observation that both ligands vary. That the Tcr varies from clone to clone is to be expected because, after all, this is part of its function. Surprising is, however, that also the Mhc molecules vary from individual to individual, that is to say, the Mhc loci are polymorphic. The polymorphism means that the same antigen may be recognized in different individuals in the context of different Mhc molecules.

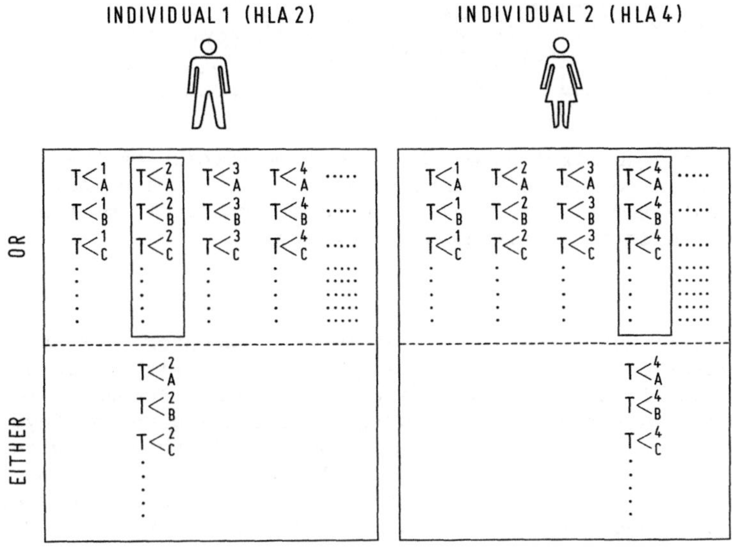

Fig. 4. Two views of ways in which the T-cell repertoire may be individualized. T indicates a T cell and < receptor specificity; numbers indicate different Mhc molecules, capital letters different antigens. For example, $T<^{1}_{A}$ is a T cell capable of recognizing antigen A in the context of the Mhc^{1} molecule. HLA = human Mhc. According to the "either" hypothesis, the periphery contains only T cells recognizing antigens in the context of self Mhc molecules. According to the "or" hypothesis, the periphery contains self- as well as nonself-restricted T cells, but uses only the former.

The Mhc polymorphism has two important consequences. The first is that the T-cell repertoires of different outbred individuals are not the same. The repertoires are individualized either qualitatively or quantitatively. There are two ways in which the individualization may occur (Figs. 4 and 5). According to one hypothesis (Zinkernagel et al., 1978), as the T lymphocytes differentiate in the thymus, they are screened for the receptors they express. The germ line contains genes coding for Tcr with the potential to recognize antigens in the context not only of self Mhc molecules, but also of the Mhc molecules that other individuals might express (nonself Mhc mole-

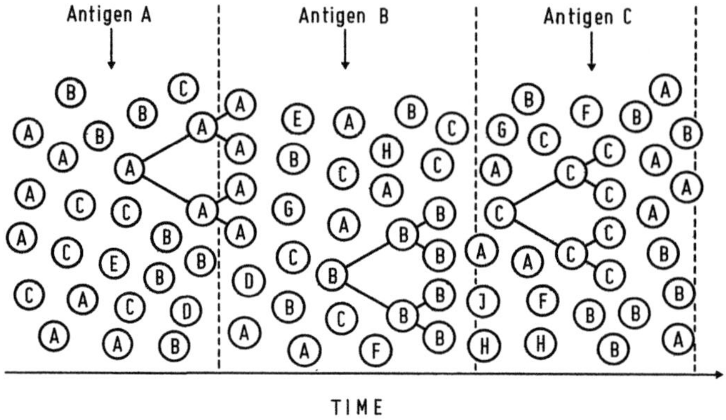

Fig. 5. Individualization of the T-cell repertoire by the expansion of self-restricted T cells. Circles indicate individual T cells; letters specificity of the T cells for antigens A, B, C, etc.

cules). But the thymus allows only T cells with receptors for antigens and self-Mhc molecules to pass into the periphery; cells with receptors for antigens and nonself Mhc molecules die in this organ. According to the second hypothesis (Klein and Nagy, 1982), the screening in the thymus is minimal, if it exists at all. In the periphery, T lymphocytes with receptors for antigens and self Mhc molecules are amplified by antigen stimulation, whereas T cells with receptors for antigen and nonself Mhc molecules are not because no nonself Mhc molecules are present in the individual. The repertoire thus drifts, with continuous antigen stimulation, toward a state in which the T cells recognizing antigens in the context of self Mhc molecules dominate.

The question of how individualization of the T-cell repertoire occurs has been left open (for discussion, see Klein 1986). Two points, however, have been established. First, the T-cell repertoire does contain lymphocytes capable of recognizing antigens in the context of nonself Mhc molecules (Ishii et al., 1981; 1982a,b; Nagy et al. 1981); what remains unclear is the frequency at which these cells occur. Second, at least some individualization of the repertoire does occur in the periphery; unclear is again the extent to which the thymus contributes to the individualization (Kast et al. 1984).

Mhc, Nonresponsiveness, and Ir Genes

The second consequence of Mhc polymorphism is the existence of nonresponder individuals in an outbred population. It so happens that certain combinations of self Mhc molecules and antigens fail to be recognized by T lymphocytes and that different individuals, carrying different Mhc molecules, fail to respond to different antigens. Were the Mhc loci not polymorphic, all the individuals would give the same patterns of responsiveness to various antigens. But because individuals differ in their Mhc molecules, some respond to antigen X and Y, but not to antigen Z, others respond to X, but not to Y and Z, others still to Z but not to X and Y, and so on, depending on the Mhc genes they carry. By mating responders with nonresponders one can show that the responsiveness is controlled by a single Immune response or Ir gene (reviewed in Klein 1986). The gene is, of course, identical with the Mhc gene because it is the Mhc that determines whether an individual will or will not respond to the particular antigen.

What is the reason for nonresponsiveness? Why are certain individuals unable to recognize the particular antigen in the context of their Mhc molecules? Two answers have been given to these questions. According to one hypothesis, a successful presentation of antigen to T cells requires the antigen to physically interact with the Mhc molecule of the APC (Babbitt et al., 1985). Not all antigens can, however, associate with all the Mhc molecules. Those antigens that fail to associate with the particular Mhc molecules are not recognized by T cells and the individual bearing these molecules is a nonresponder to the particular antigen. According to the second hypothesis, the nonresponder individuals lack functional T cells with specificity for the particular antigen and self Mhc molecules (Klein and Nagy, 1982). The reason <u>why</u> they lack them is that these T cells happen to also recognize molecules expressed in the individual itself (self molecules) in the context of self Mhc molecules. To prevent autoimmunity, such T cells are inactivated in the tolerance induction phase of development and the individual then has a <u>blind spot</u> in its T- cell repertoire for the cross-reacting foreign antigen (Klein 1984).

Evidence for both hypotheses has been put forward. Babbitt et al. (1985) have reported that Mhc molecules of responders to lysozyme bind, in a solution, lysozymal peptides with a significantly higher affinity than Mhc molecules of nonresponder individuals do. Subsequent studies have, however, indicated that the correlation between the responder status and the affinity of antigen-Mhc molecule binding is rather poor, and that in fact even autologous molecules bind autologous Mhc molecules (Phillips et al., 1986; Babbitt et al. 1986). The association hypothesis may, therefore, explain some instances of nonresponsiveness but it does not explain all the nonresponsiveness. Personally, I am convinced that even in cases in which correlation between molecular associations and nonresponsiveness has been demonstrated, the true reason for nonresponsiveness will turn out to be a blind spot in the T-cell repertoire.

We have provided evidence for the existence of blind spots in the T-cell repertoire for several antigens (Ishii et al., 1983; Vučak et al., 1983; Vidović et al., 1985). Here, I shall mention one of these, the response to the synthetic polypeptide poly($Glu^{50}Tyr^{50}$) or GT (Vidović et al., 1984). The DBA/2 strain of mice responds to GT whereas the BALB/c strain does not, although both strains carry the same Mhc haplotype (<u>$H\text{-}2^d$</u>). The F_1 hybrid between these two strains is also a nonresponder (Fig. 6) which is somewhat unusual because normally responsiveness to most antigens is dominant and nonresponsiveness recessive. The fact that the two inbred strains are Mhc identical permitted us to test antigen presentation by cells from one strain to T lymphocytes of the second strain, without running into difficulties with the T cells responding to the foreign Mhc molecules, which would normally be the case. Any response observed when the cells from the two strains are mixed and cultured in the presence of antigen should therefore be a response to GT and not to foreign Mhc molecules. The experiment showed that DBA/2 (responder) T lymphocytes can be stimulated by GT presented on BALB/c (nonresponder) APC, whereas T cells from a nonresponder are incapable of responding to GT presented on responder APC. Responsiveness or nonresponsiveness is therefore determined by the T lymphocytes and not by the APC, so that there is no defect at the antigen presentation level; the defect is in the T-cell repertoire. Furthermore, since both the DBA/2 and the BALB/c mice have the same <u>$H\text{-}2^d$</u> haplotype, it obviously cannot be the association or nonassociation of Mhc molecules with the GT that determines the nonresponsiveness to this antigen.

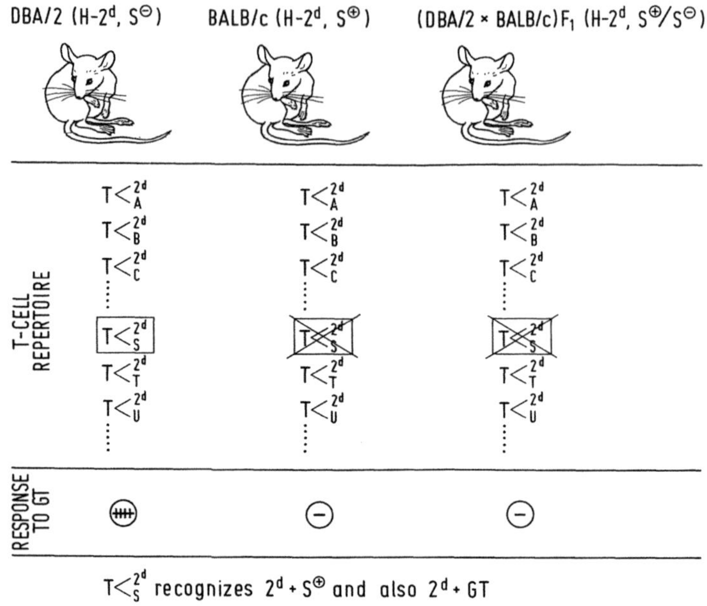

Fig. 6. T-cell repertoires and responses of mice to the synthetic polypeptide GT. $T<^{2d}_{A}$ indicates a T cell capable of recognizing antigen A in the context of an $H\text{-}2^d$ molecule. Crossed symbols indicate inactivation of T cells. Further explanation in the text.

The difference in the T-cell repertoire between the DBA/2 and BALB/c strains of mice can be explained thus (Fig. 6): The BALB/c mice express a molecule, let us call it simply S, which the T cells recognize in the context of $H\text{-}2^d$ molecules (diagrammatically, the T-cell specificity can be depicted as $T<^{2d}_{S}$). To avoid autoreactivity, these cells are inactivated during the tolerance-induction period. The $T<^{2d}_{S}$ cells, however, also recognize, by chance, GT in the context of $H\text{-}2^d$ and they are the only cells in this strain that recognize this antigen. Since they have been inactivated, the BALB/c mice are nonresponders to GT. In the DBA/2 mice, the S molecule is either not expressed or, more likely, is present in an allelic form that is not recognized by the $T<^{2d}_{S}$ cells. There is, therefore, no reason to inactivate the $T<^{2d}_{S}$ cells in these mice, and hence the DBA/2 strain is a responder to GT. In the F_1 hybrid, both allelic forms of the S molecules are expressed and the $S^{BALB/c}$ form inactivates the $T<^{2d}_{S}$ cells with the result that the F_1 hybrid is a nonresponder. Vidovič (personal communication) has now identified and mapped the locus coding for the S molecule and determined the tissue distribution of the S antigen. There can thus no longer be any doubt that the molecule exists and that the explanation of nonresponsiveness described above is correct.

I conclude that blind spots in the T-cell repertoire exist and are responsible for nonresponsiveness to at least some antigens. Whether there are other reasons for nonresponsiveness besides the blind spots is not certain. Unanswered is also the question why the Tcr recognizes Mhc molecules in addition to the antigen and why the Mhc genes are so highly polymorphic.

Acknowledgements — I thank Ms. Lynne Yakes for outstanding editorial assistance.

REFERENCES

Babbitt, B. P., Allen, P. M., Matsueda, G., Haber, E., and Unanue, E. R., 1985, Binding of immunogenic peptides to Ia histocompatibility molecules. Nature 317:359.

Babbitt, B. P., Matsueda, G., Haber, E., Unanue, E. R., and Allen, P. M., 1986, Antigenic competition at the level of peptide-Ia binding. Proc. Natl. Acad. Sci. USA 83:5509.

Baxevanis, C. N., Wernet, D., Nagy, Z. N., Maurer, P. H., and Klein, J., 1980, Genetic control of T-cell proliferative responses to poly(Glu^{40} Ala^{60}) and poly(Glu^{5}Lys^{34}Tyr^{15}): Subregion-specific inhibition of the responses with monoclonal Ia antibodies. Immunogenetics 11:617.

Carel, S., Bron, C., and Corradin, G., 1983, T-cell hybridoma specific for a cytochrome c peptide: specific antigen binding and interleukin 2 production. Proc. Natl. Acad. Sci. USA 80:4832.

Corradin, G., and Engers, H. D., 1984, Inhibition of antigen-induced T-cell clone proliferation by antigen-specific antibodies. Nature 308:547.

Grey, H. M., and Chesnut, R., 1985, Antigen processing and presentation to T cells. Immunol. Today 6:101.

Ishii, N., Baxevanis, C. N., Nagy, Z. A., and Klein, J., 1981, Responder T cells depleted of alloreactive cells react to antigen presented on allogeneic macrophages from nonresponder strains. J. Exp. Med. 154: 978.

Ishii, N., Nagy, Z. A., and Klein, J., 1982a, Absence of Ir gene control of T cells recognizing foreign antigen in the context of allogeneic MHC molecules. Nature 295:531.

Ishii, N., Nagy, Z. A., and Klein, J., 1982b, Restriction molecules involved in the interaction of T cells with allogeneic antigen-presenting cells. J. Exp. Med. 156:622.

Ishii, N., Nagy, Z. A., and Klein, J., 1983, In vitro correlate for a clonal deletion mechanism of immune response gene-controlled nonresponsiveness. J. Exp. Med. 157:998.

Kast, W. M., de Waal, L. P., and Melief, C. M., 1984, The thymus dictates MHC specificity and Ir gene phenotype of T cells restricted to class II MHC molecules but not of T cells restricted to class I MHC molecules. J. Exp. Med. 160:1752.

Klein, J., 1984, What causes immunological nonresponsiveness? Immunol. Rev. 81:177.

Klein, J., 1986, "Natural History of the Major Histocompatibility Complex," Wiley, New York.

Klein, J., and Nagy, Z. A., 1982, Mhc restriction and Ir genes, in "Advances in Cancer Research," Vol. 37, Academic Press, New York.

Klein, J., and Walden, P., 1986, Antigen presentation: Paradigm lost?, in "Immunology 1986," B. Cinader and R.G. Miller, eds., in press.

Klein, J., Walden P., and Nagy, Z. A., 1985, Antigen processing: A reevaluation, in "Immune Regulation," M. Feldman and N. A. Mitchison eds., The Humana Press, Clifton, New Jersey.

Kovač, Z., and Schwartz, R. H., 1985, The molecular basis of the requirement for antigen processing of pigeon cytochrome c prior to T cell activation. J. Immunol. 134:3233.

Lamb, J. R., Zanders, E. D., Lake, P., Webster, R. G., Eckels, D. D., Woody, J. N., Green, N., Lerner, R. A., Feldmann, M., 1984, Inhibition of T cell proliferation by antibodies to synthetic peptides. Eur. J. Immunol. 14:153.

Lerner, L. A., Matis, L. A., Janeway, Jr., C. A., Jones, P. P., Schwartz, R. H., and Murphy, D. B., 1980, Monoclonal antibody against an Ir gene product? J. Exp. Med. 152:1085.

Nagy, Z. A., Baxevanis, C. N., Ishii, N., and Klein, J., 1981, Ia antigens as restriction molecules in Ir-gene controlled T-cell proliferation Immunol. Rev. 60:59
Ohno, S., Epplen, J. T., and Suton, S., 1981, Testis-organizing H-Y antigen as a discrete protein: its MHC restricted immune recognition and the genomic environment in which H-Y gene operates. Hum. Genet. 58:37.
Phillips, M. L., Moule, M. L., Delovitch, T. L., and Yip, C. C., 1986, Class I histocompatibility antigens and insulin receptors: evidence for interactions. Proc. Natl. Acad. Sci. USA 83:3474.
Rao, A., Ko. W. W.-P., Faas, S. J., and Cantor, H., 1984a, Binding of antigen in the absence of histocompatibility proteins by arsonate-reactive T-cell clones. Cell 36:879.
Rao, A., Faas, S. J., and Cantor, H., 1984b, Analogs that compete for antigen binding to arsonate-reactive T-cell clones inhibit the functional response to arsonate. Cell 36:889.
Sherman, L.A., 1982, Recognition of conformational determinants on H-2 by cytolytic T lymphocytes. Nature 297:511.
Siliciano, R. F., Keegan, A. D., Dintzis, R.Z., Dintzis, H. M., and Shin, H. S., 1985a, The interaction of nominal antigen with T cell antigen receptors. I. Specific binding of multivalent nominal antigen to cytolytic T cell clones. J. Immunol. 135:906.
Siliciano, R. F., Colello, R. M., Keegan, A. D., Dintzis, R. Z., Dintzis, H. M., and Shin, H. S., 1985b, Antigen valence determines the binding of nominal antigen to T cell clones. J. Exp. Med. 162:768.
Siliciano, R. F., Hemesath, T. J., Pratt, J. C., Dintzis, R. Z., Dintzis, H. M., Acuto, O., Shin, H. S., and Reinherz, E. L., 1986, Direct evidence for the existence of nominal antigen binding sites on T cell surface Ti α-β heterodimers of MHC-restricted T cell clones. Cell 471:161.
Streicher, Z., Berkower, I. J., Busch, M., Gurd, F. R. N., and Berzofsky, J. A., 1984, Antigen conformation determines processing requirements for T-cell activation. Proc. Natl. Acad. Sci. USA 81:6831.
Vidović, D., Klein, J., and Nagy, Z. A., 1985, Recessive T cell response to poly(Glu^{50}Tyr^{50}) possibly caused by self tolerance. J. Immunol. 134: 3563.
Vučak, I., Raska, K., Nagy, Z. A., and Klein, J., 1983, Frequency of responsiveness to the H-Y antigen among the B10.W lines. J. Immunol. 131: 325.
Walden, P. Nagy, Z. A., and Klein, J., 1985, Induction of regulatory T-lymphocyte responses by liposomes carrying major histocompatibility complex molecules and foreign antigen. Nature 315:6017.
Walden, P., Nagy, Z. A., and Klein, J., 1986a, Antigen presentation by liposomes: inhibition with antibodies. Eur. J. Immunol. 16:717.
Walden, P., Nagy, Z. A., and Klein, J., 1986b, Major histocompatibility complex-restricted and unrestricted activation of helper T cell lines by liposome-bound antigens. J. Mol. Cell. Biol. 2:191.
Zinkernagel, R. M., and Doherty, P. C., 1974, Restriction of in vitro T cell-mediated cytotoxicity in lymphocytic choriomeningitis within a syngeneic or semiallogeneic system. Nature, 248:701.
Zinkernagel, R.M., Callahan, G. N., Althage, A., Cooper, S., Klein P. A., and Klein, J., 1978, On the thymus in the differentiation of "H-2 self recognition" by T cells: Evidence for dual recognition? J. Exp. Med. 147:882.

MURINE Ia GENES: ORGANIZATION, POLYMORPHISM AND HETEROGENEITY

Kathleen Donovan and Chella S. David

Department of Immunology, Mayo Clinic and Medical School, Rochester, MN 55905

INTRODUCTION

The genes of the major histocompatibility complex have been identified and analyzed in many species. Homology between species indicate that these genes evolved millions of years ago, and that they are part of a super-gene family. Studies in man and mouse have clearly identified at least four classes of MHC genes, class I, class II, class III and class IV. The class I genes code for the classical 'transplantation antigens' which consist of a 45,000 molecular weight chain associated with a 12,000 dalton β2 microglobulin and are expressed on all nucleated cells. The class I genes can be further subdivided into those involved in the rejection of transplants and which serve as restriction molecules for cytotoxic T lymphocytes (K, D, L in mouse and HLA-A, -B, -C in humans), and a set of class I genes with unknown function (Qa and Tla in mouse). The class II genes code for the classical 'Ia antigens' which consists of two polypeptide chains of 31,000 and 28,000 daltons in a non-covalent association and expressed predominantly on lymphoid cells. These molecules are involved in the presentation of non-self antigens and activation of the T-helper cell. The class III genes code for the classical 'complement components', C4, C2 and bf. A new set of genes involved in synthesis of certain enzymes (neuraminidase, 21-hydroxylase), tumor necrosis factor and cytochrome P450 proteins are grouped as the class IV genes. In this paper, we will concentrate primarily on the organization and polymorphism of the class II Ia genes.

GENE ORGANIZATION

The region of the chromosome coding for the Ia genes is referred to as the I region. This is due to the fact that the immune response genes identified on the basis of antibody response to synthetic polypeptides were mapped originally to this region and the products identified which also map to this region were designated as Ia antigens or Immune Response associated antigens (Shreffler and David, 1975). As shown in Figure 1, four of the Ia genes, A_α, A_β, E_β and E_α code for the polypeptide chains. The α genes code for a 34,000 dalton polypeptide while the β gene codes for a 28,000 molecular polypeptide (Cullen, et al. 1974). The difference in molecular weights of alpha and beta genes is due primarily to the presence of an additional N-linked carbohydrate side chain on the alpha molecule. On the cell surface, the Ia molecules are found as a non-covalent linkage of the alpha and beta chains, A_α and A_β forming the I-A molecule and the E_β and E_α forming the I-E molecule (Jones, et al. 1978). The Ia antigens were originally identified by serological methods, by making specific antibodies against antigenic determinants on these molecules (David, et al. 1973).

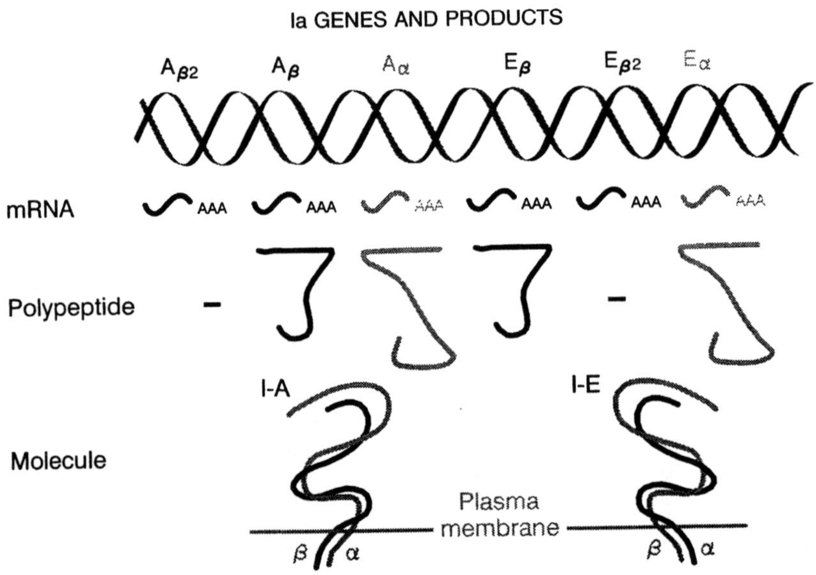

Hood and his associates (1982) identified the Ia genes by making use of cDNA clones for human class II genes that cross-hybridized with mouse class II genes as well as synthetic DNA probes whose sequences were generated from protein data. By using these probes in a chromosomal walking technique, a cosmid genomic library was constructed from BALB/c sperm DNA and approximately 200 kb of DNA was characterized. A_β, A_α, E_β and E_α lie within a 100-140 Kb of this characterized region. A second A_β-like sequence, $A_{\beta 2}$, was identified that mapped 20 Kb centromeric to the A_β gene. $A_{\beta 2}$ hybridizes only to the second external protein domain of murine and human class II β genes and upon sequencing was found to contain the features of β chain second domains and other immunoglobulin-like domains. This gene was found to be 60% homologous to three subsets of human β chains as well as the A_β chain (Larhammar et al. 1983). To determine if $A_{\beta 2}$ may be functional, the transcription of this gene was analyzed. $A_{\beta 2}$ was shown to be transcribed, polyadenylated, processed, transported to the cytoplasm and found on membrane-bound ribosomes indicating probable translation. A protein has yet to be detected. The pattern of expression of $A_{\beta 2}$ transcripts differs from the known class II genes. Transcripts were detected in spleen and a B cell hybridoma as well as in a B cell enriched spleen population. No transcripts could be found in either T cell clones or macrophages with or without induction by γ-IFN. The sizes of $A_{\beta 2}$ nuclear and cytoplasmic poly(A)$^+$ transcripts were detected by Northern blots using an oligonucleotide probe specific for $A_{\beta 2}$. Five bands approximately 5 Kb, 4.5 Kb, 3.2 Kb, 2.3 Kb and 1.3 Kb (which comigrates with $A_{\beta 1}$ mRNA) were seen. The 3.2 Kb RNA being the most abundant. Cytoplasmic poly(A)$^+$ RNA contains the smallest three species of RNA (Wake et al. 1985).

The $E_{\beta 2}$ gene was identified in a similar manner by hybridizing to 3' DQ_{β} but not 5' DQ_{β} or $E_{\beta 1}$ probes. Its location was found to be between $E_{\beta 1}$ and E_{α}. A recent study of the $E_{\beta 2}$ gene shows it to have some similarities to other class II genes. The leader peptide, two external domains and a transmembrane region are encoded by separate exons each flanked by appropriate splice sequences. The precise identification of the $E_{\beta 2}$ IC and 3' UT exons will require isolation of an $E_{\beta 2}$ cDNA. The predicted RNA contains a continuous open reading frame coding for 253 amino acids. Several conserved sequences are found in the putative promoter region 5' of exon one. Conserved sequences found up stream of most other class II genes analyzed to date (Mathis et al. 1983a; Kelly and Trowsdale, 1985), are located 158 and 123 bp upstream of the potential initiation codon. A possible CAAT box is found at position -93. No TATA sequence was found at the expected position which is similar, however, to $A_{\beta 1}$ (Malissen et al. 1983; Larhammar et al. 1983). As was seen in the $A_{\beta 2}$ sequence, the residues shared among class II β2 domains and immunoglobulin domains are retained in $E_{\beta 2}$. The overall sizes of the various protein domains are very similar as are the intradomain disulfide-linked cysteines present in the other class II β1 and β2 domains. The site which is present for the N-linked glycosylation in other β chains is absent. This would not, however, preclude its surface expression. The homology at both a nucleotide and amino acid level of exon 3 is highest with $E_{\beta 1}$. In this respect $E_{\beta 2}$ and $E_{\beta 1}$ seem like the non-allelic DR_{β} loci in comprising an isotypic family. The second exon, however, has no clear homologue. The transmembrane region shows similar divergence. An analysis of the sequences of $E_{\beta 2}$ and restriction fragment analysis of other haplotypes shows $E_{\beta 2}$ to be much less polymorphic than conventional class II β genes. A transcriptional analysis shows similarities to $A_{\beta 2}$ in the tissue distribution of expression. $E_{\beta 2}$ is expressd only at low levels in B cells and is not induced in macrophage or monocyte tumor lines by γ-interferon. This suggests that these class II molecules could have a distinct role in Ia functions or are molecules with a role in differentiation or regulatory interactions of B lymphocytes. Northern blot analysis shows four transcripts of 3.5, 2.4, 2.2 and 1.8 found in the B cell tumor CH-1, MRL lpr/lpr spleen cells, and in LPS-stimulated BALB/c and C57BL/6 spleen cells. Two additional transripts 4.1 and 1.0 Kb were found from the B cell hybridoma LK-35.2. All of the transcripts appear to be typical of mature mRNA molecules in that they were present in cytoplasmic mRNA preparations, specifically enriched by oligo (dT) purification, and do not appear to contain intron sequences (Braunstein and Germain 1986).

Two additional genes, $A_{\beta 3}$ and $E_{\beta 3}$ are thought to be pseudogenes. $A_{\beta 3}$ is located between 70 to 90 Kb telomeric from the K locus (Larhammar et al. 1983). The distance between $A_{\beta 3}$ and $A_{\beta 2}$ has recently been found to be 160 Kb thereby linking the K region to the I region (Steinmetz et al. 1986). $E_{\beta 3}$ has been mapped to the S region of the b haplotype, an unknown distance from the E_{α} gene (Flavell et al. 1985). The distance between the E_{α} gene and the S region, however, has recently been determined by pulse field electrophoresis to be 70 Kb (Steinmetz, Personal Communication). The A_{β}, $A_{\beta 2}$, E_{β} and $E_{\beta 2}$ have the same 5' to 3' orientation whereas A_{α}, E_{α} and $A_{\beta 3}$ have the opposite orientation (Flavell et al. 1985). The order of the genes are $A_{\beta 3}$-$A_{\beta 2}$-$A_{\beta 1}$-A_{α}-$E_{\beta 1}$-$E_{\beta 2}$-E_{α}-$E_{\beta 3}$ from centromere to telomere (Germain and Malisen, 1986).

Table 1. Viable Ia Genes in Independent Haplotypes

	I-A		I-E	
Haplotype	A_{β}	A_{α}	E_{β}	E_{α}
b	+	+	+	-
d	+	+	+	+
f	+	+	-	-
j	+	+	+	+
k	+	+	+	+
p	+	+	+	+
q	+	+	-	-
r	+	+	+	+
s	+	+	+	-

ALLELES OF THE Ia GENES

Table 1 lists 9 independent haplotypes of inbred mouse strains where the Ia genes have been analyzed. As shown, all of them express an intact I-A molecule which indicates that in each of them the A_{α} and the A_{β} genes code for viable alpha and beta chains. Four haplotypes, b, f, q, and s fail to express an intact I-E molecule on the cell surface. This is due to a defect in either or both of the E_{β} and E_{α} genes. In the b and s haplotype, the E_{β} gene codes for a viable beta polypeptide chain which is found in the cytoplasm and can be shown to complement in F_1 mice bearing a functional E_{α} gene to yield a normal I-E moleucle. The E_{β} genes for the f and q haplotype appear grossly normal by Southern blot analysis (Steinmetz et al. 1982) with no major insertions or deletion, but were shown not to produce viable proteins (Jones et al. 1981). They do, however, show approximately 5% of the normal level of 1.3 Kb E_{β}-hybridizing message in both cases. Whether this reflects low-level cross-hybridization of an E_{β} probe to A_{β} mRNA or low levels of E_{β} transcription has not been determined (Mengle-Gaw and McDevitt, 1985). S_1 nuclease mapping would need to be performed to rule out this possibility.

An example of an $E_\alpha^+E_\beta^-$ inbred strain is A.TFR5, an (A.CA x A.TL)F_1 heterozygote intra-I region recombinant. These mice fail to synthesize E_β polypeptide but synthesize normal levels of cytoplasmic E_α. Unexpectedly surface E_α is expressed at 10-20% of normal levels as detected by lymphocyte absorption studies with anti-I-E antisera (Murphy et al. 1980). A recent explanation for this expression proposes an association of the E_α polypeptide with A_β (Germain and Quill, 1986) based on the demonstration of such associations between A_β^d $E_\alpha^{a/k}$ molecules on the surface of L cell transfectants. The E_α gene of the b and s haplotype is present but is neither transcribed nor translated. Two independent studies utilizing restriction fragment analysis showed a deletion of 650 ± 50 bp encompassing the first exon and the promoter region of this gene explaining this phenomenon (Mathis et al. 1983b; Hyldig-Nielsen et al. 1983). The explanation for the lack of E_α polypeptide in the f and q haplotype has not been so straightforward; both genes are transcribed although there are qualitative and quantitative differences from normal. The q haplotype has low levels of message none of which are the appropriate size for mature mRNA. The f haplotype expresses normal amounts of E_α hybridizing message composed of two bands approximately 1.25 Kb and 2.8 Kb. The 1.25 Kb band corresponds with the expected size of the mature E_α mRNA predicted from the cDNA sequence. The 2.8 kb band is presumably a precursor form and was present in RNA from k, d and u haplotype mice in varying intensities. The f strain expresses predominantly the 2.8 Kb species with low amounts of the mature message present. A sequence of the cDNA for the f strain revealed no obvious deviations from the E_α^k sequence (Diane Mathis, Personal communication) suggesting that the differences seen in both f and q haplotypes may be problems in appropriate splicing.

Similar observations have been made in studies of wild mice where more than half of the t-bearing strains have been shown to be defective in their expression of cell surface I-E molecules by monoclonal and polyclonal antibody analysis (Nizetic et al. 1984). As in the laboratory inbred strains, all of the wild mice analyzed express an intact I-A molecule. A study of these wild mice at the level of transcription and Southern blot analysis divided the defect into several groups similar to those found in the inbred strains of mice (Dembic et al. 1984). Most of the strains analyzed carry the deletion pattern seen in the b and s haplotypes suggesting the E_α gene of all these strains is derived from the same ancestral gene. This mutation has possibly been maintained in the mouse population for such a long time being spread piggyback fashion by the t haplotypes. In the few strains which express the E_α message, one appears to resemble the f haplotype by having the predominant message of the 2.8 Kb size, while another appears different from both f or q.

Ia EPITOPES

As many as 51 serological specificities have been defined for the Ia loci within the MHC by using monoclonal and alloantibodies each recognizing unique determinants. Efforts have been made in recent years to assign the particular chain, and even particular amino acid sequences on individual chains, primarily responsible for the binding of particular antibodies. Due to the nearly 90% homology at the sequence level, the E_α genes cannot be distinguished serologically. They appear to express an identical antigenic determinant.

For the A_α and A_β chains, two different techniques have been useful in assigning chain specificities for anti-Ia monoclonal antibodies. These have been the generation of L cell transfectant lines of haplotype matched and mismatched Ia complexes such as A^k_α:A^k_β, A^k_α:A^b_β, A^b_α:A^k_β and A^b_α:A^b_β (Landais et al. 1986a) and the development of mutant cell lines expressing slightly altered Ia molecules (Beck et al. 1986). In screening L cell transfectants with 18 mAb reactive to A^k but not A^b and 26 reactive to A^b but not A^k it was possible to determine that most of these recognize a determinant specified by one chain: either α or β. A few determinants, however, were more complex requiring both α and β chains of the same haplotype for binding. By the analysis of mutant cell lines five distinct epitopes can be assigned to the A^k_β polypeptide including Ia.17 with three distinct epitopes for this specificity, and Ia.1. In this system, the Ia.17 specificity could not be distinguished from Ia.18. It has been proposed that Ia.18$^+$ haplotypes may be a subset of the Ia.17$^+$ haplotypes and that structurally the Ia.18 epitope may be part of the Ia.17 epitope. The relationship of the Ia.2 and Ia.19 epitopes on the A^k_α polypeptide may be of a similar nature (Beck et al., 1986). In studying an I-A^b mutant DP6 staining by mAb 25-9-3 corresponding to allospecificity, Ia.20 defines an epitope on the A^b_β-chain. Seven other monoclonal antibodies recognize epitopes on the A^b_α polypeptide divisible into three groups.

L cells expressing a hybrid gene composed of the A^k_β exons for the amino-terminal domain and β2, TM, IC exons from A^d_β together with A^k_α show staining by I-A^k specific antibodies, indicating the importance of this polymorphic domain in contributing to epitopes on the intact I-A molecules (Germain et al. 1985a). A different hybrid construct utilizing the β1 domain of A^k_β and the C2, TM, IC domains from H-$2D^d$ allows the expression of the polymorphic domain from A^k_β without an α polypeptide. This showed the ability of monoclonal antibody 10-2-16 specific for the Ia.17 specificity to bind the β^k_1 domain without A^k_α or the β2 domain. Three other antibodies were able to show significant binding but the level was diminished in comparison to a recombinant $A^k_{\beta_1}$ paired with A^k_α. Therefore the epitopes for these antibodies depended on the presence of β^k_1 but additional affinity required the context of the rest of the I-A molecule. An additional group of antibodies were unable to bind out of context of an Ia molecule, emphasizing the importance of chain tertiary structure on epitope formation (McClusky et al. 1985).

The localization of binding of monoclonal antibodies has been further dissected into particular regions of a domain and amino acids reponsible for the effect have been determined. By creating hybrid molecules between the b and k haplotype within the β1 domain, the hypervariable regions of each haplotype could be monitored for their role in antibody binding. In the case of A^b_α reactive antibodies, control for formation of the epitopes for six monoclonal antibodies can be mapped to the second hypervariable group in the first domain with residues 57 and 59 potentially being the controlling amino acids. The binding of the A^k_α monoclonals, however, appear strongly governed by the third hypervariable group. By site directed mutagenesis they were able to demonstrate the importance of glutamic acid at residue 75 in forming the Ia.19 epitope which falls in this hypervariable group (Landais et al. 1986b). This clustering of antibody sites within a domain raises questions about what determines the immunogenicity of molecules and may explain the conflicting estimates regarding the degree of polymorphism in the A_α chain. Serologically, this chain exhibits very little variability whereas sequence analyses revealed high levels of polymorphism similar to that seen in A_β. The murine immune system is just not capable of responding to all of the A_α allelic variability.

TRANSCOMPLEMENTATION

Studies by Silver et al. (1980) had shown that in (H-2^k x H-2^b)F_1 mice, four I-A molecules are expressed. The two molecules formed by cis-complementation, $A^k_\beta A^k_\alpha$, $A^b_\beta A^b_\alpha$ and two by transcomplementation, $A^b_\beta A^k_\alpha$, $A^k_\beta A^b_\alpha$. Similar analyses showed that cross-isotype pairing (e.g. $E_\beta A_\alpha$, $A_\beta E_\alpha$) does not occur (Murphy et al. 1980). These findings led to the view that there is "free association" of allelic variants within an isotype giving rise to heterozygous I-A molecules with a restriction on cross-isotype pairing. These assumptions were made despite data indicating this may not always be the case. In most F_1's involving the I-E molecule, the E_α gene can associate with most E_β chains, with one exception, the E^k_α chain failed to associate with the E^u_β chain (Lafuse et al. 1982). McNicholas et al. (1982) demonstrated an eight-fold preference for $E^u_\beta E^u_\alpha$ formation over $E^k_\beta E^u_\alpha$. In addition, immune responsiveness to pigeon cytochrome C demonstrated a defect in response due to the low quantity of hybrid molecules generated (Matis et al. 1982). An attempt to explain the anomaly of pairing involving the E^u_α and E^u_β was recently undertaken by comparing sequences for these chains with previously described sequences (Ayane et al. 1986). No glaring structural abnormalities were found, however, some u-specific residues were identified which may play some role in the selectivity for pairing observed in the u haplotype. In light of additional studies on pairing to be described below, the u haplotype may reflect one extreme of a continuum in the ability of hybrid Ia molecules to form. The demonstration of expression of mixed-isotype molecules $A^d_\beta E^{a/k}_\alpha$ in L-cell transfectants (Germain and Quill 1986), $A_\beta DR_\alpha$ pairing in transfected human Epstein-Barr virus transformed lymphoblastoid cells and the demonstration of Lerner et al. (1980) of possible $E_\beta A_\alpha$ pairing recognized by the Y-17 monoclonal antibody, all indicate a re-evaluation of inter-isotypic pairing should be undertaken to determine the degree and potential significance of such inter-isotypic molecules.

A new view of the process of Ia chain pairing and expression is developing due to recent studies by Germain et al. (1985b) using Ia gene transfected L cells showing differences in expression of various α and β chain pairs. A failure of A^d_β:A^k_α to be detected by various monoclonal antibodies or a rabbit anti-$A_\beta A_\alpha$ heteroantiserum is one extreme of the spectrum while barely significant expression of $A^k_\beta A^d_\alpha$ is detectable with the rabbit heteroantiserum. Combination of A^b_β:A^k_α are detectable with monoclonal antibodies whereas $A^b_\beta A^d_\alpha$ is barely evident. These results indicate that particular α and β alleles used in each pair can strongly influence the extent of membrane $A_\beta A_\alpha$ expression. The expression of A^k_β:A^d_α cell surface molecules was detected by the transfection of A^k_β gene into the Ia^d B lymphoma M12.4.1 (Germain et al. 1983) in contrast with the L cell data. In re-analyzing these cells, a large excess of A_α chain can be demonstrated by Northern blot analysis and flow microfluorimetric studies. In this situation there would be no competition for the A_{α}^{d} chain after transfection with A_{β}^{k}, yielding sufficient although inefficient membrane expression of the $A_{\beta}^{k}:A_{\alpha}^{d}$ molecule. All the appropriate controls by Southern and Northern analysis where done to confirm integration and transcriptional activity of the transfected genes. As has been found for T cell recognition and antibody binding sites in exon shuffled hybrid genes where the immunologically relevant A_{β} determinants of I-A^{k} maps to the highly polymorphic amino-terminal domain; the control of the haplotype preference in k:d mixes also maps to this domain. This was shown by the equivalent expression of a recombinant molecule containing the NH_{α}-terminal (β1) domain of A_{β}^{k}, with the β2, transmembrane and cytoplasmic portions of A_{β}^{d} pairing with A_{α}^{k} against $A_{\beta}^{k}:A_{\alpha}^{k}$ expression. This being distinctly different from the negative results of $A_{\beta}^{k}:A_{\alpha}^{d}$ transfectants.

According to Germain et al. (1985b) these data demonstrate a preference for the association of cis-chromosomal pairs over those composed of trans-chromosomal genes and may explain the tight linkage disequilibrium seen between these α and β genes so that each pair may co-evolve for best fit ensuring a high level of membrane Ia expression. The case of the b haplotype, which demonstrates higher efficiency of hybrid pairing, may be a case where the lack of E molecule expression has led to a sacrificing of some efficiency in cis-pairing for better trans-pairing in order to maintain some variation in total Ia molecules expressed. This would suggest other E_{α}-null haplotypes should demonstrate this same permissiveness, a testable hypothesis. The co-evolution observed between A_{α} and A_{β} has not occurred between E_{β} and E_{α} and it is possible the low level of polymorphism seen in the E_{α} gene was derived from a need for a "generalist" form of E_{α} capable of adapting to the frequent changes in its E_{β} partner. The level of these trans molecules being expressed under the influence of lymphokines known to enhance Ia expression during an inflammatory process may be of suitable levels for efficient T cell recognition. This expression is postulated to having a possible role in development of autoimmune disease following bacterial or viral infections as has been noted in HLA-DR linked diseases such as juvenile-onset diabetes where heterozygosity has been postulated to play a role (Scholz and Albert, 1983). The upregulation during an inflammatory response may increase the presentation of self antigens in a system defective of regulatory mechanisms (e.g. via suppressor T cells) capable of dampening such responses in context of these poorly expressed, unique Ia molecules. Additional data regarding T cell function in vivo will need to be obtained to further support these hypotheses.

ALLELIC POLYMORPHISM

The abundance of antigens required to be presented to T cells in conjunction with Ia molecules and the nature of immune responsiveness suggest a need for these molecules to be polymorphic in nature to optimally act as the restriction element. Analyses of Ia molecules by serology, 2-dimensional gel electrophoresis, tryptic peptide mapping, amino terminal protein sequence determination, as well as cellular assays such as MLR and CML have demonstrated a large degree of variability among alleles of the beta chains and of the A_{α} chain (Cullen, et al. 1976; Klein and Figueroa 1981; and Cecka et al. 1979).

The use of restriction fragment analyses and nucleic acid sequencing of multiple alleles of class II genes have confirmed and refined this knowledge of polymorphism. The analyses of restriction fragment length polymorphisms (RFLP) from 75 strains of laboratory inbred mice, as well as haplotypes derived from wild mice would localize particular gene loci of polymorphism as opposed to a polymorphic region containing the A_β, A_α and E_β genes due to no difference being found on the degree of polymorphism between the A_α gene and the E_α gene (Bukara et al. 1985). This controversy will require the sequencing of the A_α chains from the wild strains of mice as well as additional E_α genes to determine the actual sequence polymorphism. At this time, many of the alleles of the different class II genes have been sequenced. From this combined information, several conclusions can be drawn regarding gene organization as well as polymorphism. An interesting observation is the correlation of exon organization with functional/structural domains. The E_α and A_α genes contain 5 exons with separate exons coding for the leader peptide, α1 and α2 domains, a single exon to encode the transmembrane and cytoplasmic domains with part of the 3' untranslated region and an additional exon encoding the remaining 3' untranslated region. The A_β and E_β genes contain six exons similar in organization to the alpha genes with the distinction of separate exons coding the transmembrane and cytoplasmic domains (Germain and Malissen, 1986).

In comparing nucleotide sequences for the β chains and A_α it can be seen that nucleotide substitutions occur throughout the molecules. There is, however, a definite clustering of substitutions in the region encoding the first external domain of the mature proteins with the majority of these being productive. The sequences comparing E_α^d and E_α^k show very few nucleotide differences. There are actually a larger number of differences between the two published E_α^d sequences indicating some of the variance may be due to sequencing errors or genetic variability (Hyldig-Nielsen, et al. 1983). Comparison of the predicted protein sequences for A_α, A_β and E_β alleles shows that the variability is clustered in three or four short stretches within the first domain with conserved regions among alleles at a particular locus as well as between α or β loci. An example of this is seen particularly in the A_β loci where 8.4% of the total protein sequence contains 60% of the variability (Mengle-Gaw and McDevitt, 1985).

When the A_β is compared between haplotypes q, k, u, s and f, the homology ranges between 87-98% for the first beta domain. The rest of the gene shows a 96% or greater homology. Further, the changes in the nucleotides in the β1 lead to productive changes causing amino acid alterations while scattered nucleotide changes in the rest of the gene rarely lead to amino acid differences. This implies that the variable regions of the first domain are specifically tolerant to mutations that alter amino acid sequences compared with the rest of the molecule. The presumed functions (processing, heterodimer formation, membrane anchoring and perhaps intracytoplasmic signaling) of the conserved domains appear to be associated with limited structural heterogeneity (Estess et al. 1986). The β1 and β2 domains of A_β and E_β share 58% and 65% of residues respectively, while the leader peptide shows only 31% homology. This difference may play some role in regulating A and E region associations. The intracytoplasmic regions of I-A_β chains contain no phosphorylatable serines as compared to E_β chains. This may be a reflection of functional differences between the two types of molecules.

Figure 2 diagramatically depicts the polymorphic regions of the first domain of the A_β gene. Amino acid sequence 60-80 is the most polymorphic segment of the gene and is different in almost every haplotype studied. Antibodies made between haplotypes invariably recognize this region of the polypeptide. T cells seem to recognize this region in association with other regions depending on the conformation. T cells also recognize sequences 8-14 as well as 80-90. Sequence 26 and 28 also show some variability.

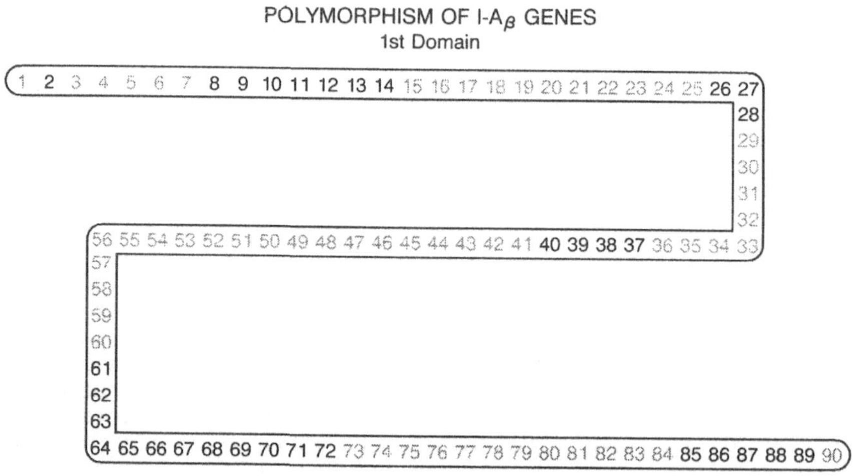

The mechanisms for the generation of this diversity have been analyzed and, the end result may be a composite of several possibilities including multiple point mutations and copy substitution mechanisms. There have been many debates on how the MHC polymorphism arose. There may be other Ia genes that do not code for viable polypeptide chains and thus are not expressed on the cell surface. Mutations may occur in these genes at random and because there is a neutral selection, these mutations will survive and accumulate. These accumulated mutations from the non-expressed genes could periodically be transferred to expressed genes by either a gene conversion-like copy mechanism or by micro-double recombination. There may be sites on the Ia genes where specific signals are transmitted for these types of interchanges. Some regions may be important in terms of antigen presentation such as sequences 65-75 and 80-90 in the first domain. Thus, unique functional determinants are generated and if there is a positive selection for the altered Ia product, they will survive and be established in the population.

Ia MUTANT B6.H-2^{bm12}

In contrast to many class I mutants which have been identified, so far only one class II mutant has been found. We believe this is because class II mutations do not give rise to drastic alterations which can be picked up by skin grafting techniques. Other methods to try to screen for class II mutants have not been successful. The one class II mutant that is known, bm12, was identified by Melvold, et al. (1982). The mutation was mapped to the I-A subregion by McKenzie et al. (1979) and eventually localized to the A_β chain by McKean, et al. (1981).

Tryptic peptide maps revealed a limited number of differences between bm12 and the parent, B6 indicating that is is not due to a single point mutation, but involves a minimum of three different amino acid substitutions. McIntyre and Seidman (1984) have cloned and sequenced the gene coding for bm12 A_β polypeptide chain. Three nucleotide substitutions resulted in three amino acid substitutions within a span of 5 amino acids; isoleucine at position 67, arginine at position 70, and threonine at position 71, are being substituted by phenylalanine, glutamine and lysine, respectively. Two of these amino acid substitutions (arginine to glutamine and threonine to lysine) are non-conservative changes in the tertiary structure of the β polypeptide chain, resulting in the observed alterations in the serology and the function of the bm12 I-A molecule. Amino acid sequence comparison also shows that two of the amino acid substitutions found in the bm12 A_β chain are found at the same positions in several human class II beta chains (McIntyre and Seidman, 1984). These comparisons suggest that the bm12 mutation in the I-A_β chain arose from a gene conversion type event in which another class II beta chain gene acted as a donor sequence. Comparison of the bm12 nucleotide substitutions to the sequence of a cosmid clone for the I-E_β^b gene have suggested that this gene may have served as a donor sequence (Widera and Flavell, 1984) where a minimum of 14 nucleotides of the A_β gene are replaced by homologous information from the E_β gene (Figure 3). The same sequence is also found in the I-$E_\beta^{s,k}$ chains.

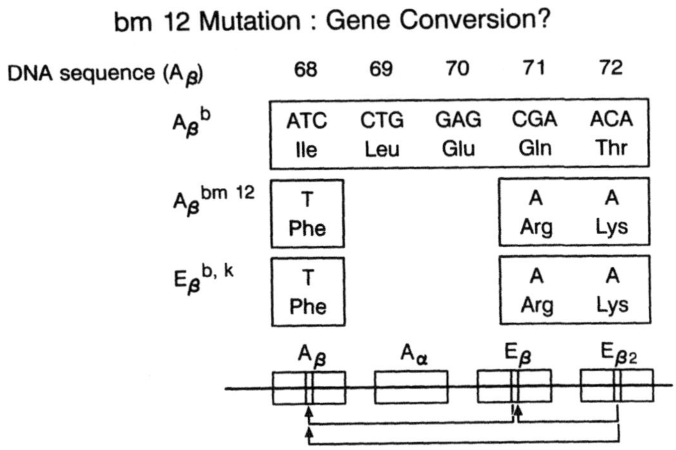

We were interested in seeing whether the identical segment of the E_β polypeptide chain and A_β^{bm12} polypeptide chains can be identified by serological methods. We produced an antibody between the B6 parent and the mutant, bm12. The antibody gave cytotoxic reactivity against bm12 and precipitated an Ia type molecule by immunoprecipitation. A survey of other strains showed that the antibody did not react with any other A_β chain but did react with E_β chains of the b, k, and s haplotypes. This indicated to us that the antigenic determinant generated in the bm12 mutation is also found in these E_β chains and we designated this specificity as Ia.51. In the bm12 mutation, antigenic determinant, Ia.51 has replaced the native determinant, Ia.8. Ancient serological studies had shown that Ia.8 is also found in haplotypes d and q. Comparison of the amino acid sequences of A_β chains between b, d, and q indicate identity between sequences 55 to 75. Further, the sequences 60-70 of the A_β chain are identical in haplotypes k, s and f, and possibly code for the Ia determinant, Ia.17 (Estess et al. 1986). Thus, this segment in these haplotypes might have all been donated from other genes by gene conversion or copy mechanism. On the other hand, they could have been generated by microrecombination between these haplotypes.

This gave us an idea to look for gene conversion type events by serological crossreactions. In the early days of Ia serology, it was assumed that the public specificities of Ia antigens are a result of serological crossreactions. We have even noticed crossreactions between the A and E molecules. Antibodies made against I-E sometimes crossreact with I-A and vice versa. We had attributed these crossreactions to evolutionary homology between haplotypes. Another explanation for these crossreactions could also be recent gene conversion type exchanges. In order to use serological crossreactions as an indication of gene conversion type events, we have recently started screening several monoclonal antibodies for crossreactions and to compare the sequence similarities between crossreacting haplotypes. One such example is given in Table 2. Two monoclonal antibodies, H39-59 and H9-15.4, react with the A_β chain of the b and d haplotypes and E_β chain of the b,d, and k haplotype. The only common residue we find between these five chains are the sequences 60-67. The A_β chain from the k haplotype differs only in position 64 and 67 and is negative for these antibodies. These findings indicate that polymorphism between different alleles for the class II genes are generated by exchange of genetic information at critical sites. At this time, we cannot show whether all of these sequences were derived from the same third party donor or were just a random exchange between different alleles.

Table 2. Crossreactions of Monoclonal Antibody

	Amino Acids		H39-459
A_β Chain	64	67	H9-15.4
b	ser	glu	+
d	ser	glu	+
k	lys	tyr	-
E_β Chain			
b,d,k	ser	glu	+

The bm12 mutant has been used by several investigators to define structure/function relationships of the Ia molecule. Hochman and Huber (1985) and Mengle-Gaw et al. (1984) have shown that functional determinants are shared between A_β^{bm12} and E_β^d polypeptides. This is based upon responsiveness of bm12 to sheep insulin. B6, the parental strain of bm12 is a nonresponder to sheep insulin. Studies by Lin, et al. (1981) have shown that a lymphoid proliferation response to beef insulin in the bm12 mutant is greatly reduced compared to the parent B6, while response to other antigens (T,G)-A--L, DNP-OVA, PPD, and pork insulin is unaffected. Using bm12, Mengle-Gaw et al. (1984) have demonstrated that the I-A subregion is responsible for Ir gene phenomenon and mixed lymphocyte reaction. They have also shown that alloreactive T cell clones recognize a determinant shared by A_β^{bm12} and E_β^b molecules. Based upon the above findings it was proposed that, the segment of gene donated by E_β^b maintains its functional determinants in bm12. However, this notion has been challenged by Tse et al. (1985), who used a number of alloreactive clones generated against Ia_β^{bm12} antigens. If bm12 inherits a functional E_β^b unit, these B6-anti-bm12 alloreactive T cells should be stimulated by E_β^b positive cells. However, in their study B10.A(5R) (E_β^b, E_α^k) failed to stimulate B6-anti-bm12 T cell clones. Recently, Hansen et al (1986) have shown that responses of B6.C-H-2^{bm12} to heterologous insulins show no correlation with the putative gene conversion but define Ia_β^{bm12} as functionally unique. These findings strongly suggest that T cells recognize conformational determinants on Ia molecules. Since activation of T cell depends on the concommitant recognition of Ia and antigen on the surface of antigen presenting cells, any change in the tertiary structure of the Ia molecule might affect the immune response.

We have used (B6 x A.TFR5)F_1 mice to characterize the mutant Ia determinant by T cells (Donovan, et al., submitted for publication). B6, being a nonexpressor of the I-E molecule does not express E_β on the cell surface. A.TFR5 has an E_β (E_β^f) gene which fails to make a protein product. However, A.TFR5 synthesizes a functional E_α polypeptide chain. The (B6 x A.TFR5)F_1 expresses a functional I-E molecule, which is comprised of E_β^b and E_α^k. This molecule carries the linear determinant which is expressed on the surface of bm12 lymphocytes. So, one would predict that if T cells do not recognize the conformational determinants, bm12 skin grafts would be accepted by (B6 x A.TFR5)F_1s. However, this is not the case. These F_1s reject the bm12 skin grafts as readily as the B6 strains do. It has been proposed that since B6 and bm12 mice fail to express E_β chains, the bm12 gene conversion resulted in the expression of a new determinant expressed by bm12 and not by B6 cells. Hence, the reciprocal grafts are rejected. Even though the E_β^b chain is expressed on the F_1 recipients, it recognizes bm12 determinants as foreign and causes the skin graft rejection.

To further characterize the role of Ia conformation, we also tested the (B6 x A.TFR5)F_1 anti-bm12 proliferative response. B6 anti-bm12 cells respond strongly to each other in a primary mixed lymphocyte response. If the conformational determinant is not important in T cell recognition of an Ia molecule, one would not expect a (B6 x A.TFR5)F_1-anti-bm12 response. However, a strong mixed lymphocyte response is observed.

The data presented here strongly supports the idea that T cells recognize predominantly the tertiary structure of Ia in both allogeneic and syngeneic responses. In the bm12 mice, the sequences from the E_β gene are flanked by the sequences from A_β. This results in a different tertiary structure than the E molecule in F_1 mice, where E_β is represented in its normal conformation. Further, there is evidence that the association of E^b_β and E^k_α chains generate new functional determinants. Thus, the combinatorial structure of $E^b_\beta E^k_\alpha$ in (B6 x A.TFR5)F_1 may be different from $A^{bm12}_\beta A^b_\alpha$ which would be seen as non-self. So, "gene conversion" like events would create entirely new restricting elements. This could explain why the F_1 mice see the Ia of bm12 as alloantigen and mount both mixed lymphocyte response and skin graft rejection.

HOT SPOTS OF RECOMBINATION

The distance between genes on the same chromosome has initially been determined based upon the percentage of recombination between genes where one map unit (or centiMorgan) equals 1% recombination. This method of determining map distances may have to be re-evaluated due to the finding of what may be hot spots of recombination. By recombinational analyses the A_β and E_α genes are approximately .1 centiMorgan apart (Snell et al. 1976). This corresponds to about 200 Kb, if recombination is random throughout the mouse genome. Mapping by aligning cosmid clones determines this distance to be more in the range of 85 Kb of DNA (Steinmetz et al. 1982). In analyzing recombination events in nine independently generated recombinant congenic mice by restriction length polymorphism, the point of recombination could be localized to within a 9.8 Kb segment of DNA (Steinmetz et al. 1982). It has since been shown that 16 recombinants map within this distance or less, and that 3 of these [B10.A(3R), B10.A(5R) and B10.GD] recombined within a 1.0 Kb region of the 3' end of the class II E_β gene (Kobori et al. 1986). Eleven recombinant mouse strains with possible crossovers in the E_β gene were also analyzed by Lafuse and David (in press) in which nine have been found to have crossed over in a 5 Kb DNA segment in the middle of the E_β gene. This segment contains the large intervening sequence between exons 2 and 3, within which the above mentioned recombinants were mapped. The crossing over in the other two recombinants maps in the DNA segment between the E_β and the E_α gene.

In laboratory mice, the recombination events between the K and I region have a very low frequency (0.02%) with only three strains described, A.TL (David and Shreffler, 1972), B10.AQR (Klein 1975) and B10.MBR (Sachs et al. 1979). In contrast, the Mus musculus molossinus MHC haplotype of the B10.MOL-GSR (H-2^{wm7}) strain when crossed with a, k or b MHC haplotypes shows a recombination frequency of 2.1% (Shiroishi et al. 1982). This suggest the presence of a genetic element in the M.m. molossinus MHC that specifically enhances recombination between K and I region genes. A similar enhancement of recombination between the K and I region involving the M.m. castaneus haplotypes (CAS3 and CAS4) crossed with k or b was analyzed using restriction length polymorphisms (Steinmetz et al. 1986). Unlike the three laboratory strains which showed different points of crossovers between the K and $A_{\beta 2}$ genes, the eight recombinants between M.m. castaneus and laboratory mice could be localized to two regions.

Three recombinants derived from CAS4 and C3H.Pgk-1^a could be mapped to a 42 Kb segment approximately 45 Kb distal to the K gene. Five recombinants derived from CAS3 were shown to have crossed over within a stretch of 9.5 Kb about 50 Kb upstream of the $A_{\beta 2}$ gene. The point of recombination in the M.m. molossinus mice will need to be analyzed to determine if they fall into one of the hot spots defined above. The finding of hot spots between K and I regions in M.m. molossinus and M.m. castaneus but not in M.m. domesticus from which most of the laboratory inbred strains of mice have been derived suggest that particular hot spot regions may be species dependent or even haplotype dependent.

In a recent study by Lafuse et al. (1986) a new potential hot spot involving the E_α gene was postulated. This was based on a study of nine recombinant mouse strains involving the k and p haplotypes by restriction fragment analysis. It was found that seven of these recombinants had crossover points in a 12 Kb DNA segment extending from a Hpa I restriction site polymorphism within the $E_{\beta 2}$ gene to a Rsa I restriction site polymorphism 1 Kb 5' of the E_α gene. In a further analysis of these recombinants by Lafuse and David (in press), this distance was narrowed to a 6 Kb distance including the E_α gene. The use of the Dra I and Pst I enzymes localizes the crossover point to the immediate E_α gene region between the Dra I and Pst I sites in the intron between exons 4 and 5 and the Rsa I and Pst I sites 5' of the E_α gene.

Of the nine recombinants looked at, none mapped to the previously described hot spot in the E_β gene. The two additional recombinants in this study had crossovers between E_α and the S region. It is possible that this new hot spot is a reflection of the B10.F(13R) which was one of the parents in all nine of these recombinants. In the E^d gene (Wake et al. 1985) and seven recombinant strains examined by Kobori et al. (1986), an imperfect four-base repeat sequence (AGGC)n was found approximately 50 bp 5' to the β2 exon of the E_β gene. This sequence is repeated 18 times in the d haplotype and 10 times in b and k haplotypes. Low homology, is found between the repeat sequence and the lambda phage chi sequence (Smith et al. 1981), which facilitates recombination in Escherichia coli. The homology to the core sequence of the hypervariable minisatellite core sequence is more striking. The hypervariable minisatellite sequences have been found at regions that are highly polymorphic in the human genome due to allelic variation in repeat copy number of the minisatellite. It has been suggested that these minisatellites are recombination hot spots generating allelic variability by frequent unequal crossing-over events during meiosis (Jeffreys et al. 1985). In addition to these observations, it was also noted that the repeat sequence of CAGG was closely related to (CGGG)8 which has been proposed to be able to form Z-DNA (Ellison et al. 1985) which may play some role in recombination events. An oligonucleotide probe complementary to part of the repeat sequence was used to probe 24 BALB/c cosmid clones to check for additional copies of the repeat sequence. The two clones containing the E_β gene hybridized strongly to the probe. Other than one clone mapping to the K region which hybridized weakly, no other clone was positive for this oligomer (Steinmetz et al. 1986). A 40 nucleotide fragment was used for the same purpose with similar results (Kabori et al. 1986). In addition, a genomic blot with the repeat region as a probe indicated a few major hybridizing bands, including one corresponding to the E_β hot spot, and a high background of weak hybridization. Due to the highly conserved nature of the E_α genes, if the sequences responsible for the increased recombination frequency seen in the E_α hot spot were the same as in the E_β hot spot, these probes would have cross hybridized to the cosmid clones containing the E_α gene. Since no such hybridization is seen, any controlling sequences are probably different for this hot spot.

Recombination hot spots are not unique to MHC genes. Similar regions of increased recombination frequencies have been found in the human β globin gene cluster (Orkin and Kazaziau, 1984; Chakravarti et al. 1984) and the human insulin loci (Lebo et al. 1983). It was found that 75% of the recombinations in the 63 kb β globin gene cluster occur within a 9.1 kb region. It was estimated that the rate in this segment was approximately 3-30 times greater than the expected rate (Chakravarti et al. 1984). Restriction fragment analysis of the human insulin gene has shown significant polymorphism in restriction fragment lengths in both the 3' and 5' regions of the insulin gene (Lebo et al. 1983). This indicated that recombination occurred 33 times more frequently than expected to generate this polymorphism.

The effect of crossover events in the E_β and E_α genes on the function of these Ia molecules is probably minimal. The crossover in the E_β gene occurs between the exons coding the first external domain which is polymorphic in different haplotypes (reviewed by Mengle-Gaw and McDevitt 1985) and the second external domain of the E_β polypeptide. Although the crossover event does create a new I-E_β polypeptide chain with a different second external domain, transmembrane domain and cytoplasmic domain, sequence analysis has shown that these domains are relatively nonpolymorphic. The E_α gene is also nonpolymorphic so that recombination within the gene should not alter the E_α polypeptide. Thus there is no obvious advantage for crossovers at these sites. However, recombination involving crossing-over in general is advantageous since it results in the formation of chiasmata during the first meiotic division, which is necessary for the proper reduction segregation of homologous chromsomes. If homologous chromsomes are joined by chiasmata they remain associated as a bivalent during the first meiotic division. However, if no chiasmata is formed the homologs may fail to remain associated and segregate randomly resulting in aneuploid gamates.

Where cross-over occurs is also of evolutionary importance. Eukaryotic genomes have transposable elements which vary in location and numbers and on an evolutionary time scale the position is not predictable. Recombination between such elements present in nonhomologous locations would generate aberrations such as duplications and deficiencies, resulting in the possibility of lethality due to genetic imbalance. Thus, it has been suggested by Carpenter (1984) that the normal recombination pathway includes a process that insures the presence of extended sequence homology before cross-over can occur. Observance of recombination hot spots in the H-2 complex may be the result of such a process.

Finally, crossovers produce new combinations of MHC genes which must be advantageous to the survival of the species. Having the crossover points at non-polymorphic regions of the gene keeps the first domain intact, thereby not disrupting the determinants involved in antigen presentation. There may be other advantages that we are not aware of at this time.

REGULATION OF Ia GENES

The tissue specific nature of class II expression has been well documented being limited primarily to macrophages, B cells, dendritic cells and thymic epithelial cells. Regulation of this selective expression has been analyzed by several different approaches. Examples of both positive and negative regulatory substances have been demonstrated to affect cell surface expression of class II antigens. IFN-γ has been shown to have a stimulatory effect for both class I and class II molecules in macrophages (King and Jones, 1983), where as in B cells there is no observable effect by this lymphokine (Roehm et al. 1984). Nuclear run-on experiments in WEHI-3 cells indicate that IFN-γ induces the transcription of Ia genes through a complex induction process as indicated by the long lag phase before increases are observed (Jones et al., Personal Communication). In addition, protein synthesis inhibitors show a need for de novo protein synthesis in the induction of HLA-DR genes indicating that γ-interferon induces the synthesis of a regulatory protein which induces transcription of class II genes (Armaldi et al., Personal Communication). Preliminary experiments using DNA fragments from the region 5' of the E^d_α structural gene have been analyzed by 'gel retardation' assays utilizing nuclear protein extracts from various cell lines. These experiments have shown at least one protein from extracts of both IFN-γ induced and uninduced WEHI-3 cells that bind specifically to a region approximately 400 nucleotides 5' of the ATG of exon 1 (Blanar et al., Personal Communication). This finding is being examined for its relationship to E_α expression. In contrast, LPS stimulation of macrophages inhibits the expression of Ia, presumably by stimulating the production of prostaglandins known to be inhibitory to class II expression (Steeg et al. 1982). The level of Ia expression on normal B cells is heterogeneous and may be dependent on the maturational state of the cells which are Ia negative in the pre-B cell as well as the plasma cell stage. In addition to IFN-γ, neither IL-2 nor IL-3 has any enhancing effect on B cell Ia expression. BSF-1, however, does (Roehm et al. 1984; Polla et al. 1986). The effect of BSF-1 is mediated by an induction of transcription of class II genes within one hour by a mechanism independent of protein synthesis. It is not thought that this effect is mediated through calcium fluxes or activation of protein kinase C since treatment with agents such as PMA or the calcium inophore A23187 did not result in class II expression. Together these data indicate that class II expression is regulated at different levels in various cell types.

Several studies have shown the existence of interspecies trans-acting factors having a role in expression of class II genes. This has been done by fusing a class II negative human B-lymphoma cell line with murine Ia-positive B lymphoma cell line (Accolla et al. 1985). This factor is supplied by a murine locus that maps to chromosome 16 (Accolla et al. 1986).

Structural studies have been undertaken in the class I genes to determine regulatory regions of importance. In an analysis of the K^b gene by Israel et al. (1986), sequenes responsible for the effect seen by IFN-γ have been localized. Using a series of deletion mutants attached to the bacterial chloramphenicol acetyltransferase (CAT) gene, they were able to demonstrate a need for both interferon response sequences and enhancer A for the IFN effect to occur. The interferon response sequences are similar to the concensus sequence determined by Friedman and Stark (1985) for IFN responsiveness. A similar study in the miniature swine localizes an interferon responsiveness region to within 400 bp of the promoter (Ehrlich and Singer, Personal Communication). In addition a negative regulatory element 5' of this region has also been identified. The analysis of sequences in the IFN responsive region, however, does not correlate well with the consensus sequence. Further studies will have to be done in class II genes to determine the regions responsible for IFN responsiveness. A cell type specific enhancer element was identified by Gillies et al. (1984) in the E_β gene by analyzing 28 Kb of E_β coding and flanking sequences in a plasmid containing the gpt gene. A 2.0 Kb region 5' of the E_β gene 600 bp from the promoter region was shown to contain the enhancing capability and functioned in either orientation as has been shown for other enhancer elements. This region does not contain the two short sequences shown previously to be conserved between E_α, human DR_α genes and the E_β gene (Saito et al. 1983). Studies in the E_α gene have identified sequences and factors responsible for the expression of this gene (Mathis, Personal Communication). Using mutants transfected into cells or in transgenic mice, the role of the conserved "class II boxes" x and y have been studied. The need of sequences 5' of the E_α gene for appropriate tissue expression was demonstrated by transgenic mice containing various constructs of the gene. The use of an E_α^d construct which contained only 1.4 Kb 5' of the gene, showed that tissue expression was altered. Expression was found only in the thymus and in splenic adherent cells, and was inducible in peritoneal exudate cells by IFN-γ. This construct appears to have separated sequences necessary for normal B cell expression from those required for macrophages and in the thymus (Blanar et al., Personal Communication). Other constructs such as an 8.2 Kb Bgl1 fragment containing the E_α^k gene plus 2 Kb of DNA 5' to the cap site and 1.5 Kb 3' to the polyadenylation site gave rise to normal tissue distribution (leMeur et al. 1985) as well as mice made with an E_α^d construct containing less of the 3' region but more of the 5' region (Pinkert et al. 1985). On the basis of these observations more defined sequences can be identified for their role in class II gene regulation.

In the past five years DNA studies have shown us many interesting aspects of Ia genes. The in vitro studies have indicated many restrictions and gene control. The functional studies are still a black box. There are many controversies and contradictions. Regardless of what elegant in vitro studies we do, eventually these results have to be tested in vivo. We believe in the next decade, transgenic mice expressing injected Ia genes will be the tool of immunogenetic research in this area. We have embarked on a major effort to produce transgenic mice. We do not have any data to share at this time, but we will show you the picture of the first transgenic mice from our lab.

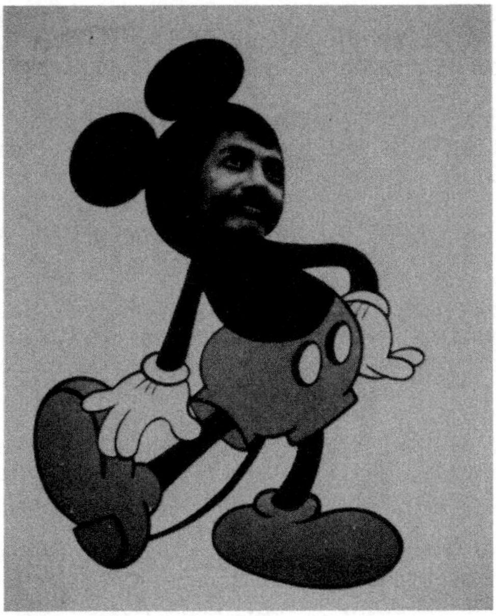

Figure 1

ACKNOWLEDGEMENTS

The authors thank Mary Brandt for patient and skillful preparation of this manuscript. The studies cited in this paper from the authors' laboratory were supported by NIH grants AI-14764 and CA-24473.

REFERENCES

Accolla, R.S., Carra, G. and Guardiola, J.: Reactivation by a trans-acting factor of human MHC-Ia gene expression in interspecies hybrids between an Ia-negative human B-cell variant and an Ia-positive mouse B-cell lymphoma. Proc. Natl. Acad. Sci. USA 82:5145, 1985.

Accolla, R.S., Jotteraud-Bellomo, M., Scarpellino, L., Maffei, A., Carra, G. and Guardiola, J.: aIr-1, a newly found locus on mouse chromsome 16 encoding a trans-acting factor for MHC class II gene expression. J. Exp. Med. 164:369, 1986.

Ayane, M., Mengle-Gaw, L., McDevitt, H.O., Benoist, C. and Mathis, D.: E^u_α and E^u_β chain association: where lies the anomaly. J. Immunol. 137:948, 1986.

Beck, B.N., Buerstedde, J-M., Krco, C.J., Hilson, A.E., Chase, C.G. and McKean, D.J.: Characterization of cell lines expressing mutant I-A^b and I-A^k molecules allows the definition of distinct serologic epitopes on A_α and A_β polypeptides. J. Immunol. 136:2953, 1986.

Braunstein, N.S. and Germain, R.N.: The mouse $E_{\beta 2}$ gene: a class II MHC β gene with limited intraspecies polymorphism and an unusual pattern of transcription. EMBO J. 5:2469, 1986.

Bukara, M., Vincek, V., Figueroa, F. and Klein, J. How polymorphic are class II loci of the mouse H-2 complex? Immunogenetics 21:569, 1985.

Carpenter, A.T.C.: Meiotic roles of crossing-over and of gene conversion. Cold Spring Harbor Symp. Quant. Biol. 49:23, 1984.

Cecka, J., McMillan, M., Murphy, D.B., McDevitt, H.O. and Hood, L.: Partial N-terminal amino acid sequence analyses and comparative tryptic peptide maps of murine Ia molecules encoded by the I-A subregion. Eur. J. Immunol. 9:944, 1979.

Chakravarti, A., Beutow, K., Antonarakis, S.E., Waber, P.G., Boehm, C.D. and Kazaziau, H.H.: Non-uniform recombination within the human β-globin gene cluster. Am. J. Hum. Genet. 36:129, 1984.

Cullen, S.E., David, C.S., Shreffler, D.C. and Nathenson, S.G.: Isolation of membrane molecules determined by the H-2 associated immune response region. Proc. Natl. Acad. Sci. 71:811, 1974.

Cullen, S.E., Freed, J., nathenson, S.G.: Structural and serological properties of murine Ia alloantigens. Transplant. Rev. 30:236, 1976.

David, C.S. and Shreffler, D.C.: Studies on recombination within the mouse H-2 complex. II. Serological analyses of four recombinants, $H\text{-}2^{al}$, $H\text{-}2^{ol}$, $H\text{-}2^{tl}$ and $H\text{-}2^{th}$. Tissue Antigens 2:241, 1972.

David, C.S., Shreffler, D.C. and Frelinger, J.A.: New lymphocyte antigen system (Lna) controlled by the Ir region of the mouse H-2 complex. Proc. Natl. Acad. Sci. (USA) 70:2509, 1973.

Dembic, Z., Singer, P.A. and Klein, J.: E^{o}: a history of a mutation. EMBO J. 3:1647, 1984.

Donovan, K.A., Singh, S.K. and David, C.J.: T cell recognition of conformational Ia determinants. Submitted.

Ellison, M.J., Kelleher, R.M. III, Wang, A. H-J, Habener, J.F. and Rich, A.: Sequence-dependent energetics of the B-Z transition in superoided DNA containing nonalternating purine-pyrimidine sequences. Proc. Natl. Acad. Sci. USA 82:8320, 1985.

Estess, P., Begovich, A.B., Koo, M., Jones, P.P., McDevitt, H.O.: Sequence analysis and structure-function correlations of murine q, k, u, s and f haplotype $I\text{-}A_{\beta}$ cDNA clones. Proc. Natl. Acad. Sci. USA 83:3594, 1986.

Flavell, R.A., Allen, H., Huber, B., Wake, C. and Widera, G.: Organization and expression of the MHC of the C57Black/10 mouse. Immunological Reviews 84:29, 1985.

Friedman, R.L. and Stark, G.R.: α-interferon-induced transcription of HLA and metallothionein genes containing homologous upstream sequences. Nature 314:637, 1985.

Germain, R.N., Norcross, M.A. and Margulies, D.M.: Functional expression of a transfected murine class II MHC gene. Nature 306:190, 1983.

Germain, R.N., Ashwell, J.D., Lechler, R.I., Margulies, D.H., Nickerson, K.M., Suzuki, G. and Tou, J.Y.E.: "Exon-shuffling" maps control of antibody- and T-cell-recognition sites to the NH_2-terminal domain of the class II major histocompatibility polypeptide A_β. Proc. Natl. Acad. Sci. USA 82:2940, 1985.

Germain, R.N., Bentley, D.M. and Quill, H.: Influence of allelic polymorphism on the assembly and surface expression of class II MHC (Ia) molecules. Cell 43:233, 1985.

Germain, R.N. and Quill, H.: Unexpected expression of a unique mixed-isotope class II MHC molecule by transfected L-cells. Nature 320:72, 1986.

Germain, R.N. and Malissen, B.: Analysis of the expression and function of class II major histocompatibility complex-encoded molecules by DNA-mediated gene transfer. Ann. Rev. Immunol. 4:281, 1986.

Gillies, S.D., Folsom, V. and Tonegawa, S.: Cell type-specific enhancer element associated with a mouse MHC gene, E_β. Nature 310:594, 1984.

Hansen, T.H., Walsh, W.D., Rubocki, R.J. and Kapp, J.A.: Responses of B6.C-H-2^{bm12} to heterologous insulins show no correlation with the putative gene conversion but define Ia^{bm12} as functionally unique. J. Mol. Cell. Immunology 2:359, 1986.

Hochman, P.S. and Huber, B.T.: A class II gene-conversion event defines an antigen-specific Ir gene epitope. J. Exp. Med. 160:1925-1930, 1984.

Hyldig-Nielsen, J.J., Schenning, L., Hammerling, U., Widmark, E., Heldiu, E., Lind, P., Servenis, B., Lund, T., Flavell, R., Lee, J.S., Trowsdale, J., Schreier, P., Zablilzky, F., Larhammar, D., Peterson, P.A. and Rask, L.: The complete nucleotide sequence of the I-E_α^d immune response gene. Nucleic Acids Research 11:5055, 1983.

Israel, A., Kimura, A., Fournier, A., Fellous, M. and Kourilsky, P.: Interferon response sequence potentiates activity of an enhancer in the promoter region of a mouse H-2 gene. Nature 322:743, 1986.

Jeffreys, A.J., Wilson, V., and Theiu, S.L.: Hypervariable minisatellite regions in human DNA. Nature 314:67, 1985.

Jones, P.P., Murphy, D.B. and McDevitt, H.O.: Two-gene control of the expression of a murine Ia antigen. J. Exp. Med. 148:925, 1978.

Jones, P.P., Murphy, D.B. and McDevitt, H.O.: Variable synthesis and expression of E_{α} and A_{e} (E_{β}) Ia polypeptide chains in mice of different H-2 haplotypes. Immunogenetics 12:321, 1981.

Kelly, A. and Trowsdale, J.: Complete nucleotide sequence of a functional HLA DP^{β} gene, and the region between $DP_{\beta 1}$ and $DP_{\alpha 1}$ genes: comparison of the 5' ends of the HLA class II genes. Nucleic Acids Res. 13:1607, 1985.

King, D.P. and Jones, P.P.: Induction of Ia and H-2 antigens on a macrophage cell line by immune interferon. J. Immunol. 131:315, 1983.

Klein, J.: Biology of the mouse histocompatibility complex. Berlin: Springer Verlag, 1975.

Klein, J. and Figueroa, F.: Polymorphism of the mouse H-2 loci. Immunol. Rev. 60:23, 1981.

Kobori, J.A., Strauss, E., Minard, K. and Hood, L. Molecular analysis of the hot spot of recombination in the murine major histocompatibility complex. Science 234:173, 1986.

Lafuse, W.P., mcCormick, J.F., Corser, P.S. and David, C.S.: Hybrid (combinatorial) Ia specificities: gene complementations to generate Ia.22. Immunogenetics 13:115, 1981.

Lafuse, W.P., Berg, N., Savarirayan, S. and David, C.S.: Mapping of a second recombination hot spot within the I-E region of the mouse H-2 gene complex. J. Exp. Med. 163:1518, 1986.

Lafuse, W.P. and David, C.S.: Recombination hot spots within the I region of the mouse H-2 complex map to the E_{β} and E_{α} genes. Immunogenetics (in press).

Landais, D., Beck, B.N., Buerstedde, J-M., Degraw, S., Klein, D., Koch, N., Murphy, D., Pierres, M., Tada, T., Yamamoto, K., Benoist, C. and Mathis, D.: The assignment of chain specificities for anti-Ia monoclonal antibodies using L cell transfectants. J. Immunol. 137:3002, 1986.

Landais, D., Waltzinger, C., Beck, B.N., Staub, A., mcKean, D.J., Benoist, C. and Mathis, D.: Functional sites on Ia molecules: A molecular dissection of A_{α} immunogenicity. Cell 47:173, 1986.

Larhammar, D., Hammerling, U., Denaro, M., Lund, T., Flavell, R.A., Rask, L. and Peterson, P.A.: Structure of the murine immune response I-A_{β} locus: Sequence of the I-A_{β} gene and an adjacent β-chain second domain exon. Cell 34:179, 1983.

Lebo, R.V., Chakravarti, A., Beutow, K.H., Cheung, M.C., Cann, H., Cordell, B. and Goodman, H.: Recombination within and between the human insulin and β globin gene loci. Proc. Natl. Acad. Sci. USA 80:4808, 1983.

LeMeur, M., Gerlinger, P., Benoist, C. and Mathis, D.: Correcting an immune response deficiency by creating E_{α} gene transgenic mice. Nature 316:38, 1985.

Lerner, E.A., Matis, L.A., Janeway, C.A. Jr., Jones, P.P., Schwartz, R.H. and Murphy, D.B.: Monoclonal antibody against an Ir gene product? J. Exp. Med. 152:1085, 1980.

Lin, C.S., Rosenthal, A.S., Passmore, H.C. and Hansen, T.H.: Selective loss of antigen-specific Ir gene function in Ia mutant B6.C-H-2^{bm12} is an antigen-presenting cell defect. Proc. Natl. Acad. Sci. USA 78:6406, 1981.

Malissen, M., Hunkapiller, T. and Hood, L.: Nucleotide sequences of a light chain gene of the mouse I-A subregion. Science 221:750, 1983.

Mathis, D.J., Benoist, D.O., Williams, V.E. II, Kanter, M.R., McDevitt, H.O.: The murine E_{α} immune response gene. Cell 32:745, 1983.

Mathis, D.J., Benoist, C., Williams, V.E. II, Kanter, M. and McDevitt, H.O.: Several mechanisms can account for defective E_{α} gene expression in different mouse haplotypes. Proc. Natl. Acad. Sci. USA 80:273, 1983.

Matis, L.A., Jones, P.P., Murphy, D.B., Hedrick, S.M., Lerner, E.A., Janeway, C.A. Jr., McNicholas, J.M. and Schwartz, R.H.: Immune response gene function correlates with expression of an Ia antigen. II. A quantitative deficiency in Ae:Eα complex expression causes a corresponding defect in antigen-presenting cell function. J. Exp. Med. 155:508, 1982.

McCluskey, J., Germain, R.N. and Margulies, D.H.: Cell surface expression of an in vitro recombinant class II/class I major histocompatibility complex gene product. Cell 40:247, 1985.

McIntyure, K.R. and Seidman, J.G.: Nucleotide sequence of the mutant I-A^{bm12} genes is evidence for genetic exchange between mouse immune response genes. Nature 308:551, 1984.

McKean, D.J., Melvold, R.N. and David, C.: Tryptic peptide comparison of Ir antigens and polypeptides from the I-A mutant B6.C-H-2^{bm12} and its congenic parental strain B6. Immunogenetics 14:41, 1981.

McKenzie, I.F.C., Morgan, B.M., Saudrin, M.S., Michaelides, M.M., Melvold, R.W. and Kohn, H.I.: B6.C-H-2^{bm12}. A new H-2 mutation in the I region in the mouse. J. Exp. Med. 150:1323, 1979.

McNicholas, J.M., Murphy, D.B., Matis, L.A., Schwartz, R.H., Lerner, E.A., Janeway, C.A. Jr. and Jones, P.P.: Immune response gene function correlates with the expression of an Ia antigen: 1. Preferential associaiton of certain A_e and E_{α} chains results in a quantitative deficiency in expression of an Ae:Aα complex. J. Exp. Md. 155:490, 1982.

Melvold, R., Kohn, H. and Dunn, G.: History and genology of the H-2K^b mutants from the C57BL/6kh colony. Immunogenetics 15:177, 1982.

Mengle-Gaw, L., Conner, S., McDevitt, H.O., Fathman, C.G.: Gene conversion between murine class II major histocompatibility complex loci. Functional and molecular evidence from the bm12 mutant. J. Exp. Med. 160:1184, 1984.

Mengle-Gaw, L. and McDevitt, H.O.: Genetics and expression of mouse Ia antigens. Ann. Rev. Immunol. 3:367, 1985.

Murphy, D., Jones, P.P., Loken, M., McDevitt, H.O.: Interaction between I region major histocompatibility complex loci. Functional and molecular evidence from the bm12 mutant. J. Exp. Med. 160:1184, 1984.

Nizetic, D., Figueroa, F. and Klein, J.: Evolutionary relationships between the t and H-2 haplotypes in the house mouse. Immunogenetics 19:311, 1984.

Orkin, S.H. and Kazaziau, H.H. Jr.: The mutation and polymorphism of the human β-globin gene and its surrounding DNA. Ann. Rev. Genel. 18:131, 1984.

Pinkert, C.A., Widera, G., Cowing, C., Heber-Katz, E., Palmiter, R.D., Flavell, R.A. and Brinster, R.L.: Tissue-specific, inducible, and functional expression of the E_α^d MHC class II gene in transgenic mice. EMBO J. 4:2225, 1985.

Polla, B.S., Poljak, A., Geier, S.G., Nathenson, S.C., Ohara, J., Paul, W.E. and Glimcher, L.H.: Three distinct signals can induce class II gene expression in a murine pre-B-cell line. Proc. Natl. Acad. Sci. USA 83:4878, 1986.

Roehm, N.W., Leibson, H.J., Zlotnik, A., Kappler, J., Marrack, P. and Cambier, J.C.: Interleukin-induced increase in Ia expression by normal mouse B cells. J. Exp. Med. 160:679, 1984.

Sachs, D.H., Arn, J.S. and Hansen, T.H.: Two new recombinant H-2 haplotypes, one of which juxtaposes K^b and I^k alleles. J. Immunol. 123:1965, 1979.

Saito, H., Maki, R.A., Clayton, L.K., Tonegawa, S.: Complete primary structures of the E_β chain and gene of the mouse major histocompatibility complex. Proc. Natl. Acad. Sci. USA 80:5520, 1983.

Scholz, S. and Albertl, E.: HLA and diseases: involvement of more than one HLA-linked determinant of disease susceptibility. Immunol. Rev. 70:77, 1983.

Shiroishi, T., Sagai, T. and Moriwaki, K.: A new wild-derived H-2 haplotype enhancing K-IA recombination. Nature 300:370, 1982.

Shreffler, D.C. and David, C.S.: The _H-2_ major histocompatibility complex and the _I_ immune response region: genetic variation, function and organization. Advances in Immunology 20:125, 1975.

Silver, J., Wsain, S. and Hubert, J.: Small subunit of I-A subregion determines the allospecificity recognized by a monoclonal antibody. Nature 286:272, 1980.

Smith, G.B., Kunes, S.M., Schultz, D.N., Taylor, A. and Trinau, K.L.: Structure of chi hot spots of generalized recombination. Cell 24:249, 1981.

Snell, G.D., Dausset, J. and Nathenson, S.: Histocompatibility (academic, New York, 1976).

Steeg, P.S., Johnson, H.M. and Oppenheim, J.J.: Regulation of murine macrophage Ia antigen expression by an immune interferon-like lymphokine: inhibitory effect of endotoxin. J. Immunol. 129:2402., 1982.

Steinmetz, M., Minard, K., Howath, S., McNicholas, J., Frelinger, J., Wake, C., Long, E., Mach, B. and Hood, L.: A molecular map of the immune response region from the major histocompatibility complex of the mouse. Nature 300:35, 1982.

Steinmetz, M., Stephen, D. and Lindahl, K.F.: Gene organization and recombinational hot spots in the murine major histocompatibility complex. Cell 44:895, 1986.

Tse, H.Y., Kanamori, S., Walsh, D. and Hansen, T.H.: The murine bm12 gene conversion provides evidence that T cells recognize predominantly Ia conformation. Proc. Natl. Acad. Sci. USA 82:7058, 1985.

Wake, C.T. and Flavell, R.A.: Multiple mechanisms regulate the expression of murine immune response genes. Cell 42:623, 1985.

Widera, G., Flavell, R.A.: The nucleotide sequence of the murine I-E_{β}^{b} immune response gene: Evidence for gene conversion events in class II genes of the major histocompatibility complex. EMBO J. 3:1221, 1984.

INTERMEDIATES IN CLASS II HLA ANTIGEN BIOSYNTHESIS

Peter Cresswell, Drew N. Kelner, and Michael S. Marks
Department of Microbiology and Immunology
Duke University Medical Center
Durham, N.C.

INTRODUCTION

It has been appreciated for a number of years that the biosynthesis and intracellular transport of class II HLA antigens is unusual compared to that of the majority of membrane glycoproteins studied. The α and β subunits which make up the mature class II antigen dimer are known to be associated with a third glycoprotein, the invariant or I chain, during their intracellular transport (Jones, et al., 1978; Machamer and Cresswell, 1982). The nature of this intracellular complex has been difficult to elucidate because of its transient nature. We have used the sodium ionophore monensin (Tartakoff, 1983) to arrest class II antigen transport in human B-lymphoblastoid cell lines (B-LCL), and have successfully isolated accumulated class II antigen biosynthetic intermediates using monoclonal antibody affinity columns (Kelner and Cresswell, 1986). This report summarizes our current understanding of the nature of these intermediates.

PURIFICATION OF CLASS II ANTIGEN BIOSYNTHETIC INTERMEDIATES

Incubation of B-LCL for 24 hr in 1μM or 10μM monensin results in no change in cell surface expression of HLA-DR antigens as determined by quantitative antibody binding assays. However, when extracts of the cells in the non-ionic detergent Triton X-100 were assayed for HLA-DR antigens by a competitive radioimmunoassay, 1μM monensin was found to have caused a two-fold, and 10μM monensin a five-fold, increase in the total class II antigen content (Machamer and Cresswell, 1984). By analogy with other studies (reviewed in Tartakoff, 1983) we assumed that this accumulation resulted from a block in intracellular transport through the Golgi apparatus.

B-LCL cultured for 24 hr with 10μM monensin were extracted with the non-ionic detergent polyoxyethylene-9-lauryl ether ($C_{12}E_9$), and class II antigens isolated from the extracts by affinity chromatography using monoclonal antibody columns. Class II antigen complexes were eluted at pH11.0 and subjected to gel filtration chromatography using Sephacryl S300 equilibrated in 0.5% (w/v) sodium deoxycholate, 0.15M NaCl, 0.01M Tris, pH8.0. The predominant species, detected by radioimmunoassay, eluted in the position of a 270,000 dalton globular protein (Kelner and Cresswell, 1986). This was a minor species in similar extracts from control B-LCL cultured without monensin, where the major species had an apparent Mr of approximately 90,000.

CHARACTERIZATION OF THE CLASS II ANTIGEN COMPLEXES

Two dimensional gel electrophoretic analysis of the high molecular weight class II complexes from monensin-treated B-LCL followed by silver staining revealed the 35,000 dalton α subunit, the 27,000 dalton β subunit, and the 31,000 dalton I chain. The processed form of the I chain, characterized by its increased Mr of 35,000 caused by O-linked glycan addition and its increased acidity due to sialic acid addition (Machamer and Cresswell, 1984) was not apparent. These data are consistent with the interpretation that the high molecular weight complexes correspond to biosynthetic intermediates arrested during transport through the Golgi apparatus. Surprisingly, no other components were detectable which might account for the large apparent size of the accumulated complex.

Following the reports of Sant et al. (1983, 1984) that a chondroitin-sulfate proteoglycan could be detected in immune precipitates of both human and murine class II antigens, we investigated the possible presence of such a molecule in the 270,000 dalton complexes isolated from monensin-treated B-LCL. Class II antigen complexes isolated by affinity chromatography from extracts of B-LCL labeled with ^{35}S-sulfate had the same apparent Mr of 270,000 when analysed by gel filtration. The ^{35}S-sulfate labeled component was dissociated from the class II complex by either 6M urea or 6M quanidine-HCl treatment and analysed by gel filtration chromatography. The mean apparent Mr by gel filtration in either 0.5% (w/v) deoxycholate on Sephacryl S300 or 6M guanidine HCl on Sephacryl S200 was approximately 180,000 (Kelner and Cresswell, 1986). Thus it was concluded that the sulfate-containing component was a major contributor to the apparent size of the 270,000 dalton class II antigen biosynthetic intermediate. The sulfate-containing component had a lower apparent Mr of 70,000 - 110,000 when analysed by SDS-polyacrylamide gel electrophoresis (SDS-PAGE). The difference between the two size estimates presumably reflects the fact that the molecule is not a conventional globular protein. We were able to confirm that the sulfate-containing species is a proteoglycan by demonstrating the susceptibility of the ^{35}S-sulfate-labeled side chains to hyaluronidase (Kelner and Cresswell, 1986).

Because of the substantial contribution of the proteoglycan to the size of the class II antigen biosynthetic intermediate, we reasoned that the entire complex was likely to contain a single proteoglycan molecule in association with α , β and I chain subunits. To determine the stoichiometric ratio of the α, β and I chains, HLA-DR complexes were isolated from B-LCL labeled with ^{3}H-leucine in the presence of monensin, and separated by two dimensional gel electrophoresis. Fluorographs of the gel were scanned by laser densitometry. The relative amounts of the three subunits were determined using their respective leucine contents, which were calculated from published cDNA sequences. The results of this analysis indicated that the α , β and I chain subunits were present in equimolar amounts (Kelner and Cresswell, 1986). On the basis of this data we believe that the HLA-DR antigen biosynthetic intermediate isolated from monensin-treated B-LCL is a tetrameric species containing a proteoglycan molecule and an I chain molecule in association with an αβ heterodimer.

THE NATURE OF THE I CHAIN ASSOCIATION WITH THE CLASS II ANTIGEN COMPLEX

The ability of monensin to induce the accumulation of biosynthetic intermediates of class II antigens containing I chain prompted us to investigate the susceptibility of such complexes to protease digestion. Triton X-100 extracts of B-LCL labeled with ^{35}S-methionine in the presence of 1μM monensin were treated on ice for various periods of time with the non-specific protease proteinase K at 10μg/ml. Proteolysis was terminated by the addition of the serine protease inhibitor phenyl methyl sulfonyl fluoride. Class II antigens were isolated from the extracts by immunoprecipitation and analysed by two-dimensional gel electrophoresis and fluorography.

After only 30 seconds of exposure to proteinase K the I chain was virtually quantitatively degraded to a major fragment of 25,000 daltons. Further digestion reduced the size of the fragment to 19,500 daltons, and ultimately to a stable size of approximately 18,000 daltons (Marks and Cresswell, 1986). All three proteolytic products retained reactivity with the I chain-specific monoclonal antibody VIC-Y1 (Quaranta et al., 1984), and all retained the capacity to interact with class II antigens, since they were coprecipitated by both monoclonal and rabbit antibodies to class II antigens with no I chain reactivity.

The I chain fragments were extensively characterized to determine from which region of the I chain they arose. All three fragments retained both of the N-linked oligosaccharide side chains of the I chain, determined by susceptibility the enzyme endoglycosidase H. The larger fragment retained the O-linked glycans of the I chain, but the 18,000 dalton limit digestion product clearly did not. This was determined by neuraminidase treatment of similar fragments isolated from non-monensin treated B-LCL followed by two dimensional electrophoresis, and also by determining the ability of the fragments to be bound by the lectin _Bandeireae simplicifolia_, isolectin 1, which binds intact I chain via its O-linked glycans (Marks and

Cresswell, 1986; Machamer and Cresswell, 1984).

None of the I chain-derived fragments remained associated with the plasma membrane following dissociation from the class II antigens themselves. This was shown by digesting intact membranes from ^{35}S-methionine-labeled B-LCL with proteinase K in the absence of detergent. After removing the insoluble membrane pellet by ultracentrifugation the I chain fragments, but not intact I chain, were precipitable from the aqueous supernatant by rabbit antibodies to the I chain (Marks and Cresswell, 1986). This suggests that the fragments have lost the transmembrane region responsible for integrating the I chain into the membrane. Lack of the transmembrane sequence was confirmed on the 18,000 dalton fragment by site specific cleavage at tryptophanyl residues using the reagent o-iodosobenzoic acid, which demonstrated that a substantial portion of the C-terminal extracytoplasmic portion of the I chain beyond trp 162 was retained. Taken together, the data suggests that the I chain interacts with the class II antigen complex via its extracytoplasmic region.

DISCUSSION

The tetrameric class II antigen complex containing I chain and proteoglycan has been most completely characterized following isolation from monensin-treated cells. In these complexes the N-linked glycans of the α, β and I chain subunits are sensitive to the enzyme endoglycosidase H (Machamer and Cresswell, 1984), consistent with a block early in Golgi transport. Clearly then, the proteoglycan becomes associated with class II antigens at a relatively early stage in biosynthesis. Sulfation of the chondroitin sulfate side chains is not inhibited by monensin, arguing that the synthesis of this particular proteoglycan in B-LCL is completed in the <u>cis</u> or <u>medial</u> Golgi apparatus. Since similar high molecular weight complexes are found in non-monensin treated B-LCL labeled for four hours with ^{35}S-methionine, and in these complexes processing of the N-linked glycans to the complex form is evident, it would appear that the tetrameric species is transported intact through the <u>trans</u> Golgi region.

At some point between the <u>trans</u> Golgi and the plasma membrane the I chain appears to dissociate from the HLA-DR antigen complex. Evidence for this is that the I chain cannot be readily detected on the surface of B-LCL by either monoclonal antibodies (Quaranta et al., 1984) or rabbit antibodies (Accolla et al., 1985). The mechanisms involved in this dissociation are unknown, although exposure to an acidic environment may be involved since the lysosomotropic agent chloroquine has been shown to inhibit the dissociation step (Nowell and Quaranta, 1985). The fate of the proteoglycan remains to be determined, although evidence in the murine system suggests that some cell surface Ia antigens remain associated with proteoglycan (Sant et al., 1985a).

The core protein of the class II antigen-associated proteoglycan is either identical to, or very closely related to, the I chain itself (Sant et al., 1985b, Giacoletto et al., 1986). Evidence for this is that the core protein, isolated following removal of the chondroitin sulfate side chains by chondroitinase digestion reacts with a monoclonal antibodies to the I chain. In addition, peptide maps of the genuine I chain and the core protein are very similar. Precisely how the I chain can simultaneously exhibit these two forms, i.e. proteoglycan and conventional trans-membrane glycoprotein, in a single tetrameric complex with class II antigen dimers has not been elucidated, and is currently under intensive investigation.

The function of the I chain and its proteoglycan derivative remain completely unknown. The I chain does not appear to be required for assembly of class II antigen αβ dimers or their subsequent cell surface expression (Miller and Germain, 1986; Sekaly et al., 1986). We have speculated that the I chain may play a role in the antigen presentation function of class II glycoproteins (Cresswell et al., 1986), perhaps regulating the kinetics of transport of the class II antigen complex through an intracellular compartment where critical interactions between the class II molecules and endocytosed antigens occur. Evidence for intracellular interactions between class II molecules still associated with I chain and the endocytic pathway followed by the transferrin receptor has been obtained (Cresswell, 1985). Since proteolysis of internalized foreign antigens may be an important component of the antigen processing mechanism of antigen presenting cells (Unanue, 1984), it is conceivable that the proteoglycan component of the intracellular class II complex may be involved in protecting the class II molecule from degradation. Evidence for proteases in endosomal compartments of macrophages has in fact been obtained (Diment and Stahl, 1985), and such a compartment could be that in which the class II antigen interaction with the endocytic pathway occurs.

REFERENCES

Accolla, R. S., Carra, G., Buchegger, F., Carrell, S., and Mach, J. P., 1985, The human Ia-associated invariant chain is synthesized in Ia-negative B cell variants and is not expressed on the cell surface of both Ia-negative and Ia-positive parental cells, J. Immunol., 134:3265.

Cresswell, P., 1985, Intracellular class II HLA antigens are accessible to transferrin-neuraminidase conjugates internalized by receptor-mediated endocytosis, Proc. Natl. Acad. Sci. U.S.A., 82:8188.

Cresswell, P., Blum, J. S., Kelner, D. N., and Marks, M. S., 1986, Biosynthesis and processing of class II histocompatibility antigens, CRC Critical Reviews in Immunol., in press.

Diment, S., and Stahl, P., 1985, Macrophage endososomes contain proteases which degrade endocytosed protein ligands, J. Biol. Chem., 260:15311.

Giacoletto, K. S., Sant, A. J., Bono, C., Gorka, J., O'Sullivan, D. M., Quaranta, V., and Schwartz, B. D., 1986, The human invariant chain is the core protein of the human class II associated proteoglycan, J. Exp. Med. 164:1422.
Jones, P. P., Murphy, D. B., Hewgill, D., and McDevitt, H. O., 1978, Detection of a common polypeptide chain in I-A and I-E subregion immunoprecipitation, Mol. Immunol., 16:51.
Kelner, D. N., and Cresswell, P., 1986, Biosynthetic intermediates of HLA class II antigens from B lymphoblastoid cell lines, J. Immunol., 137:2632.
Machamer, C. E., and Cresswell, P., 1982, Biosynthesis and glycosylation of the invariant chain associated with HLA-DR antigens, J. Immunol., 129:2564.
Machamer, C. E., and Cresswell, P., 1984, Monensin prevents terminal glycosylation of the N- and O-linked oligosaccharides of the HLA-DR-associated invariant chain and inhibits its dissociation from the α-β chain complex, Proc. Natl. Acad. Sci. U.S.A., 81:1287.
Marks, M. S., and Cresswell, P., 1986, Invariant chain associates with HLA class II antigens via its extracytoplasmic region, J. Immunol., 136:2519.
Miller, J., and Germain, R. N., 1986, Efficient cell surface expression of class II MHC molecules in the absence of associated invariant chain, J. Exp. Med., 164:1478.
Nowell, J., and Quaranta, V., 1985, Chloroquine affects biosynthesis of Ia molecules by inhibiting dissociation of invariant (gamma) chains from alpha-beta dimers in B cells, J. Exp. Med., 162:1371.
Quaranta, V., Majdic, O., Stingl, G., Liszka, K., Honigsmann, H., and Knapp, W., 1984, A human Ia cytoplasmic determinant located on multiple forms of invariant chain (γ_1, γ_2, γ_3), J. Immunol., 132:1900.
Sant, A., Schwartz, B. D., and Cullen, S. E., 1983, Identification of a new component in the murine Ia molecular complex, J. Exp. Med., 158:1979.
Sant, A. J., Cullen, S. E., and Schwartz, B. D., 1984, Identification of a sulfate-bearing molecule associated with HLA class II antigens, Proc. Natl. Acad. Sci. U.S.A., 81:1534.
Sant, A. J., Cullen, S. E., and Schwartz, B. D., 1985a, Biosynthetic relationships of the chondroitin sulfate proteoglycan with Ia and invariant chain glycoproteins, J. Immunol., 135:416.
Sant, A. J., Cullen, S. E., Giacoletto, K. S., and Schwartz, B. D., 1985b, Invariant chain is the core protein of the Ia-associated chondroitin sulfate proteoglycan, J. Exp. Med., 162:1916.
Sekaly, R. P., Tonnelle, C., Strubin, M., Mach, B., and Long, E. O., 1986, Cell surface expression of class II histocompatibility antigens occurs in the absence of the invariant chain, J. Exp. Med., 164:1490.
Tartakoff, A. M., 1983, Perturbation of vesicular traffic with the carboxylic ionophore monensin, Cell, 32:1026.
Unanue, E. R., 1984, Antigen presenting function of the macrophage, Ann. Rev. Immunol., 2:395.

TRINITROPHENYL REACTIVE T-CELL CLONES IN FUNCTIONAL AND MOLECULAR ANALYSIS OF THE HLA-D REGION

Robert R. Rich, Jeffrey H. Hanke and Richard G. Cook

Howard Hughes Medical Institute
Department of Microbiology and Immunology
Baylor College of Medicine
Houston, TX

A central role for major histocompatibility complex (MHC) molecules in presentation of non-MHC antigens to T lymphocytes is generally acknowledged. Among the seminal studies demonstrating this phenomenon were those of Shearer and associates demonstrating that recognition of mouse target cells by trinitrophenyl (TNP)-specific cytolytic T cells required genetic homologies between the killer and target cells at H-2 class I loci (rev., Shearer et al., 1976). This system, employing target cells surface modified by hapten conjugation, has proven particularly useful in subsequent studies of MHC restrictions on antigen recognition by human T lymphocytes. As in the mouse, recognition of TNP-modified target cells by hapten-specific cytotoxic T lymphocytes has appeared to involve restrictions for class I HLA homology (Shaw and Shearer, 1978). The data in human systems have been substantially less compelling, however, with evidence in some instances for effective interactions between target and killer cells that did not involve obvious class I HLA homologies (Shaw and Shearer, 1978; Seldin et al., 1979). In contrast to target cell recognition by cytolytic T-cells, recognition of antigen by helper T-cells has generally required genetic homology between antigen-presenting cells and helper T cells (or B cells and helper T cells) for class II loci of the MHC (rev., Thomas et al., 1977). Subsequently, clear exceptions have been documented with respect to correlations between functional activity and MHC restrictions for antigen recognition (rev., Rich et al., 1986). On the other hand, identification of a dichotomy of T lymphocytes, one subset of which expresses the CD4 molecule (L3T4 in mice) and the other of which expresses the CD8 molecule (Ly2 in mice), has led to a more convincing correlation between T-cell subset and MHC recognition requirements in antigen presentation. That is, recognition of non-MHC antigens by $CD4^+$ ($L3T4^+$) cells requires class II MHC homologies between T-cells and antigen presenting cells, whereas recognition by $CD8^+$ ($Ly2^+$) T-cells is MHC class I restricted (rev., Swain, 1983).

HLA CLASS II-RESTRICTED TNP RECOGNITION

Initial studies in human systems demonstrated a distinct preference in hapten-specific proliferative responses of TNP-primed T cells for recognition of antigen when presented by hapten-modified cells that were HLA-D region homologous with the TNP-specific T cell responders (Figure 1). It is noteworthy, however, that although proliferation of a population of primed hapten-specific T-cells was optimal when hapten-modified allogeneic stimulators shared defined HLA-D region homologies, significant proliferative responses were also observed in instances where no such homologies were defined. In the interval since those initial studies, several major advances have permitted a reexamination of the issue of class II-restricted recognition by human T-cells. These have included the development of T-cell cloning technology, which has permitted assessment of MHC restrictions for antigen recognition at the clonal level rather than with bulk cultures; the identification of three distinct genetic regions of the HLA-D region that encode molecules represented on the surfaces of antigen-presenting cells (designated from the centromere DP, DQ, and DR); and the development of monoclonal antibodies (mAb) with specificity for framework or polymorphic determinants of each of the distinct class II molecular species.

T Cell Clones in Analysis of Class II Restrictions

Utilizing cloned $CD4^+$ T-cell lines (TCL), antigen recognition in the context of each of these class II antigenic systems has been clearly demonstrated. For example, Qvigstad et al. (1984a, 1984b) reported that antigen-specific TCL recognized Chlamydia trachomatis antigens in association with specific DR or DP allodeterminants. Eckels and coworkers (1983) showed that T-cell clones could respond to influenza A viral antigens when presented in the context of DP-encoded antigens. In addition, the DRβ2-associated epitope DRw53 has been shown to function in the presentation of mumps virus antigen (Ball and Stastny, 1984a) and HLA-DQ restricted TCL specific for the

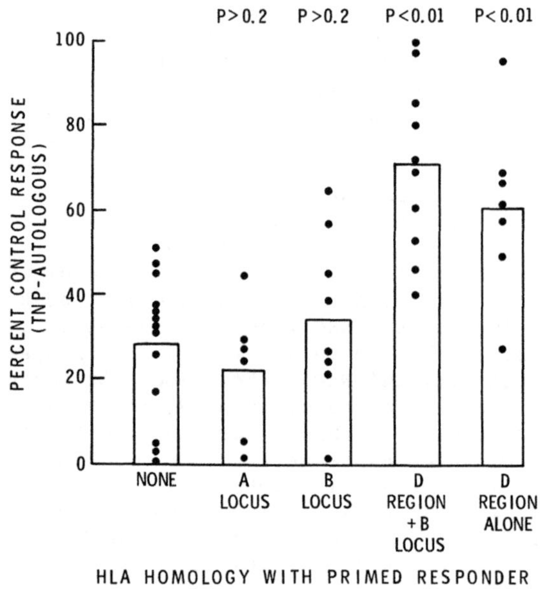

Fig. 1. D region determinant sharing between primed responder and stimulators correlates with the magnitude of the secondary TNP-conjugate proliferative responses. D region homology was determined on the basis of DR antigens (●), or responses to homozygous typing cells, Dw (▲). The p values given above represent a comparison between responses induced by allogeneic stimulators, which shared HLA determinants with the primed responder, and responses induced by allogeneic stimulators, which did not share HLA antigens. From Seldin et al., 1979.

synthetic peptide GAT have been identified (Ball and Stastny, 1984b). Such antigen-specific TCL, as well as allospecific TCL, have often recognized class II determinants that did not appear closely associated with serologically defined allospecificities; it has been suggested that HLA-Dw specificities, defined by alloantigen recognition in mixed leukocyte cultures, may correlate better than serologically defined specificities with restriction elements for T-cell recognition of non-MHC antigens (Fleischer et al., 1985). Furthermore, it has appeared that the majority of class II-restricted TCL recognize determinants associated with Dw/DR-associated determinants, rather than with DP or DQ (Ottenhoff et al., 1985).

Initial studies defining HLA-D region restriction elements employed in T-cell recognition were based upon patterns of responsiveness to panels of allogeneic antigen-presenting cells with defined HLA homologies to the responder TCL. More recently such studies have been extended by utilization of mAb with specificity for particular D region molecules. For example, Ball and Stastny (1984b) defined the restriction specificity of a GAT-specific TCL to DQ based on preferential inhibition with a DQ-specific mAb and Pawelec et al. (1985) used mAb blocking to define TCL specific for DP-related allodeterminants that strongly suppressed proliferative responses of cloned alloantigen-specific cell lines. Qvigstad et al. (1984b) utilized mAb to analyze DR- and DP-related determinants recognized by TCL specific for <u>Chlamydia</u> <u>trachomatis</u> antigen. These investigators reported that although DR-specific mAb inhibited TCL with putative specificity for both DRβ1- and DRβ2-encoded epitopes, DP-restricted TCL were not significantly inhibited by any tested mAb including two putatively DP-specific antibodies. Thus, although the mAb inhibition patterns generally correlated well with DR restriction specificity, they found this not to be the case with respect to HLA-DP.

The involvement of both DR and non-DR associated HLA epitopes in restriction of hapten recognition by TNP-specific TCL has similarly been demonstrated in studies from our laboratory (Hanke et al., 1985). Figure 2 illustrates restriction specificities of two such cell lines employing a panel of allogeneic stimulator cells. Proliferation of TCL 1B6 (top panel) was induced with few exceptions by hapten-modified stimulators that shared the DRw53 specificity of the cell line. In contrast, no DRw53$^-$ allogeneic stimulators were capable of presenting TNP effectively to this TCL. On the other hand, TCL 2H10 (lower panel), derived from the same cell donor, demonstrated apparent restriction for recognition of a DP-associated determinant. That is, allogeneic cells that shared the DP4 specificity with the cell donor were generally efficacious in hapten presentation when TNP modified, whereas hapten-conjugated DP4$^-$ stimulators were ineffective.

<u>Possible Nonpolymorphic DP-Associated Restricting Element</u>

In analysis of HLA specificities employed by a panel of >50 TCL, an additional novel pattern was established that may in part explain the responsiveness in bulk cultures in responder stimulator cell combinations lacking defined HLA-D region homologies (Hanke et al., 1985). This was the identification of a novel TCL that appeared to recognize TNP on all stimulator cells tested (Table 1). Thus, although the hapten specificity of this cell line was readily demonstrable, APC entirely lacking HLA homology with the cell line were not consistently less effective stimulators than were hapten-modified HLA-matched or autologous stimulators. To ascertain whether this reactivity pattern was the result of more than one clone of cells within the TCL, responses of two subclones derived utilizing an autoclone attachment to a Coulter EPICS V flow cytometer were characterized. Both subclones (e.g., 3A1.1) responded to all haptenated stimulators tested, leading us to conclude that this TCL either recognized TNP in an HLA-nonrestricted fashion or recognized the hapten in the context of a highly

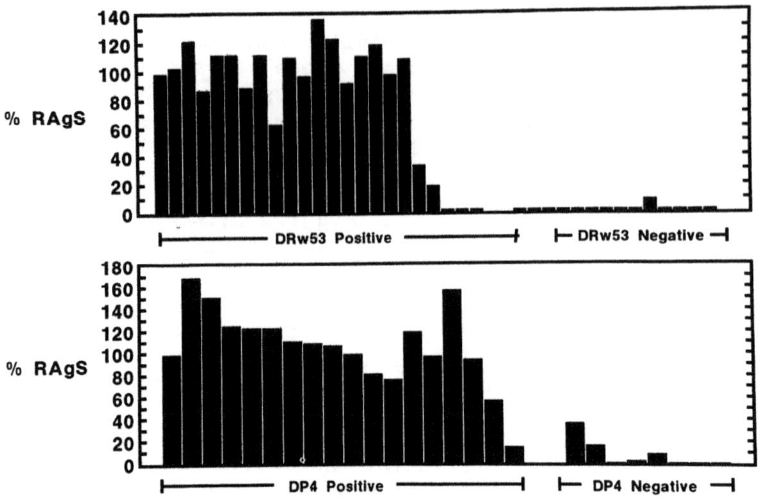

Fig. 2. Restriction specificity analysis of TLC G1-1B6 and G1-2H10 that recognize TNP in the context of determinants closely associated with DRw53 and DP4, respectively. The correlation values for G1-1B6 (top panel) were: DR1 (0.19), DR7 (0.76), DRw53 (0.92), DQw1 (0.24), DQw2 (0.81), DP2 (0.63), DP4 (0.37). The data represent four separate experiments with autologous net responses of 23,335 34,063, 14,473, and 10,147 cpm. The correlation values for G1-2H10 (lower panel) were: DR1 (0.38), DR7 (0.35), DRw53 (0.50), DQw1 (0.54), DQw2 (0.46), DP2 (0.35), DP4 (0.96). The data are from four representative experiments with autologous net responses of 26,054, 31,200, 28,565, and 21,355 cpm. Adapted from Hanke et al., 1985.

nonpolymorphic HLA determinant. Clearly, this determinant could not be identified utilizing allogeneic panel analysis. Moreover, proliferation of this cell line was not inhibited by the DR-specific mAbs, L243 and L227. In contrast, the mAbs Tü35, Tü39 and 2D6, each of which reacts with both DR and DP epitopes, all strongly inhibited the clone suggesting that the TCL was recognizing a nonpolymorphic determinant on the DP molecule. To test this hypothesis, we attempted to block the reactivity of this cell line with the DP-specific mAbs, B7/21 and Tü39, as well as mAbs with specificities for DP and DR shared determinants (Figure 3). The DP-specific mAb significantly inhibited responses of this TCL, although they did not inhibit proliferative responses of any TCL restricted to DR1, DR2, DR5 or DRw53 (data not shown). Hence, it appears that this T-cell clone recognized a nonpolymorphic restricting element on the DP molecule. This conclusion was further supported by the fact that this clone reacted to a hapten-modified lymphoblastoid mutant cell line (variant 526.12.81; Nicklas et al., 1984) that had deletions of one complete HLA haplotype and DR on the other haplotype (data not shown).

Uncertainty regarding the molecular structure recognized by this clone, however, leads to two alternative mechanistic interpretations. It is possible that TCL 3A1 recognizes a direct hapten modification of the DP molecule. If so, TNP recognition may be mechanistically indistinguishable from recognition of an MHC alloantigen, presumably reflecting conjugation of TNP to an essentially invarient DP residue. On the other hand, TNP recognition in this instance may reflect hapten modification of a non-MHC cell surface molecule. If so, it would be expected to obey the usual rules for recogni-

Table 1. A TNP-Specific Clone Recognizing a Nonpolymorphic Determinant

Stimulator cells	HLA-D Region Phenotype DR	DQ	DRw52,53	DP	Clone 3A1 %RAgS[a]	Subclone 3A1.1 %RAgS[b]
SJ	2,5	1,3	52	2,4	100	100
TF	2,4	1,3	53	4	94	59
EF	4,7	2,3	53	NT	106	90
FB	4	3	53	1,4	66	163
RM	2,7	1,2	53	1,4	150	229
SR	3	2	52	1	152	165
RI	1,2	1		NT	92	74
MC	5	3	52	3	61	56
JM	4,5	3	52,53	2,4	NT	169
BB	2,7	1,2	53	4	93	
MT	4,7	2,3	53	NT	106	
RS	5,7	2,3	52,53	6	98	
FS	2,4	1,3	53	4	175	
F1	2,4	1,3	53	3,4	83	
MR	2,w6(6.3)	1,3	52	4	97	
VM	7	2	53	4	239	
CG	1,5	1,3	52	2,3	83	
RD	3	2	52	1,4	136	
GM	1,7	1,2	53	2,4	385	
MW	2,3	1,2	52	1,4	178	
GG	1,w8	1,3	52	1	103	
RC	2,4	1,3	53	2,4	119	
DH	3,7	2	52,53	1,4	76	
DL	3	2	52	4	96	
PM	4,7	2,3	53	4	317	
MA	w6	1	52	3,4	170	
RR	2,w6	1	52	2,3	76	
SC	2	1		3	143	

a The antigen-specific response is expressed as a percentage of the relative antigen stimulation (% RAgS) where:

$$\%RAgS = \frac{\text{net cpm to TNP-modified minus unmodified allogeneic stimulators}}{\text{net cpm to TNP-modified minus unmodified autologous stimulators}} \times 100$$

The data represent three separate experiments with autologous net responses of 56,941, 33,906, and 14,435 cpm.

b The data represent one experiment with an autologous net response of 14,680 cpm. From Hanke et al., 1985.

tion by $CD4^+$ lymphocytes in the context of autologous class II molecules. This alternative would thus suggest that nonpolymorphic areas of class II molecules, at least DP, may act as T-cell restricting elements.

FUNCTIONAL AND MOLECULAR DQ SUBTYPES

The phenomenon of linkage disequilibrium, particularly the very strong positive linkage disequilibrium between specific DR and DQ alleles, may also lead to substantial difficulties in assignment of T cell restriction specificities. This is largely because characterization of DR serological polymorphism has been significantly more detailed than that of DQ molecules.

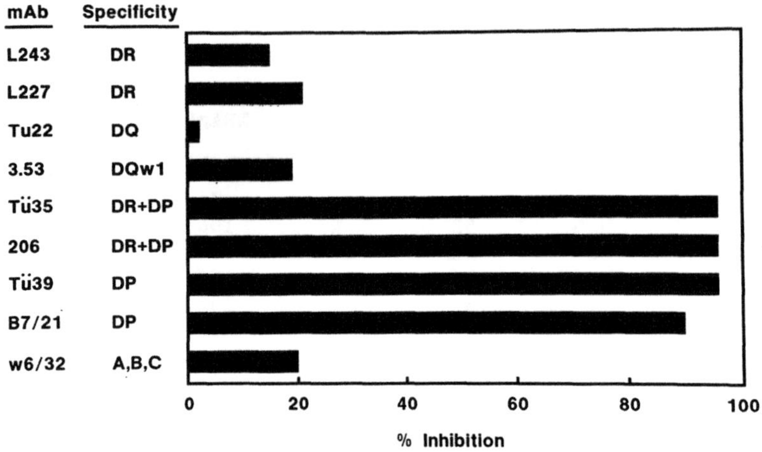

Fig. 3. Proliferative responses of TCL 2A1 are inhibited by mAb with specificity for HLA-DP. Each TCL was cultured with an equal number of irradiated autologous, TNP-modified PBMC for 2 days in the presence or absence of antibody. Proliferation was assessed by the addition of ^{3}H-thymidine for the last 20 h of culture. Data are expressed as mean percent inhibition of control responses from four experiments in the absence of antibody.

For example, the DQw1 specificity represents a serologically defined specificity on DQ molecules (Tosi et al., 1978) that is inherited in strong linkage disequilibrium with DR1, 2, w6, w8, and w10 (Bodmer, 1977; Betuel et al., 1984; Ferrara et al., 1984). Nevertheless, several studies have indicated that the DQw1 specificity may comprise subtypic specificities (Giles et al., 1985; Trowsdale et al., 1985; Shackelford et al., 1981; Cohen et al., 1984) that may separately be specifically associated with different DR alleles. Thus, Southern blot hybridization studies of Cohen et al. (1984) and Trowsdale et al. (1985) have indicated that DQw1 can be split into at least two alleles, one of which is associated with DR1 and the other with DR2, DRw6 and untyped DR alleles.

In studies of class II restricted hapten presentation we have investigated whether in some instances TCL apparently employing DR-associated restricting elements, as assessed utilizing allogeneic stimulator cell panels, may instead require recognition of DQ epitopes inherited in linkage disequilibrium with particular DR specificities (Hanke et al., 1986). Support for this hypothesis was obtained by detailed analysis of restriction specificities of four TNP-specific TCL for which effective antigen presentation was highly correlated with the expression of DR2 (Table 2). It is noteworthy, however, that two of the four cell lines (T1C5 and T3G4) also responded strongly to haptenated stimulators GG (DRw1,w8) and KR (DR3,w6), but not to other DR1$^+$, DRw6$^+$ or DRw8$^+$ stimulators that did not express DR2. Furthermore, none of these four cell lines could clearly be associated with a DQ restriction specificity based upon serologically defined DQ polymorphisms of the stimulator panel.

To gain insight into the molecular nature of the class II determinants recognized by these TCL, mAb blocking studies were performed on lines T3F6 and T3G4 (Figure 4;). As shown in panel A, TCL T3F6 was inhibited by the DR-specific mAbs L243, L227 and 2D6, but not by the DQ-specific mAbs Genox 3.53 (anti-DQw1) or Leu10. In contrast, TCL T3G4 (panel B) was only inhibited by the DQ-specific mAbs Genox 3.53 and Leu10, although the reac-

Table 2. DR2 and DQ-Restricted TNP-Specific TCL Derived From Individual TF[a]

Stimulator cells	Phenotype DR	DQ	Percent RAgS[b] in T cell lines T1B10[c]	T3F6[d]	T1C5[e]	T3G4[f]
DR2 positive						
TF	2,4	1,3	100	100	100	100
SJ	2,5	1,3	263	282	93	38
BB	2,7	1,2	348	161	170	227
FS	2,4	1,3	277	145	210	279
MR	2,w6	1,3	65	165	195	258
RM	2,7	1,2	300	NT	131	NT
R1	1,2	1	35	452	16	NT
SC	2	1	157	148	449	117
SF	2,4	1,3	171	109	87	121
RC	2,4	1,3	130	109	197	100
RR	2,w6	1	NT	138	NT	107
CR	2,3	1,2	NT	NT	NT	133
DR2 negative						
GM	1,7	1,2	3	19	2	5
EF	4,7	2,3	<1	<1	<1	1
RS	5,7	2,3	<1	6	<1	4
FB	4	3	<1	<1	<1	<1
CG	1,5	1,3	<1	20	<1	4
RD	3	2	<1	<1	<1	<1
OM	1,7	1,3	NT	<1	NT	<1
GG	1,w8	1	<1	<1	156	91
AG	1,3	1	NT	13	NT	<1
IG	1,3	1	NT	<1	NT	<1
PS	1,w8	1,3	<1	3	<1	<1
WF	5,w8	3	<1	<1	4	<1
RO	7,w8	2	4	5	5	<1
SR	3	2	<1	5	<1	9
DL	3	2	<1	13	<1	4
MC	5	3	<1	NT	<1	NT
RJ	3,4	2,3	<1	9	<1	18
JM	4,5	3	<1	1	<1	1
KR	3,w6	1,2	NT	NT	NT	148
MA	w6	1	<1	9	10	4
PM	4,7	2,3	NT	5	NT	4
MT	4,7	2,3	NT	10	NT	8
SQ	5,w9	2,3	NT	8	<1	4
MP	5,7	2,3	<1	<1	NT	NT

a From Hanke et al., 1986.
b The antigen specific responses of four TF derived TCL are expressed as a percentage of the relative antigen stimulation (% RAgS) value as described in Table 1. The data are pooled from different representative experiments with:
c Net autologous responses equal to 11,932, 12,573, 16,577, and 14,964 cpm.
d Net autologous responses equal to 3,341, 11,317, 33,264, and 31,071 cpm.
e Net autologous responses equal to 2,190, 2,379, 4,166 and 4,897 cpm.
f Net autologous responses equal to 8,852, 6,210, 19,540 and 7,024 cpm.

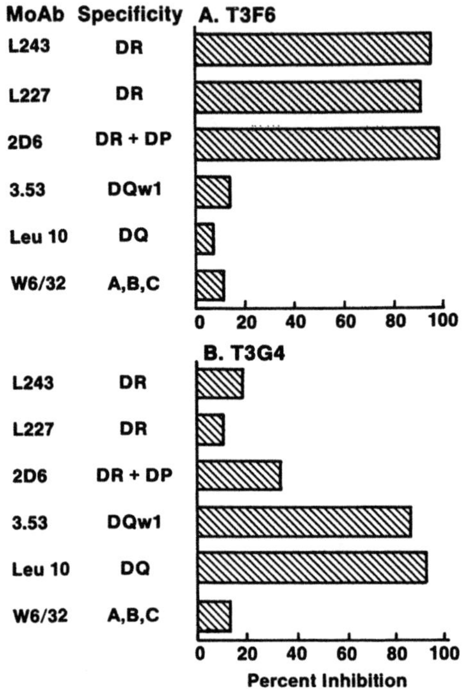

Fig. 4. MoAb blocking of two autologous TNP-specific TCL restricted to determinants associated with the expression of DR2. Each TCL was cultured with an equal number of irradiated, autologous, TNP-modified PBMC for 2 days in the presence or absence of antibody. Proliferation was assessed by the addition of ^{3}H-thymidine for the last 20 h of culture. The control responses were 40,402 $\pm$ 2,197 cpm for TCL T3F6 and 26,573 $\pm$ 882 cpm for TCL T3G4. The data are presented as percent inhibition of the response obtained in the absence of antibody. From Hanke et al., 1986.

tivity of this line correlated better with DR2 (correlation of 0.94) than with DQw1 (correlation of 0.78). Antibody blocking studies with TCL T1B10 and T1C5 demonstrated similar inhibition patterns to lines T3F6 and T3G4, respectively (data not shown). These results suggested that TCL T3F6 and T1B10 recognized a DR2-related determinant on the DR molecule while T3G4 and T1C5 recognized a DQ molecule inherited in linkage disequilibrium with DR2 (and with some DRw6 and DRw8 haplotypes), but distinct from DQ found in association with DR1. Moreover, this latter T cell recognition epitope appeared to be on the same molecule as the DQw1 determinant because Genox 3.53 inhibited both of these cell lines.

Detection of a subtype of DQw1 associated with DR2 could account for the discrepancy between apparent HLA restrictions assessed by correlation on allogeneic panel analysis and by mAb blocking. A panel of DQw1$^+$ Epstein-Barr virus transformed B-cell line stimulators was therefore used to analyze possible structural differences in the DQw1 molecules expressed by DR1, DR2, and DRw8 cells. Selected lines were metabolically labeled with [^{3}H]-tyrosine and immunoprecipitated with the DQw1-specific mAb Genox 3.53. Isolated DQα and DQβ chains were then analyzed for tyrosine residues. The DQα chains from all the lines examined had tyrosines at positions 9, 16 and 25 (data not shown). In contrast, differences associated with functional heterogeneity were detected in the DQw1 β chains precipitated from

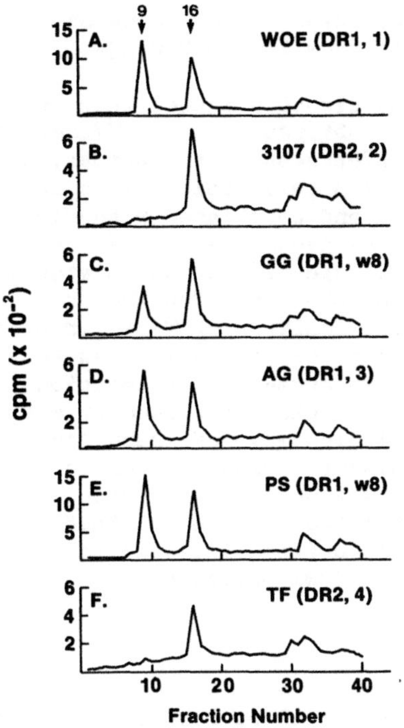

Fig. 5. Partial amino-terminal amino acid sequences of Genox 3.53-reactive β chains. Selected EBV-transformed stimulator B-cell lines were labeled with ^{3}H-Tyr, and the Genox 3.53 (anti-DQw1) reactive DQ β-chain molecules were isolated. The Tyr positions were determined by measuring radioactivity in sequential fractions eluted from an amino acid sequencer. From Hanke et al., 1986.

these B-cell lines (Figure 5). The DQβ chains precipiated from two DR2$^+$ cell lines that were effective stimulators of TCL T1C5 and T3G4 contained Tyr at position 16 (panels B and F), whereas DQβ chains from a nonstimulatory DR1 homozygous line (panel A) and a nonstimulatory DR1,w8 line (panel E) had Tyr at position 9 as well as 16. As shown in panel C, the DQβ chain sequence from the effective stimulator GG (DR1,w8) also contained Tyr at positions 9 and 16, but the Tyr peak at position 16 was higher than at position 9, demonstrating, on the basis of expected repetitive yield analysis, that two distinct DQβ polypeptides were being sequenced. There are two possible explanations for these data. The first is that one DQβ chain had a Tyr at position 9 and the other a Tyr at position 16. This is unlikely, however, because the DQβ chain from subject AG, an offspring of GG who inherited the DR1 haplotype from GG, also had Tyr at positions 9 and 16 (panel D). The second and more likely possibility is that one DQβ chain from GG encoded on the nonstimulatory DR1-associated haplotype had Tyr at 9 and 16, while the stimulatory DQ molecule associated with the DRw8 haplotype had Tyr only at position 16. Further evidence for a functionally important DQw1-associated polymorphism correlating with stimulatory capacity for the DQw1-restricted TCL T3G4 and T1C5 was provided by genomic analysis with a DQβ probe (Wiman et al., 1982). Utilizing both the Taql and EcoR1 restriction enzymes, particular restriction fragment length polymorphism patterns that correlated with the stimulatory capacity of these cell lines were identified (data not shown). Unique restriction fragments associated with both effective antigen presentation and a DQβ tyrosine residue at position 16, but not at position 9, were present in four DQw1$^+$ stimulatory cell lines and were absent from four other DQw1$^+$ nonstimulatory lines.

These studies provide direct evidence that the DQw1 specificity may be divided into at least two subtypes that are differentially recognized by antigen-specific TCL. Differences in the primary sequence of the NH2-terminal region of the DQw1 β chain molecule isolated from DR2$^+$ and DR1$^+$ lines were identified and correlated with distinct restriction fragment length polymorphisms by genomic analysis. More importantly, these molecular subtypes of DQw1 were clearly associated with distinct differences in patterns of antigen presentation. Together these findings strongly supported the possibility that analysis of T-cell restriction specificities based exclusively on patterns of responsiveness to allogeneic stimulator cell panels could lead to incorrect interpretations. They lead us to conclude, moreover, that the relative frequency with which DQ molecules are utilized for T-cell stimulation may have been significantly underestimated due to the inability to discern, with serological techniques, polymorphic determinants on DQ that may also correlate with TCL reactivity. Indeed, our data have demonstrated that two of five TCL that appeared putatively restricted to serologically-defined DR2-associated determinants, in fact, recognized a determinant on DQw1 molecules.

SUMMARY

We believe that the approach we have utilized contributes to more complete understanding of the role of HLA class II molecules in presentation of antigen to T lymphocytes and helps to resolve paradoxes presented by earlier studies in which class II-associated restrictions were not apparent. The approach has depended upon development of a library of cloned TCL reactive to a particular haptenic determinant in various class II MHC contexts. It employed initial screening for MHC restriction by analysis on allogeneic stimulator cell panels that could be confirmed or clarified by antibody blocking experiments employing mAb of defined specificities. This has led to clear identification of TCL restricted to recognition of TNP in the context of each of the major class II molecular species, DR, DQ and DP. It has also raised the intriguing and novel possibility that in some instances, at least for DP, T-cells may employ restricting elements, as revealed by mAb blocking, that are either nonpolymorphic or of very low polymorphism. Finally, where important functional polymorphisms have been identified at apparent variance from defined serological specificities, it has been possible to correlate antigen recognition with molecular polymorphisms defined at both the protein level, by amino acid sequencing, and the genomic level by restriction enzyme polymorphisms. As these approaches are combined with new molecular genetic techniques for generation of novel class II constructs, it seems likely that important, but as yet unresolved, questions relating to the nature of the ternary complex involving antigen, MHC molecule and T-cell receptor will be resolved.

Supported in part by U.S.P.H.S. Research Grants AI15394 and AI21289.

REFERENCES

Ball, E. J., and Stastny, P., 1984a, Antigen-specific HLA-restricted human T-cell lines. I. An MT3-like restriction determinant distinct from HLA-DR, Immunogenetics, 19:13.

Ball, E. J., and Stastny, P., 1984b, Antigen-specific HLA-restricted human T-cell lines. II. A GAT-specific T-cell line restricted by a determinant carried by an HLA-DQ molecule, Immunogenetics, 20:547.

Betuel, H., Gebuhrer, L., Schreuder, G. M. T., Layrisse, Z., Villena, A. A., and Goldman, S. F., 1984, HLA-DRw8, in: "Histocompatibility Testing 1984," E. D. Albert, M. P. Baur, and W. R. Mayr, eds., Springer-Verlag, New York.
Bodmer, J. G., 1977, Ia serology, in: "Histocompatibility Testing 1977," W. F. Bodmer, J. R. Batchelor, J. G., Bodmer, H. Festenstein, and P. J. Morris, eds., Munksgaard, Copenhagen.
Cohen, D., LeGall, I., Marcadet, A., Font, M., Lalouel, J., and Dausset, J., 1984, Clusters of HLA class II β restriction fragments describe allelic series, Proc. Natl. Acad. Sci. U.S.A., 81:7870.
Eckels, D. D., Lake, P., Lamb, J. R., Johnson, A. H., Shaw, S., Woody, J. N., and Hartzman, R. J., 1983, SB-restricted presentation of influenza and herpes simplex virus antigens to human T-lymphocyte clones, Nature, 301:716.
Ferrara, G. B., Park, M. S., Tanigaki, N., and Terasaki, P. I., 1984, HLA-DQw1, in: "Histocompatibility Testing 1984," E. D. Albert, M. P. Baur, and W. R. Mayr, eds., Springer-Verlag, New York.
Fleischer, B., Pawelec, G., and Wernet, P., 1985, Homozygous typing cell-defined HLA-Dw specificities correlate better than serologically defined HLA-DR specificities with restriction elements for influenza virus-specific proliferative human T lymphocyte clones, Human Immunol., 14:37.
Giles, R. C., DeMars, R., Chang, C. C., and Capra, J. D., 1985, Allelic polymorphism and transassociation of molecules encoded by the HLA-DQ subregion, Proc. Natl. Acad. Sci. U.S.A., 82:1776.
Hanke, J. H., Brown, M. F., Pollack, M. S., and Rich, R. R., 1985, Class II determinants recognized by TNP-specific cloned human T cell lines, Human Immunol., 14:59.
Hanke, J. H., Cook, R. G., Leone, J. W., Van, M., and Rich, R. R., 1986, Molecular characterization of a subtype of DQw1 recognized by hapten-specific T cells, Immunogenetics, 24:209.
Nicklas, J. A., Miyachi, Y., Taurog, J. D., Wee, S., Chen, L., Grumet, F. C., and Bach, F. H., 1984, HLA loss varients of a $B27^+$ lymphoblastoid cell line: Genetic and cellular characterization, Human Immunol., 11:19.
Ottenhoff, T. H., M., Elferink, D. G., Hermans, J., and DeVries, R. R., 1985, HLA class II restriction repertoire of antigen-specific T cells. I. The main restriction determinants for antigen presentation are associated with HLA D/DR and not with DP and DQ, Human Immunol., 13:105.
Pawelec, G., Ziegler, A., and Wernet, P., 1985, Dissection of human allostimulatory determinants with cloned T cells: Stimulation inhibition by monoclonal antibodies Tü22, 34, 35, 36, 37, 39, 43, and 58 against distinct human MHC class II molecules, Human Immunol., 12:165.
Qvigstad, E., Moen, T., and Thorsby, E., 1984a, T-cell clones with similar antigen specificity may be restricted by DR, MT (DC), or SB class II HLA molecules, Immunogenetics, 19:455.
Qvigstad, E., Gaudernack, G., and Thorsby, E., 1984b, Antigen-specific T cell clones restricted by DR, DRw53 (MT3), or DP (SB) class II HLA molecules. Inhibition studies with monoclonal HLA-specific antibodies, Human Immunol., 11:207.
Rich, R. R., ElMasry, M. N., and Fox, E. J., 1986, Human suppressor T cells: Induction, differentiation, and regulatory functions, Human Immunol., 17:369.
Seldin, M. F., Rich, R. R., and Dupont, B., 1979, Human immune responses to hapten-conjugated cells. II. The roles of autologous and allogeneic histocompatibility determinants in proliferative responses in vitro, J. Immunol., 122:1828.
Shackelford, D. A., Mann, D. L., van Rood, J. J., Ferrara, G. B., and Strominger, J. L., 1981, Human B-cell alloantigens DC1, MT1, and LB12 are identical to each other but distinct from the HLA-DR antigen,

Proc. Natl. Acad. Sci. U.S.A., 78:4566.
Shaw, S., and Shearer, G. H., 1978, Human cytotoxic responses in vitro to trinitrophenyl-modified autologous cells. II. Diversity of self determinants recognized in association with TNP, J. Immunol., 121:290.
Shearer, G. M., Rehn, T. G., and Schmitt-Verhulst, A.-M., 1976, Role of the murine major histocompatibility complex in the specificity of in vitro T cell-mediated lympholysis against chemically-modified autologous lymphocytes, Transplant. Rev., 29:222.
Swain, S. L., 1983, T cell subsets and the recognition of MHC class, Immunol. Rev., 74:129.
Thomas, D. W., Yamashita, U., and Shevach, E. M., 1977, The role of Ia antigens in T cell activation, Immunol. Rev., 35:97.
Tosi, R., Tanigaki, N., Centis, D., Ferrara, G. B., and Pressman, D., 1978, Immunological dissection of human Ia molecules, J. Exp. Med., 148:1592.
Trowsdale, J., Young, J. A. T., Kelly, A. P., Austin, P. J., Carson, S., Meunier, H., So, A., Erlich, H. A., Spielman, R. S., Bodmer, J., and Bodmer, W. F., 1985, Structure, sequence and polymorphism in the HLA-D region, Immunol. Rev., 85:5.
Wiman, K., Larhammar, D., Claesson, L., Gustafsson, K., Schenning, L., Bill, P., Böhme, J., Denaro, M., Dobberstein, B., Hammerling, U., Kvist, S., Servenius, B., Sundelin, J., Peterson, P. A., and Rask, L., 1982, Isolation and identification of a cDNA clone corresponding to an HLA-DR antigen β chain, Proc. Natl. Acad. Sci. U.S.A., 79:1703.

T-CELLS RECOGNIZE IA CONFORMATION IN THE INTERACTION WITH ANTIGEN PRESENTING CELLS

Harley Y. Tse, Ted H. Hansen, Shirley C-C. Lin
and Alan S. Rosenthal

Department of Immunology and Microbiology, Wayne State University School of Medicine, Detroit, MI., Department of Genetics, Washington University School of Medicine, St. Louis, MO., Department of Immunology, Merck, Sharp & Dohme Research Lab., Rahway, NJ., and Research and Development, Boehringer Ingelheim Pharmaceutical, Inc., Ridgefield, CT.

INTRODUCTION

The presentation of soluble antigens by antigen presenting cell (APC) to T-cells requires that the antigen be recognized in the context of an Ia determinant (Shevach and Rosenthal, 1973). Although the T cell antigen receptor has been identified and sequenced (Hedrick et al., 1984; Fink et al., 1986), the nature of the ligand that triggers the T cells remains unclear. The early experiments of Lin et al. (1981) and Michaelides et al. (1983) using the IA mutant strain of mouse B6.C-$\underline{H\text{-}2}^{bm12}$ (bm12) demonstrated that limited alteration of the Ia molecule concomitantly led to changes in the response pattern of T-cells to soluble antigens. Specifically, it was shown that bm12 lost immune responsiveness to the antigens beef insulin and H-Y while their responses to other antigens remained normal when compared to the wild type C57BL/6. Besides providing convincing evidence equating Ia to the Ir gene product, these experiments also suggest that there are multiple funcitonal domains (Beck et al., 1983) on the Ia molecule that by some unknown mechanisms determine responsiveness to certain antigens. Indeed, this conclusion is consistent with other studies using a variety of approaches such as monoclonal antibody blocking (Frelinger et al., 1984), site-directed mutagenesis (Cohen et al., 1986), *in vitro* selection of variant APC lines (Glimcher et al., 1983b) and inhibition of specific antigen response with structurally related co-polymers (Benacerraf and Rock, 1984). More recently, Babbitt and coworkers (1985) using biochemical methods demonstrated a weak but measurable physical association between a hen egg lysozyme antigenic fragment and purified Ia molecules. This association was demonstrated for Ia derived from responder strains but not that from non-responder strains. In another analysis, Ashwell and Schwartz (1986) also provided arguments that antigen and Ia physically interacted to form a ternary complex recognizable by the T-cell antigen receptor.

With the notion that there are indeed multiple functional domains on the Ia molecule, we performed experiments to investigate the relative importance of these association sites in determining immune responsiveness. Our results demonstrate that the T-cell receptor recognizes a structural form of an Ia epitope rather than its sequence. In this communication, we will first summarize the results of a series of experiments establishing the bml2 mutation site as the predominant site on the Ia molecule for interaction with the T-cell receptor and then provide evidence leading to the concept of T-cell recognition of Ia conformation.

CLONAL ANALYSIS OF ANTIGEN-SPECIFIC, Ia-RESTRICTED T-CELL RECOGNITION

As discussed earlier, bml2 mice was found to have an altered immune response to a selected group of antigens under I-A^b gene control. Conceptually, the most straightforward prediction would be that, in such responses an Ia determinant was used that was affected by the bml2 mutation. Since it had been shown biochemically that the bml2 mutation involved limited alteration in the Aβ chain (McKean et a., 1981; Lee et al., 1982; McIntyre and Seidman, 1984), the fact that bml2 responded to other antigens such as GAT and TGAL at levels as high as B6 was taken to mean that the Ia determinant used to associate with these antigens lied outside the bml2 mutation site. If this were the case, then B6 T cells responding to such antigens could be presented antigens in association with either B6 or bml2 APC via a conserved Ia determinant. This hypothesis was tested by raising a series of antigen-specific T-cell clones. T-cell clones were used in order to avoid allogeneic stimulation in in vitro cultures. In our studies, T cell clones were isoalted by the soft agar method as described by Sredni et al. (1981). Briefly, animals were immunized to antigen in complete Freund's adjuvant in the hind foot-pads and at the base of the tail. After 7-10 days, the popliteal, inguinal and para-aortic draining lymph nodes were isolated, teased into single cell suspension and passed over nylon-wool columns. The T cells so obtained were cultured in 24-well plates in the presence of antigen and APC. After 5 days, cells were harvested and seeded in soft agar containing syngeneic irradiated spleen cells and antigen. Colonies were picked between days 3 to 5 and were cultured in complete RPMI medium supplemented with IL-2 together with antigen and irradiated spleen cells in 96-well round-bottomed microculture plates. Colonies thus generated were tested for activities in the T cell cell proliferative assay.

In the first series of experiments, six B6 PPD-specific T-cell clones were established (Kanamori et al., 1984). These clones were tested for their ability to proliferate in the presence of PPD presented by either B6 or bml2 APC. Results showed that five of the six clones proliferated only when B6 APC were present (type 1 clones). There was absolutely no response when bml2 APC were used. The sixth clone, however, did respond to antigen presented by either APC (type 2 clones). Thus, certain but not all antigen specific T-cell clones have the capability to discriminate between B6 and bml2 presenting cells. The number of clones obtained was too few to allow a meaningful statistical analysis.

It had previously been shown that bml2 expressed two to three times less surface Ia when compared to B6 cells (Melino et al., 1983). This quantitative difference of Ia expression may account for the fewer number of clones capable of responding to bml2 APC. To investigate this possibility, antigne-specific T-cell clones from bml2 mcie have also been established. bml2 mice, like B6, are responders to the antigen GAT. In this paticular experiment, bml2 mice were immunized to GAT and a total of 27 clones were isolated. These clones were all specific for the antigen. The clones were similarly tested for their ability to respond to antigen in the context of Ia^b and Ia^{bml2}. Not surprisingly, the 27 clones could again be distinctly categorized into two groups. As exemplified in Table I, type 1 clones represented by clones #91F7 required that the antigen be associated with Ia^{bml2} and not Ia^b. On the other hand, type 2 clones represented by clone #87F11 did not distinguish Ia^b from Ia^{bml2}.

Table I. Proliferative responses of two types of bml2 GAT-specific T lymphocyte clones to antigen presented by various APC

Clone #	Source of APC	H-2 K	A	J	E	S	D	Proliferative Responses (cpm) Medium	GAT
91F7	---							821	922
	B6	b	b	b	b	b	b	1035	1355
	bml2	b	b*	b	b	b	b	1124	88463
	B10.A(4R)	k	k	b	b	b	b	496	572
	B10.A(5R)	b	b	k	k	d	d	665	869
	B10.BR	k	k	k	k	k	k	1003	1232
	B10.D2	d	d	d	d	d	d	433	513
87F11	---							449	656
	B6	b	b	b	b	b	b	670	31048
	bml2	b	b*	b	b	b	b	1231	36395
	B10.A(4R)	k	k	b	b	b	b	1085	1188
	B10.A(5R)	b	b	k	k	d	d	639	29329
	B10.BR	k	k	k	k	k	k	659	736
	B10.D2	d	d	d	d	d	d	784	876

The ratio of type 1 to type 2 clones was 16:11. Again the majority responded only to the priming APC. In addition, because a reciprocal pattern of reactivity with B6 and bml2 APC was obtained from this analysis, it was concluded that structural and not quantitative difference in Ia appeared accountable.

Our initial interpretation of the data was that the experiments now demonstrated at the clonal level multiple antigen associated sites on the Ia molecule. Type 1 clones, in this instance, utilized association sites located within bml2 mutation site and hence could only respond to antigen in association with the APC used in priming. Type 2 clones, on the other hand, utilized association sites outside of the bml2 mutation site which were indistinguishable on the two Ia molecules.

However, the fact that there are always more type 1 clones than type 2 clones warrants further investigation. In order to generalize the observation, experiments were set up to generate T-cell clones from B6 specific for the antigens GAT and TGAL and from bml2 responding to TGAL. In all cases, results similar to those of Table I were obtained, i.e. clones could be identified as either type 1 or type 2. The frequency distribution of the two types of clones responding to three different antigens are summarized in Table II. As can be seen, the skew is towards type 1 clones. In fact, except for the bml2 clones specific for GAT, less than 25% of the clones could be stimulated with APC other than the one used for priming. This has been the experience of other investigators as well. For example, Hathcock et al. (1983) characterized B6 KLH clones and reported 14 of 15 used B6 and not bml2 APC. Bikoff and Birshstein (1986) also characterized B6 Igh-1a clones and reported that 12 of 12 used B6 and not bml2 APC. These data together show that for responses to antgiens where both B6 and bml2 are responders, T cell predominantly recognize the polymorphic portions of Ia^{b} and Ia^{bml2} involved in the mutation. If there are indeed as many as four sites per Ia molecule as suggested by the

Table II. Frequency distribution of two types of antigen-specific T cell clones from B6 and bml2 responding to various antigens

Strain	Antigen	Frequencies	
		Type 1 clones[a]	Type 2 clones[b]
B6	PPD	5/6	1/6
B6	GAT	16/21	5/21
bml2	GAT	16/27	11/27
B6	TGAL	21/24	3/24
bml2	TGAL	29/35	6/35

[a]Type 1: clones intearcting only with the priming APC.
[b]Type 2: clones not discriminating between B6 and bml2 APC.

monoclonal antibody blocking studies of Frelinger et al. (1984), then the bml2 site is by far the most frequently used.

THE BM12 MUTATION SITE AS A UNIQUE DETERMINANT RECOGNIZED BY ALLOREACTIVE T CELLS

The precise structural definition of the bml2 mutation was recently made by using molecular biological techniques (McIntyre and Seidman, 1984; Mengle-Gaw et al., 1984; Widera and Flavell, 1984). The A_β gene of bml2 and B6 were found to differ by three productive nucleotides within a stretch of 14 nucleotides in the exon encoding the first extracellular domain (β_1). Allelic comparisons of several sequences of different β_1 domains, have defined four regions of hypervariability, HV1 to HV4 and the bml2 was found to be located in the HV3 region. Furthermore, gene transfer and nucleotide sequencing studies (Cohn et al., 1986; Brown et al., 1986) on two of the several somatic Ia variant cell lines derived through mutagenesis and selected by complement mediated lysis using an anti-Ia monoclonal antibody indicated that the functional and phenotypic changes could be acounted for by a single amino acid substitution (glu → lys) at position 67 of the A^k polypeptide chain. All available molecular data thus suggest that the sequence from positions 63 to 75 in which the bml2 mutation lies is the most critical site for T cell recognition. This segment of the bml2 $A_\beta$chain when analyzed by comparison with other β chains unexpectedly revealed complete homology with an E^b_β sequence at this region (Widera and Flavell, 1984; Mengle-Gaw et al., 1984). It is thus proposed that the bml2 mutation can be accounted for by a gene conversion event in which the E^b_β gene provides the donor sequence that replaces homologous information in the A^b_β gene. In the study of Mengle-Gaw et al. (1984), an A anti-(A x B6)F_1 T cell clone which recognized a determinant associated with the E^k_β:E^b_α hybrid molecule could be stimulated by bml2 cells. It was concluded that gene conversion "shift functionally important mini genes between active sites to interact with antigen or the T cell receptor". Similar argument was used by Hochman and Huber (1984) who reported that while B6 was a nonresponder to sheep insulin, both bml2 and B10.A(5R) reponded. Because the response to sheep insulin was mapped to IE genes, these authors felt that the Ia^{bml2} molecules conferred responsiveness as the result of receiving genetic information from E^b_β via the gene conversion event. It was thus concluded that the bml2 mutation defined the functional epitope on Ia for immune responses to sheep insulin. This conclusion, however, appears somewhat obscure since 1) B6 was found in other studies to be responder to sheep insulin (Hansen et al., 1986; Keck, 1981) and 2) we have previously demonstrated that the bml2 "gain" epitope appears to be a unique determinant not shared with other standard strains (Tse et al., 1985). In those experiments, B6 anti-bml2 alloreactive T-cell clones were raised using the soft agar methodology and two, four, and six months after the establishment of the clones, they were tested in mixed lymphocyte cultures for crossreactivity with stimulators from the b, bml2, d, k, r, q, or s haplotypes. Crossreactivity was defined as proliferation that was minimally 10% that of the responses to the Ia antigen. This definition was based on the fact that the standard error of the mean of control culture responses were usually less than 10%. Based on this criteria, the majority of the 17 B6 anti-bml2 clones were found to be specific for the bml2 determinant and exhibited no extensive cross-reaction with other haplotypes. Three of the four clones (51E5, 52E8, 53G6 and 54B8) that initially showed some degree of crossreactivity became specific for bml2 when tested again after 4 months in culture. These false positives could have arisen from the fact that the soft-agar colonies were not recloned and might in addition to the bml2 specific cells, contain other alloreactive cells that were also propagated due to nonspecific recruitment (Tse et al., 1980). These nonspecific contaminants were eventually diluted out as the specific cells constituted the majority and increased in number faster than the nonspecific cells. One of the 17 clones, however, did persistently show crossreactivity with Ia^d after six months in culture. Representative data of two experiments are shown in Table III. Taken together, we concluded that the "gain" antigenic determinant on bml2 Ia represents a private specificity. The minor crossreactivity with Ia^d was only 1 of 17, suggesting that 51E5 was a rare clone.

If the bml2 determinant represents the transfer of a functional unit from E_β^b to A_β^{bm12}, one would predict that B6 anti-bml2 alloreactive T cells should also be stimulted by E_β^k- or E_β^b-bearing cells. To test this prediction, we chose to use the intra-I region recombinant mouse strain B10.A(5R) which express both cell surface Ia dimer A_α^b:A_β^b and E_α^k:$E_\beta^{b/k}$.

Table III. Alloantigen specificity of B6 anti-bml2 T-cell colonies

Exp.	T-cell colonies	Proliferative response in culture with stimulators (cpm)							
		Medium	B6	bml2	B10.BR	B10.D2	B10.S	B10.G	B10.RIII
1	63F5	134	177	9992	337	358	261	292	367
	51B9	1152	1304	11554	1341	1633	1858	1882	1889
	53G11	76	249	11542	302	316	358	222	195
	54E10	121	130	10815	383	270	275	203	204
2	51E5	-	651	32171	683	6079	145	213	228
	52E8	-	124	8241	95	65	245	101	49
	53G6	-	62	14139	141	29	81	99	95
	54B8	-	103	12330	196	110	99	180	36

Experiment 1 was performed two months after establishment of colonies.
Experiment 2 was performed six months after establishment of colonies.

Table IV. Mixed lymphocyte reaction of a B6 anti-bml2 T-cell line

# of responding cells (x 10^{-3})	Proliferative response in cultures with stimulator (cpm)				
	B6	bml2	(B10.A5R)	B10.BR	B10.D2
5	148	41654	247	463	155
10	663	51031	538	2160	722

Since the B1 exon of the E_β gene of B10.A(5R) was derived from the b haplotype, bml2 and B10.A(5R) both express the same Ia sequence involved in the conversion event, albeit bml2 in the context of A and B10.A(5R) in the context of E . As a consequence, B10.A(5R) cells should serve to stimulate B6 anti-bml2 T-cell clones and B10.A(5R) itself should show no alloreactivity against bml2 cells. To determine whether T-cells see the site of the bml2 mutation as a separate functional domain, we generated a B6 anti-bml2 alloreactive T-cell line by the method of Kimoto and Fathman (1981). This line was repeatedly stimulated with bml2 cells for 3 months and then was tested for responses against bml2 or B10.A(5R) stimulator cells. As shown in Table IV, while the line showed a strong response to bml2 stimulators, only background levels of response were observed with the B10.A(5R) stimulator cells. This suggests that the bml2 mutation is seen by T cells not as a linear sequence as B10.A(5R) Ia which contains the sequence failed to stimulate the bml2-specific T cells. To further explore the role of Ia conformation, we also set up primary mixed lymphocyte cultures between bml2 and B10.A(5R) cells. We observed that B10.A(5R) mounted a strong primary MLR against bml2. These cultures were eventually developed into a B10.A(5R) anti-bml2 cell line, which as shown in Table V, was found to be highly specific for the Ia^{bml2} antigen. Since B10.A(5R) cells are incapable of recognizing the primary sequence of the bml2 mutation, these data further underscore the importance of conformation in T-cell recognition of Ia.

CONCLUSIONS

The T-cell receptors that recognize allogeneic Ia are apparently a subset of those that recognize nominal antigen in the context of self Ia. Therefore, the results reported here raise important questions regarding functional recognition of Ia in the immune response. Several lines of evidence are presented indicating that Ia molecules have multiple functional sites and a high proportion of relevant T-cell clones can

Table V. Mixed lymphocyte reaction of a B10.A(5R) anti-bml2 T-cell line

# of responding cells (x 10^{-3})	Proliferative response in cultures with stimulator (cpm)				
	B6	bml2	B10.A(5R)	B10.BR	B10.D2
5	652	161930	456	3111	988
10	412	240113	827	3246	2215

discriminate between Ia^b and Ia^{bm12} molecules in either antigen-specific or allogeneic immune responses. The high frequency of T-cells that can distinguish mutant from wild type Ia may be a reflection of the extent of the conformational change ensuing from the bm12 mutation rather than the importance of the primary structure of this region of the molecule. Studies using T cells immune to cytochrome c (Buchmiller and Corradin, 1982), myoglobin (Berkower et al., 1983) or insulin (Glimcher et al., 1983a) also suggested that Ia-restricted T-cells see conformational determinants on nominal antigen. Taken with the data presented here, we feel the evidence supports the conclusion that T-cells recognize predominantly the conformation of Ia in both allogeneic and syngeneic responses. This conclusion is also consistent with previous studies using K^b mutants that demonstrated that cytotoxic T-cells see conformational determinant on class I major histocompatibility complex molecules (Sherman, 1982).

REFERENCES

Ashwell, J. D., and Schwartz, R. H., 1986, T-cell recognition of antigen and Ia molecule as a ternary complex, Nature, 230:176.

Babbitt, B. P., Allen, P. M., Matsueda, G., Haber, E., and Unanue, E. R., 1985, Binding of immunogenic peptides to Ia histocompatibility molecules, Nature, 317:359.

Beck, B. N., Nelson, P. A., and Fathman, C. G., 1983, The $I\text{-}A^b$ $B6.C\text{-}H\text{-}2^{bm12}$ allows definition of multiple T cell epitopes on I-A molecules, J. Exp. Med., 157:1396.

Benacerraf, B., and Rock, K. L., 1984, Cellular expression and function of Ir genes, in: "Immunogenetics: Its Application to Clinical Medicine", T. Sasazuki and T. Tada, ed., Academic Press, Inc., Tokyo.

Berkower, I., Buckenmeyer, G. K., Gard, R. N., and Berzofsky, J. A., 1982, A possible immunodominant epitope recognized by murine T lymphocytes immune to different myoglobins, Proc. Natl. Acad. Sci. USA, 79:4723.

Bikoff, E., and Birshstein, B. K., 1986, T cell clones specific for IgG2a of the allotype: direct evidence for presentation of endogenous antigen, J. Immunol., 137:28.

Brown, M. A., Glimcher, L. A., Nielsen, E. A., Paul, W. E., and German, R. N., 1986, T cell recognition of Ia molecule selectively altered by a single amino acid substitution, Science, 231:255.

Buchmiller, Y., and Corradin, G., 1982, Lymphocyte specificity to protein antigens. V. Conformational dependence of activation of cytochrome C-specific T cells, Eur. J. Immunol., 12:412.

Cohn, L. E., Glimcher, L. H., Waldman, R. A., Smith, J. A., Ben-Nun, A., Seidman, J. B., and Choi, E., 1986, Identification of functional regions of the $I\text{-}A^b$ molecule by site-directed mutagenesis, Proc. Natl. Acad. Sci. USA, 83:747.

Fink, P. J., Matis, L. A., McElligott, D. L., Bookman, M., Hedrick, S. M., 1986, Correlations between T-cell specificity and the structure of the antigen receptor, Nature, 321:219.

Frelinger, J. G., Shigeta, M., Infante, A.J., Nelson, P. A., Pierres, M., and Fathman, C. G., 1984, Multiple functional sites on a single Ia molecule define dusing T cell clones and antibodies with chain-determined specificity, J. Exp. Med., 159:704.

Glimcher, L. H., Schroer, J. A., Chan, C., and Shevach, E. M., 1983a, Fine specificty of cloned insulin-specific T cell hybridoma: evidence supporting a role of tertiary conformation, J. Immunol., 131:2868.

Glimcher, L. H., Sharrow, S. D., and Paul, W. E., 1983b, Serologic and functional characterization of a panel of antigen-presenting cell lines expressing mutant I-A class II molecules, J. Exp. Med., 158:1573.

Hansen, T. H., Walsh, W. D., Rubocki, R. J., and Kapp, J. A., 1986, Responses of B6.C-H-2^{bm12} to heterologous insulins show no correlation with the putative gene conversion but define Ia^{bm12} as functionally unique, J. Cell Mol. Immunol., 2:359.
Hathcock, K. S., Singer, A., Davis, M., Longo, D., and Hodes, R. J., 1983, The role of polymorphic MHC products in determining the T cell self-recognition repertoire, in: "Intercellular Communication in Leucocyte Function", J. W. Parker and R. L. O'Brien, ed., John Wiley & Sons Ltd.
Hedrick, S. M., Cohen, D. I., Nielsen, E. A., and Davis, M. M., 1984, Isolation of cDNA clones encoding T cell-specific membrane-associated proteins, Nature, 308:149.
Hochman, P. S., and Huber, B. T., 1984, A class II gene conversion event defines an antigen-specific Ir gene epitope, J. Exp. Med., 160: 1925.
Kanamori, S., Walsh, W. D., Hansen, T. H., and Tse, H. Y., 1984, Assessment of antigne-specific restriction sites on Ia molecules as defined by the bml2 mutation, J. Immunol., 133:2811.
Keck, K., 1981, Insulin as a tool for the study of immunologic problems, in: "Basic and Clinical Aspects of Immunity to Insulin", K. Keck and D. Erb, ed., deGruyter Berlin, New York.
Kimoto, M. S., and Fathman, C. G., 1981, Antigen reactive T cell clones. I. Transcomplementing hybrid I-A region gene products functions effectively in antigen presentation, J. Exp. Med., 152:759.
Lee, D. R., Hansen, T. H., and Cullen, S. E., 1982, Detection of an altered I-A polypeptide in the murine Ir mutant B6.C-H-2^{bm12}, J. Immunol., 129:245.
Lin, C-C. S., Rosenthal, A. S., Passmore, H. C., and Hansen, T. H., 1981, Selective loss of antigen-specific Ir gene function in IA mutant B6.C-H-2^{bm12} is an antigen presenting cell defect. Proc. Natl. Acad. Sci. USA, 78:6406.
MyIntyre, K. R., and Seidman, J. G., 1984, Nucleotide sequence of mutant I-A^{bm12} gene is evident for genetic exchange between mouse immune response genes, Nature, 308:551.
McKean, D. J., Melvold, R. W., and David, C. S., 1981, Tryptic peptide comparisons of Ia antigen alpha and beta polypeptides from the I-A mutant B6.C-H-2^{bm12} and its congenic parental strain B6, Immunogenetics, 14:41.
Melino, M. R., Epstein, S. L., Sachs, D. H., and Hansen, T. H., 1983, Idiotypic and fluorometric analysis of the antibodies that distinguish the lesion of the I-A mutant B6.C-H-2^{bm12}, J. Immunol., 131:359.
Mengle-Gaw, L., Conner, S., McDevitt, H. O., and Fathman, C. G., 1984, Gene conversion between murine class II major histocompatibility complex loci, J. Exp. Med., 160:1184.
Michaelides, M., Sandrin, M., Morgan, G., McKenzie, I. F. C., Ashman, R., and Melvold, R. W., 1981, Ir gene function in an I-A subregion mutant B6.C-H-2^{bm12}, J. Exp. Med., 153:464.
Sherman, L. A., 1982, Recognition of conformational determinants on H-2 by cytotoxic T lymphocytes, Nature, 297:511.
Shevach, E. M., and Rosenthal, A. S., 1973, The function of macrophages in antigen recognition of guinea pig T lymphocytes. II. Role of the macrophage in regulation of genetic control of the immune response, J. Exp. Med., 138:1312.
Sredni, B., Tse, H. Y., Chen, C., and Schwartz, R. H., 1981, Antigen-specific clones of proliferating T lymphocytes. I. Methodology, specificity, and MHC restriction, J. Immunol., 126:341.
Tse, H., Schwartz, R. H., and Paul, W. E., 1980, Cell-cell interactions in the T cell proliferative response. I. Analysis of the cell types involved and evidence for nonspecific T cell recruitment, J. Immunol., 125:491.

Tse, H. Y., Kanamori, S., Walsh, W. D., and Hansen, T. H., 1985, The murine bm12 gene conversion provides evidence that T cells recognize predominantly Ia conformation, Proc. Natl. Acad. Sci. USA, 82:7058.

Widera, G., and Flavell, R. A., 1984, The nucleotide sequence of the murine I-E^b immune repsonse gene: evidence for gene conversion events in class II gens of the major histocompatibility complex, EMBO Journal, 3:1221.

T-CELL RECOGNITION AND ANTIGEN PRESENTAION OF MYOGLOBIN

M.Z. Atassi and Garvin S. Bixler, Jr.

Marrs McLean Department of Biochemistry
Baylor College of Medicine
Houston, Texas 77030, U.S.A.

ABSTRACT

Determination of the T-cell recognition profile of Mb by the overlapping peptide strategy revealed that the protein has six T sites. Five of these coincide with the antigenic sites while one site was recognized exclusively by T cells and not by any detectable levels of antibody. Recognition of the synthetic T sites by protein-primed T cell lines or clones indicated that T cells display an unusual peptide size requirement beyond the essential contact residues of the T site. The antigen presentation of Mb has been examined with the significant advantage of knowing the full profiles of T- and B-cell recognition of this multi-determinant antigen. Significant differences in the patterns of T-cell recognition were observed following protein-priming as compared to peptide-priming. The absence of a clear relationship between these patterns of recognition presents a strong evidence against a mechanism of antigen presentation which is dependent on the generation of peptide fragments with the latter being the 'presented' species. From this new perspective, the protein molecule must be predominantly presented in its intact form.

INTRODUCTION

Definition of the submolecular features involved in antibody recognition (i.e. antigenic structures) of proteins has rendered a profound understanding of the molecular basis of antibody (and presumably, therefore, B-cell) recognition of proteins. Myoglobin was the first protein for which the antigenic structure was determined (Atassi, 1975). Subsequently, the antigenic structures of several protein antigens have been determined in this laboratory (Atassi, 1975, 1978, 1980, 1984, 1982; Atassi et al., 1979, 1987; Kazim and Atassi, 1980, Yoshioka and Atassi, 1983, 1986; Atassi and Atassi, 1986; Atassi and Kurisaki, 1984). Myoglobin has served as an excellent model for probing the mechanism and molecular and cellular factors which regulate and control the immune recognition and responses of protein antigens (for reviews, see Atassi, 1984; David and Atassi, 1982; Atassi and Young, 1985; Atassi and Bixler, 1987). The antigenic structure of myoglobin has also established basic concepts and charted comprehensive synthetic strategies (Kazim and Atassi, 1980) that rendered the determination of protein antigenic sites more feasible within a reasonable time.

It is well known that the immune responses to protein antigens involve recognition by T cells as well as antibodies. In fact it was shown over 8 years ago (Okuda et al., 1979) that the synthetic antigenic sites of myoglobin that are the target of antibody recognition are also recognized by T cells. But, generally, in contrast to our extensive knowledge on antibody recognition of proteins, the submolecular details of T-cell recognition have not, until recently, been defined for a protein. Using a comprehensive synthetic approach for the delineation of antigenic (antibody binding) sites, first introduced by Kazim and Atassi (1980) we have scanned the entire polypeptide chain of sperm whale myoglobin, and determined the first full profile of T-cell recognition for a protein (Bixler and Atassi, 1983,1984). The localization, for the first time, of the full profile of the regions that are recognized by T cells on a protein, for which the antigenic sites are also known, has enabled the comparison of immune recognition at the submolecular level by T cells and by antibodies. The sites for these two aspects of immune recognition were first determined for myoglobin (Bixler and Atassi, 1983, 1984a), followed by hen egg lysozyme (Bixler et al., 1984a,b). Since the T-cell recognition profiles of myoglobin and lysozyme were reported, the full T-cell recognition profiles of several other proteins have been reported (Yoshioka et al., 1986; Kurisaki et al., 1986; Atassi and Kurisaki, 1984, 1986; Yokoi et al., 1987). The sites of antibody and T-cell recognition on myoglobin will be outlined here and compared.

It is frequently proposed that antigen presentation must proceed via internalization of the antigen by the antigen presenting cell, its fragmentation and then re-appearance in smaller fragments on the cell surface (Ziegler and Unanue, 1981, 1982; Allen et al., 1984, Unanue and Allen, 1987; Chestnut et al., 1982). The complexity of "processing" and presentation of the antigen has not been clearly resolved due to the fact that the immune recognition features of the protein models employed have been, at best, only partially delineated. Thus, an antigen whose profiles of B- and T- cell recognition are known offers a significant advantage in unravelling the complexities of antigen presentation. Since the antibody and T-cell recognition profiles of Mb have been determined, this protein affords a unique opportunity to examine antigen presentation from an entirely new perspective.

In a recent communication (Bixler and Atassi, 1985) using synthetic overlapping peptides which encompass the entire protein chain, the T-cell proliferative responses after priming with the peptides, either individually or in equimolar mixture, were compared with those resulting from protein priming. Significantly, we have found that the pattern of recognition obtained after peptide priming differs from that obtained after priming with the native protein.

ANTIBODY RECOGNITION OF MYOGLOBIN

The elucidation of the antigenic structure of myoglobin (for a comprehensive review, see Atassi, 1975) required a complex strategy that consisted of a variety of chemical approaches that ultimately led to the definition of five conformationally sensitive antigenic sites. Each of the sites occupies a discrete surface region of the molecule and consists of amino acid residues directly linked by peptide bonds. The term continuous antigenic sites was introduced (Atassi and Smith, 1978) to describe the architecture of such sites. The antigenic sites are small (6-7 residues, approximately 19-23 Å in their extended direction), have sharply defined boundaries, and reside exclusively on exposed surface regions of the protein. Although slight shifts (1-2 residues) in the boundaries have been observed with some antisera, the sites occupy regions 15-22, 56-62, 94-99, 113-119, and 145-146, regardless of the species immunized. Together, these sites account for the vast majority (>98 %) of the antibodies found in anti-myoglobin serum. Historically, myoglobin was the first protein for which the full profile of antibody recognition was described.

T-CELL RECOGNITION OF MYOGLOBIN

By application of the overlapping synthetic peptide strategy, previously introduced by this laboratory (Kazim and Atassi, 1980), a series of synthetic consecutive overlapping peptides (Figure 1) were examined for their capacity to stimulate *in vitro* proliferation of protein-primed lymph node cells or protein-specific long term T-cell cultures (Bixler and Atassi, 1983, 1984). This enabled the localization of the full profile of the Mb regions containing the continuous sites of T-cell recognition.

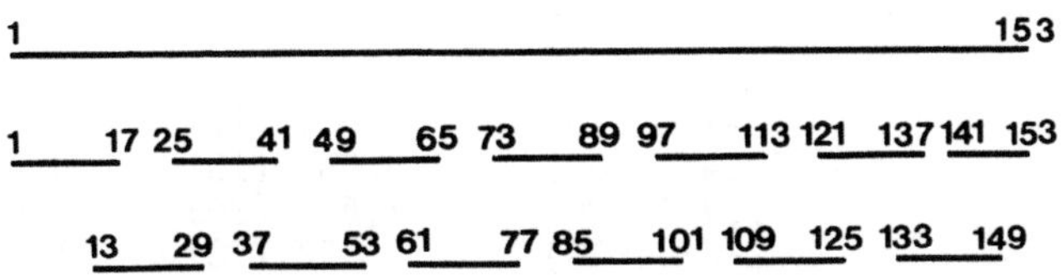

Fig. 1. Synthetic overlapping peptides employed for the delineation of the continuous T sites of sperm whale myoglobin (Bixler and Atassi, 1983,1984). The strategy relied on the synthesis of the entire molecule 17-residue peptides (except for the C-terminal region 141-153), each overlapping its two adjacent neighbors by 5 residues on both sides. (From Bixler and Atassi, 1983).

Studies with Mb-primed lymph node cells from three mouse strains showed that six regions of Mb (Table 1 and Figure 2) are capable of stimulating T-cell proliferative responses (Bixler and Atassi, 1983, 1984). Myoglobin-primed lymph node cells from DBA/2 and Balb/c mice, representing H-2^{d} haplotypes, responded to six continuous T sites localized within the regions: 10-22, 46-63, 69-80, 87-100, 107-120 and 137-151 (Bixler and Atassi, 1984). Although of the same haplotype, lymph node cells from DBA/2 mice recognized a region which was slightly shifted relative to that recognized by Balb/c lymph node cells. The minor shift occurred in the second T site from the N-terminal where T cells of DBA/2 recognized region 46-59 while T cells of Balb/c recognized 51-63. Similarly, Mb-primed lymph node cells from SJL mice (H-2^{s} haplotype) recognized T sites residing within the regions: 10-22, 46-59, 71-82, 111-124 and 138-152 (Bixler and Atassi, 1984). Thus, shifts in the location of the T sites from strain to strain of different haplotypes were also observed. Of the Mb regions that were recognized by T cells, the sites within peptides 61-77, 109-125 and 133-149 had a high level of activity in the strains studied. The site within region 109-125 was immunodominant.

It should be noted, however, that the overlapping peptide strategy is not designed to give the precise boundaries of the sites. Thus, the T sites derived by this strategy were not implied to comprise the entire regions shown in Figure 2. Rather, the T sites are expected to reside within those regions (Bixler and Atassi, 1984). Indeed, the regions containing T sites were made intentionally larger than the expected size of the site in order to avoid assignment errors stemming from close delineation at this early stage.

Table 1

The proliferative response of Mb-primed lymph node cells to synthetic peptides, proteins or mitogens

Antigens	Δ cpm*(optimum dose in μg/ml) DBA/2	BALB/c	SJL
Peptides:			
1-17	-465 (40)	-650 (10)	-324 (20)
10-22	12,459 (80)	6,981 (10)	4,210 (40)
13-29	7,747 (80)	1,673 (80)	874 (40)
25-41	2,680 (80)	373 (20)	1,409 (10)
37-53	12,494 (80)	1,600 (40)	4,275 (40)
49-65	12,587 (80)	5,685 (20)	3,446 (10)
61-77	19,049 (40)	5,265 (10)	1,979 (10)
73-89	5,361 (80)	2,778 (80)	8,019 (80)
85-101	-609 (40)	-69 (20)	2,275 (10)
87-100	7,363 (80)	1,625 (80)	1,290 (10)
97-113	391 (10)	-390 (10)	1,803 (10)
107-120	154,318 (80)	26,858 (80)	5,608 (10)
109-125	36,895 (80)	12,305 (80)	30,774 (80)
121-137	3,852 (40)	295 (80)	3,894 (10)
133-149	20,810 (80)	8,368 (40)	6,874 (40)
141-153	6,570 (80)	1,583 (80)	5,917 (80)
Controls			
Myoglobin	58,235 (5)	24,308 (10)	17,762 (20)
Con A	87,665 (1)	62,516 (1)	52,220 (1)
PPD	129,191 (100)	130,190 (100)	66,043 (100)
LPS	50,300 (500)	137,760 (500)	102,621 (500)
Haemoglobin	2,459 (50)	1,482 (50)	2,814 (50)
Lysozyme	459 (50)	51 (50)	ND
Lysozyme (31-50)	2,175 (40)	1,804 (10)	1,567 (80)
Lysozyme (109-129	2,583 (80)	2,367 (20)	2,035 (10)

* The results are reported at optimum dose of challenge antigen, although the studies were carried out in the dose range 1-100 μg/ml. Cultures containing unstimulated DBA/2, BALB/c, or SJL lymph node cells and backgrounds of 4126, 4762, and 2361 cpm respectively.
‡ND = Not done.

Table is from Bixler and Atassi (1984).

Of the six T sites in Mb, five were found to coincide with the known (Atassi, 1975) antigenic (antibody binding) sites while the remaining site was exclusively T-cell specific. The latter site was located within region 69-80 in the H-2^d haplotypes and within region 71-82 in the H-2^s haplotype. It should be noted that a slight, but reproducible, response to region 33-44 was also observed (Bixler and Atassi, 1984). Clearly, studies with the overlapping peptides of Mb have shown, in agreement with earlier studies (Okuda et al., 1979; Young and Atassi, 1982, 1983; Yoshioka et al., 1983), that this protein contains sites that are recognized by both B and T cells. Those earlier studies, however, only examined the regions containing the antigenic (antibody binding) sites for their T-cell activity. It is noteworthy that Mb contains, in addition, other regions which are recognized only by T cells but to which no antibody response is detectable.

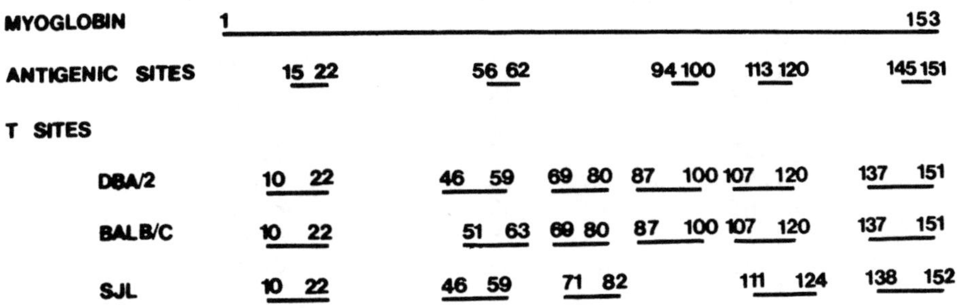

Fig. 2. Schematic diagram showing the full profile of the regions of sperm-whale myoglobin that carry the continuous sites of T-cell recognition (T-sites) in three mouse strains. It is not implied that the entire regions shown comprise the T site, rather that the sites reside within these regions. Indeed, in the localization by the overlapping peptide strategy (Figure 1), the T sites are localized within intentionally larger regions than their expected size. (From Bixler and Atassi, 1983, 1984).

Although the proliferative assay employed in the localization of the T sites of Mb is generally accepted to be indicative of T-cell function, the lymph node population, nonetheless, represents a mixture of cell types. Further, some minor T-cell specificities may be present in low quantities. Long-term T-cell cultures, that were selectively enriched for Mb-specific T cells, were also examined (Bixler and Atassi, 1984) in order to circumvent these minor objections. The examination of the proliferative response of these Mb-specific T-cell cultures with the overlapping peptides revealed that the profile of T-cell recognition was essentially the same [Table 2] as that obtained with the lymph node cells. However, T cells obtained from long-term culture had a more pronounced response to the peptides 13-29, 73-89 and 109-125 (Bixler and Atassi, 1984).

Definition of the boundaries of a T site and effect of peptide size on in vitro responses of T-cell bulk cultures

Earlier studies on T-cell recognition (Bixler and Atassi, 1983, 1984; Yoshioka et al., 1983) suggested that the carboxyl end of the T site within region 107-120 was in close proximity to reside 120, probably residue 120 itself or, at the most, plus or minus one or two residues. In order to define the carboxyl end of this T site, we compared the responses of several mouse strains to the peptides 107-119 and 107-120 [Figure 3]. From the differences in the responses and studies with peptides extended to residue 125, we were able to map the carboxyl boundary of the T site to residues 119 or 120 depending on the mouse strain examined (Bixler et al., 1986).

Table 2

The proliferative response of BALB/c T-cell long-term cultures to synthetic peptides, proteins or mitogens

Antigens	Optimum dose * (μg/ml)	cpm
Peptides		
1-17	10	4,498
10-22	40	2,767
13-29	40	8,106
25-41	5	2,262
37-53	10	1,227
49-65	5	2,110
61-77	5	3,609
73-89	40	8,587
85-101	5	1,850
87-100	5	1,119
97-113	5	25
107-120	40	30,482
109-125	10	28,897
121-137	40	2,703
133-149	10	10,843
141-153	40	3,301
Controls		
Myoglobin	40	51,784
Con A	1	76,314
PPD	100	1,244
LPS	500	0
Haemoglobin	40	0
Lysoyzme	40	4
Lysozyme (31-50)	5	258
Lysozyme (109-129)	5	419

*Studies were carried out in the dose range 1-100 μg/ml. The table summarizes the responses at the optimum dose for each antigen. The T cells were harvested from a culture in the fifth *in vitro* passage and had a background proliferation of 4,881 cpm.

Table is from Bixler and Atassi (1984).

In order to accurately map the other boundary of the T site and determine the effect of peptide size on its ability to activate T cells a new strategy had to be introduced (Bixler et al., 1986). The obvious approach to the definition of the boundaries of a T site is through the step-wise addition (or deletion) of residues on one end of the indicated region while holding the other end constant. The resulting set of peptides would represent varying lengths or the natural sequence of the protein [Figure 4]. Since earlier studies on B-cell recognition showed that deletion of a single residue at the boundary end of an antigenic site can cause complete abrogation of the binding activity (Koketsu and Atassi, 1973; Atassi, 1975), this approach would seem to be promising. However, recent studies from this laboratory suggested that peptide size by itself may have an effect on the ability of a given peptide to stimulate T-cell response, both in protein-primed lymph node cells (Young and Atassi, 1983) and in peptide driven T-cell lines and clones (Yoshioka et al., 1983). In both these studies, the response to longer peptides appeared to be improved.

These studies suggested the possibility that a peptide containing the essential 'contact' residues for T-cell stimulation would possess higher activity if it were lengthened, even though the additional segments may contain no recognition features. The T site residing within the segment 107-120 (Bixler and Atassi, 1983, 1984) was selected to examine this idea. The strategy formulated employed synthetic peptides increasing in size by one residue increments from His-113, the known N-terminal boundary of the antigenic (i.e. antibody binding) site (Atassi and Pai, 1975). The increase in size was done in two ways: (1) by addition of residues (one at a time) corresponding to the natural Mb sequence, up to residue 107 and designated by the sequence locations of the first and last residues, or (2) by addition of one-residue increments corresponding to the natural Mb sequence plus further extension of the peptide up to a uniform size of 14 residues by addition of a nonsense sequence that is not in any way related to Mb in this region or anywhere else in the molecule (Twining and Atassi, 1979). These peptides are also designated by the location of the region in the Mb sequence and, in addition, are prefixed by 'N' to denote the nonsense extension. The nonsense structure has been shown not to bind anti-Mb antibodies (Twining and Atassi, 1979; Twining et al., 1981; Allen et al., 1985) and also has no effect on Mb-primed T cells (Okuda et al., 1979; Young and Atassi, 1983). It is, therefore, ideally suited to study pure size effects. Thus, regardless of whether or not peptide size influenced T-cell responses, the strategy adopted should permit, in addition, to clarification of this point, the precise definition of the boundaries of the site. It would distinguish between those residue additions which contribute size effects alone versus those which are essential contact residues of the site.

These studies revealed unambiguously the significant contribution made by peptide size to the stimulation of Mb-primed T cells. From the dose response curves [Figure 5], the larger peptides consistently provoked a detectable proliferative response in protein-primed T cells at lower concentrations and also elicited greater maximal responses than the corresponding peptides containing only the natural Mb sequence (Bixler et al., 1986). In five of the six strains examined [Figure 6], the peptides extended by nonsense sequence elicited higher proliferative responses than their counterparts that contain only natural Mb sequence. Clearly, the greater stimulatory capacity is not related to nonspecific stimulation by the nonsense sequence extension, since those peptides containing the largest segment of nonsense residues (and correspondingly, the shortest segment of natural sequence), provoked very weak or no responses above baseline. Thus, the increase in proliferative activity of the nonsense-extended peptides, when compared to the appropriate natural sequence peptides, was attributed to a non-specific effect of peptide size (Bixler et al., 1986). These observations are consistent with earlier reports (Young and Atassi, 1983; Yoshioka et al., 1983) which initially indicated the potential role of size in the recognition of free peptides by protein-primed T cells.

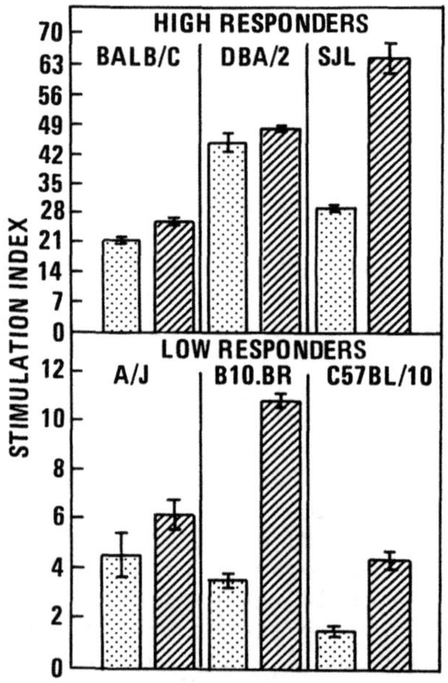

Fig. 3. Summary of proliferative responses of lymph node cells obtained from six mouse strains to in vitro challenge with peptides representing the natural Mb sequences 107-119 (stippled bar) and 107-120 (hatched bar). The responses were tested, over a wide dose range (3-300 μg/ml) and the maximum responses are shown for both the high responders (Balb/c at an optimum dose of 50 μg/ml for both peptides, DBA/2 at an optimum dose of 300 μg/ml for both peptides and SJL at optimum doses of 300 and 200 μg/ml for peptides 107-119 and 107-120, respectively), B10.BR and C57 BL/10 at an optimum dose in both strains of 200 μg/ml for both peptides) to Mb. Stimulation index is the ratio: cpm of stimulated cells /cpm of unstimulated cells. The background responses for unstimulated cells ranged from 4,999 cpm to 7,166 cpm except for cells from BALB/c mice which had a background response of 10,880 cpm. (From Bixler et al., 1986).

These synthetic peptides, which carefully dissect the region 107-120 of Mb, allow the precise definition of the boundaries of a major T site. In the three low responder mouse strains, A/J, C57BL/10 and B10.BR, the T site consists of 13 residues extending from Ser-108 to Pro-120. In two of the three high responder mouse strains, Balb/c and (*a*) Mb peptides having increasing size of natural sequence

107-120	Ile-Ser-Glu-Ala-Ile-Ile-His-Val-Leu-His-Ser-Arg-His-Pro
108-120	Ser-Glu-Ala-Ile-Ile-His-Val-Leu-His-Ser-Arg-His-Pro
109-120	Glu-Ala-Ile-Ile-His-Val-Leu-His-Ser-Arg-His-Pro
110-120	Ala-Ile-Ile-His-Val-Leu-His-Ser-Arg-His-Pro
111-120	Ile-Ile-His-Val-Leu-His-Ser-Arg-His-Pro
112-120	Ile-His-Val-Leu-His-Ser-Arg-His-Pro
113-120	His-Val-Leu-His-Ser-Arg-His-Pro

(*b*) Natural MB sequences extended by nonsense sequence to a uniform size

N(108-120)	Gly-Ser-Glu-Ala-Ile-Ile-His-Val-Leu-His-Ser-Arg-His-Pro
N(109-120)	Gly-Ala-Glu-Ala-Ile-Ile-His-Val-Leu-His-Ser-Arg-His-Pro
N(110-120)	Gly-Ala-Ser-Ala-Ile-Ile-His-Val-Leu-His-Ser-Arg-His-Pro
N(111-120)	Gly-Ala-Ser-Gly-Ile-Ile-His-Val-Leu-His-Ser-Arg-His-Pro
N(112-120)	Gly-Ala-Ser-Gly-Thr-Ile-His-Val-Leu-His-Ser-Arg-His-Pro
N(113-120)	Gly-Ala-Ser-Gly-Thr-Gly-His-Val-Leu-His-Ser-Arg-His-Pro

Fig. 4. The primary structure of the synthetic peptides employed the definition of the T site previously found to localize within region 107-120 of sperm whale Mb (Bixler and Atassi, 1983, 1984; Yoshioka et al., 1983). (a) Peptides representing step-wise extensions by one-residue of the natural Mb sequence from His-113 to Pro-120. Peptide 113-120 coincidentally corresponds to the previously defined (Atassi, 1975) antigenic (antibody binding) site 4 of Mb. (b) Peptides in which the structures shown in (A)are extended by a 'nonsense' sequence to a uniform size of 14residue by addition of an appropriate segment of the 'nonsense' sequence Gly-Ala-Ser-Gly-Thr-Gly (underlined region). (From Bixler et al., 1986).

DBA/2, the site consists of the 11 residues (Glu-109 through His-119). In the remaining high responder mouse strain, SJL, the T site comprises the residues Ala-110 through Pro-120. Thus, the T site in this region was mapped [For summary, see Figure 7] to a relatively small (11-13 residues), continuous, discrete surface region of the polypeptide chain of Mb (Bixler et al, 1986).

It should be stressed that these boundaries reflect the average of the maximal responses of a polyclonal T-cell population whose specificity is directed to this region and that the boundary residues define the minimum continuous segment of Mb which elicits an optimum proliferative response. It should be noted, however, that although the identity of the residues which define the boundaries is very clear, the differences in activity between peptides changing by one residue increments are not always dramatic. This was attributed (Bixler et al., 1986) to the polyclonal nature of the lymph node cell response. It was noted that studies with T cell clones should yield, for each clone, sharply demarcated boundary residues.

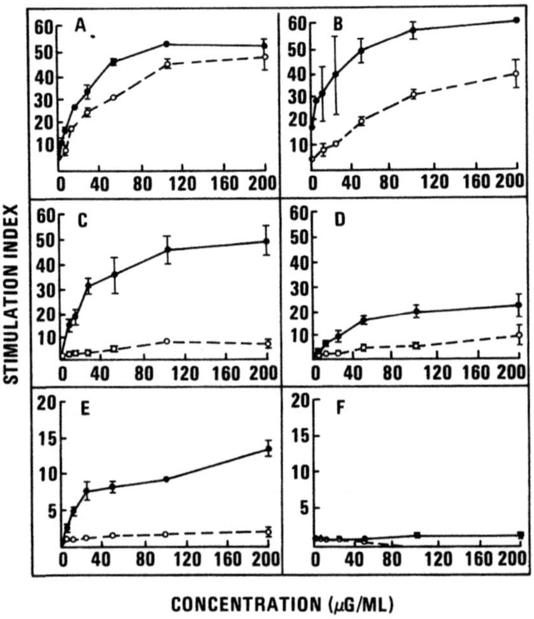

Fig. 5. Representative dose response curves to peptides of the natural sequence (o) or peptides extended by 'nonsense' sequence to a uniform size (o) in lymph-node cells obtained from Mb-primed DBA/2 mice. The responses, which were examined over a broad dose range, are shown in the panels as follows: (A) peptides 108-120 and N (108-120), (B) peptides 109-120 and N (109-120), (C) peptides 110-120 and N (110-120), (D) peptides 111-120 and N (111-120), (E) peptides 112-120 and N (112-120), (F) peptides 113-120 and N (112-120). Stimulation index is defined in the legend to Fig. 3. The background response of unstimulated cells was 3,412 cpm. (From Bixler et al., 1986).

Non-specific peptide size effect in the recognition by site-specific T-cell clones

The enhancing effect on T-cell activity observed by addition of a 'non-sense' sequence to maintain peptide size was unexpected and most dramatic. These observations, however, were made with lymph node cells and, because of the heterogeneity of such a cell population, some degree of uncertainty remained whether this peculiar phenomenon is indeed associated with T-cell recognition or is caused by some unknown parameters in the complex culture of lymph node cells. The question must then be answered with precise reagents. For this purpose T-cell clones of pre-determined specificity, derived from DBA/2 and SJL mice that had been primed with Mb, were used in more recent studies (Atassi et al., 1987). Two DBA/2 and five SJL T cell clones were isolated from T-cell lines derived from Mb-primed lymph node cells that were driven in culture by periodic passage with peptide 107-120. These cell lines were entirely specific to the driving peptide and, recognized no other regions of Mb (Yoshioka et al., 1983). The recognition was imparted to the cells by priming the mice with Mb and the specificity desired was selected by driving with the peptide. It would then be expected that the driving peptide, and hence its structural features, would be best suited for stimulation of the T-cell clones. Thus, these clones would be the most precise reagents to examine whether size effects of a non-specific and otherwise unrecognizable structure (at least by these T-cell clones) play a role in T-cell recognition. In addition, one clone which was obtained from a Mb-driven long term T-cell culture was also specific to region 107-120. The two sets of peptides (one set extended incrementally by natural Mb sequence and the other represents analogs that are extended to a uniform size by a nonsense sequence) in Figure 4 were used for these studies (Atassi et al., 1987). The peptide design (Figure 4) is such that the incremental one-residue addition of the 'nonsense' sequence would be capable of answering the above question and also of defining the left-hand boundary of the T site for each of the T-cell clones.

The results showed (Atassi et al., 1987) that peptide size exerted a dramatic effect on T-cell recognition at the clonal level. In every clone, a non-sense-extended peptide achieved maximum stimulating activity at a lower optimum peptide dose than its natural sequence (but shorter) analogue (Figure 8). In addition, removal of natural sequence by one residue increments caused loss of proliferative activity whereas the nonsense-extended analogues retained full activity until a critical 'contact' residue was removed (Figures 9 and 10). Figure 11 summarizes the boundaries of the site as perceived by the various clones. Thus, in the DBA/2 clone E4.15.15 the activity of the natural sequence peptides decreased steadily upon shortening and was drastically lost upon removal of residue 109. However, the nonsense-extended peptides retained the full activity until residue 112 was removed, thus indicating the Ile-112 defines the left-hand boundary of the T site. Similarly, the DBA/2 clone E4.8.19 revealed a left-hand boundary at Ala-100 or Ile-111 with the natural sequence peptides, whereas, with the nonsense-extended peptides, its boundary falls very sharply at Ile-112. With the five SJL clones obtained from cell lines passaged with peptide 107-120, the left-hand site boundary, as summarized in Figure 11, was precisely defined with the nonsense-extended peptides at Ile-112 (clones No. V1.E4.5.1; No. E4.5.6; No. E4.4.8 and No. E4.10) or Ile-111 (clone No. V1.E4.5.4). Even with the clone derived with Mb passage, the left-hand boundary of the site was at Ile-112, thus indicating a comparable structural requirement for the recognition by this clone. In contrast, with the natural sequence peptides, the site boundary was very poorly defined (and more of the natural Mb sequence was required) for most of the clones.

The aforementioned size effects are remarkable in view of the fact that seven of the eight clones were obtained by driving the parent T-cell lines with peptide 107-120. Yet, clearly, not all the residues of the peptide are needed for T-cell recognition. Previously, we had observed (Yoshioka et al., 1983) that peptides that were shorter than 107-120 were not capable of maintaining and driving long-term cultures to obtain mono-specific T-cell lines. Thus, the above findings provided a rational explanation (Bixler et al., 1986; Atassi et al., 1987) for this observation. The size effects observed showed that, in addition to the essential 'contact' residues, there is a decided advantage in increasing peptide size, even by an unrelated sequence. The larger peptide size (by addition of unrelated residues) may prolong its survival in the culture during T-cell stimulation. Furthermore, it may have been a reflection of the lower affinity of the T-cell receptor (relative to antibody affinity) since the 'contact' region required for optimal T-cell recognition is somewhat larger than that needed for binding to antibody. Should the binding energy of the T-cell receptor be less than, or even the same as, that of the antibody, the additional residues may assist in increasing the binding energy of the receptor-peptide complex and association with the Ia molecule. Alternative or additional influences of size may be through conformational effects. The added residues may assist the peptide to approximate more closely, the shape of its corresponding region in the native protein (Atassi and Saplin, 1968; Epand and Scheraga, 1968; Singhal and Atassi, 1970; Atassi and Singhal, 1970). It should be noted, however, that the addition of large bulky side chains at an end of a site may result in steric interference with the binding of the site (Koketsu and Atassi, 1974; Atassi and Pai, 1975; Young and Atassi, 1983). Therefore, attention was paid, in the above studies (Bixler et al., 1986; Atassi et al., 1987) to the unrelated 'nonsense' sequence which, while maintaining solubility, carried no bulky side chains that may potentially exert a steric hindrance on the 'binding part' of the peptide.

The recognition of the T site at the clonal level (Atassi et al., 1987) revealed, for a given clone, a sharper boundary for the site than was obtained with bulk cultures (Bixler et al., 1986). Also, it was apparent that the boundary of the T site shifts slightly from clone to clone. So, it should be expected that the response registered with bulk cultures will naturally define an 'average' boundary recognized by the numerous clones in the cultures (Bixler et al., 1986). The C-terminal boundary of the T site recognized by each of these clones was not determined. However, it was shown (Bixler et al., 1986) that the C-terminal 'average' boundary of the T site with T-cell bulk cultures was His-119 for DBA/2 and Pro-120 for the SJL strain. Therefore, the peptides studied were all terminated at residue 120 in order to stimulate the activity of both sets of clones. It should be noted that the T site defined at the clonal level (Atassi et al., 1987) coincides with antigenic (i.e. antibody binding) site 4 which occupies residues 113-119 (Atassi and Pai, 1975).

It has been proposed, from studies with Mb mutants, that the T-cell recognition of Mb involves a determinant "centering" on residue 109 (Berkower et al., 1982) which is different from the antigenic (i.e. antibody recognition) site and does not extend as far as residue 118 (Berkower et al., 1984). On the other hand, previous studies from this laboratory (Bixler and Atassi, 1983, 1984; Yoshioka et al., 1983) have shown that peptide 107-120 exhibited strong proliferative activity with Mb-primed T-cell bulk cultures and/or clones and a T site was localized to reside within, but not including all of, region 107-120. Recently, Berkower and colleagues (Cease et al., 1986) have examined the responses of two T-cell clones using synthetic peptides rather than protein variants and reported T-cell responses to peptide 106-118. Although extensions to the right of residue 118 were not tested to determine whether Arg-118 was in fact the C-terminal boundary for their clones, the results of Cease et al., (1986) clearly confirm our previous reports that a T site is localized within region 107-120 (Bixler and Atassi, 1983, 1984) and included the residues 113-120 (Okuda et al., 1979). The present work with clones and recent studies with T-cell cultures (Bixler et al., 1986) have shown that the T site superimposes very well with antigenic site 4 (residues 113-119) of Mb (Atassi and Pai, 1975; Atassi, 1975).

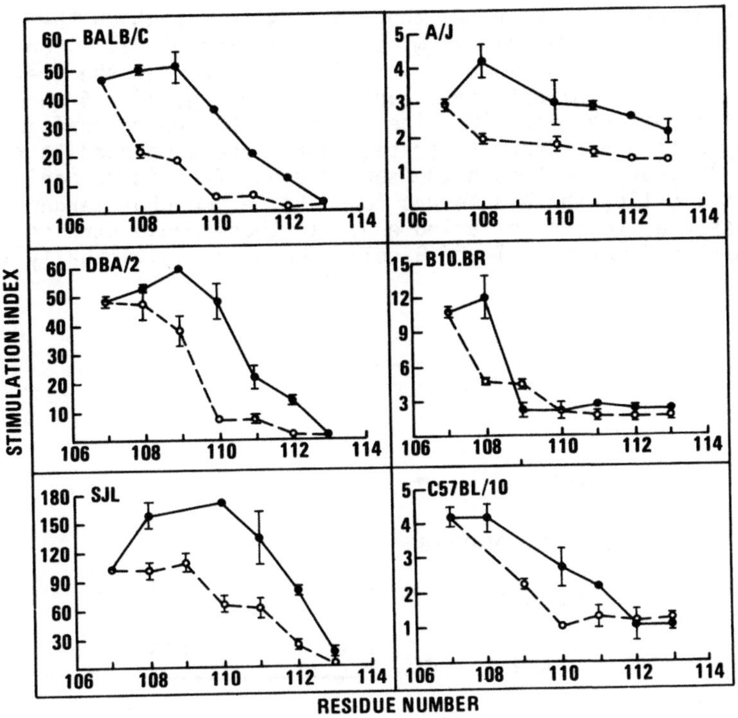

Fig. 6. Summary of proliferative responses of lymph node cells obtained from six mouse strains in vitro challenge with peptides of the natural sequence (o) or peptides extended by 'nonsense' sequence to a uniform size (•). The maximum proliferative responses obtained are plotted against the Mb residue added. Mouse strains were characterized as either high (BALB/c, DBA/2 and SJL) or low (A/J, B10.BR and C57 BL/10) responders to Mb. Stimulation index is defined in the legend to Fig. 3. Background responses for the unstimulated cells ranged from 1,094 cpm to 4,680 cpm. (From Bixler et al., 1986).

Recent speculations (Benjamin et al., 1984) have advanced the views that the sites of T-cell recognition are different from, and more diffuse than, the sites of B-cell recognition. Although these views have remained popular (Simpson, 1986; Unanue and Allen, 1987), they are not confirmed by the present and previous studies (Okuda et al., 1979; Atassi and Young, 1982; Yoshioka et al, 1983; Bixler and Atassi, 1983, 1984a,b) which show that the major T sites of a protein occupy discrete areas which very frequently [but not always (Bixler et al., 1984a,b; Bixler and Atassi, 1984)] coincide with sites of B-cell recognition.

Comparison of sites T- and B- cell recognition

It is now clear that the regions of a molecule recognized by B cells (antibody binding) can also be recognized by T cells. T cells, however, may recognize additional areas of the molecule to which no detectable antibody responses have been observed. Therefore, contrary to recent opinions (Benjamin et al, 1984; Simpson, 1986; Unanue and Allen, 1987), the fine specificity of T cells is neither limited in number nor necessarily different from that of B cells.

It is interesting to note, that the T site for which the precise boundaries have been defined in myoglobin (Bixler et al., 1986; Atassi, 1987) coincides with the same region of the protein as the previously defined (Atassi, 1975) antigenic (antibody binding) site 4 which occupies the residues 113–120. The T and B sites were localized and defined by entirely different strategies and are separated in time by more than 10 years. Although the same region of Mb is recognized by both B and T cells, the T site was found to be somewhat larger extending several residues toward the amino end. In those mouse strains examined, the carboxyl end for both T and B cells, however, is virtually identical

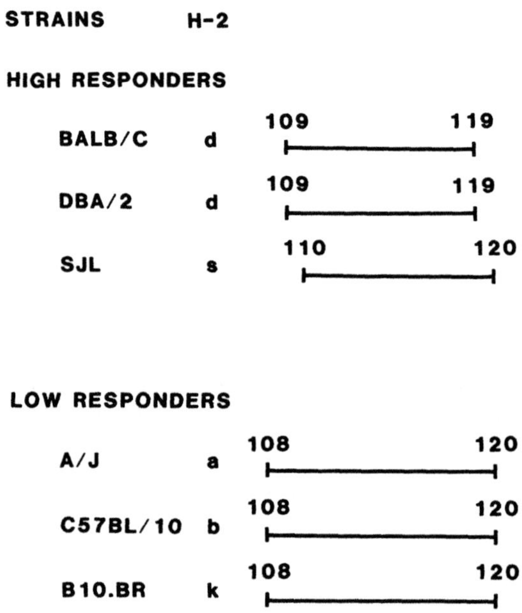

Fig. 7. Summary of the precise boundaries of the T site within region 107–120 of sperm whale Mb as defined in six mouse strains which were either high or low responders to Mb. (From Bixler et al., 1986).

since both map to residues 119 and 120. Although it is tempting to conclude that these observations may portray a general property of T-cell recognition of proteins, it must be cautioned that, at the present time, it is premature to generalize to other T sites of Mb or other proteins. Clearly, additional detailed, submolecular studies of other Mb T sites, at both the clonal and polyclonal level, and similar studies with other proteins must be performed before a general picture will emerge.

The T-cell recognition of each of the T sites probably reflects the responses of numerous T-cell subpopulations, each of which perceives the

T site somewhat differently. Thus, various T-cell clones recognize different overlapping parts of a site (i.e. shifting to the right or to the left) and the maximal effective response, which is the average of all of these reactivities, is the detected T site. This would be consistent with a heterogeneous nature of the T-cell response at the clonal level with regard to the fine submolecular specificities as has been demonstrated during B-cell recognition (Atassi, 1975, 1978, 1980, 1984). In view of the heterogencity, the possibility exists that T-cell clones with specificity for a region outside of a known T site, and which are present in traces and would not therefore be detected in T-cell proliferative assays of lymph node cells or bulk cultures, could be isolated and expanded. For example, in the case of B-cell recognition of myoglobin, monoclonal antibodies which recognize regions outside of the five major antigenic sites have been isolated (Schmitz et al., 1983). The biological significance and the immune role, if any, of such very minor T-cell and B-cell clones whose specificity is directed toward non-dominant regions is not known.

ANTIGEN PRESENTATION OF MYOBLOBIN

The crucial role of the macrophage or other accessory cells in the initial events of immune recognition is now well established (For reviews, see Moller, 1978; Rosenthal, 1980). The involvement of Ia molecules in H-2 restricted recognition (Keck, 1975; Melchers et al., 1973; Lozner et al., 1974; Okuda et al., 1978) and the association of antigenic sites of a multi-determinant protein with a particular Ia subregion (Okuda et al., 1979) is also clearly established. It is widely believed that antigen presentation must proceed via internalization of the antigen, its fragmentation and then reappearance in smaller more recognizable components on the cell surface (Ziegler and Unanue, 1981, 1982; Chestnut et al., 1982; Shimonkevitz et al., 1983; Lee et a;., 1982; Allen et al., 1984). The antigenic complexity of the protein models employed and the lack of full knowledge of their T- and B-cell recognition has made the investigation of this question most difficult. Thus, an antigen such as Mb whose full profiles of B- and T-cell recognition are known offers a unique advantage in unravelling the complexities of antigen presentation.

The synthetic strategy which was instrumental in localizing the sites of T-cell recognition of Mb (Bixler and Atassi, 1983,1984) has been employed (Bixler and Atassi, 1985) to investigate its presentation. The thirteen synthetic overlapping peptides of Mb were used (Bixler and Atassi, 1985) either individually or in a mixture to prime three high responder mouse strains in which the T sites of Mb had been previously localized (Bixler and Atassi, 1983, 1984). Thus, the pattern of T-cell recognition following protein or peptide priming could be compared. The results are summarized in Table 3.

If antigen presentation proceeds via fragmentation of the protein, similarity in the patterns of peptide recognition would be expected. In contrast to the patterns of recognition observed (Bixler and Atassi, 1985) in protein-primed mice, those mice primed with individual peptides responded to all of the peptides (Table 3) with a few exceptions (in Balb/c, peptides, 49-65, 97-113, 121-137, and 141-153; in DBA/2, peptide 49-65, 97-113, 112-137, and 141-153; in DBA/2, peptide 49-65; in SJL, peptides 1-17, 49-65, and 121-137). Thus, the patterns of recognition obtained after peptide-priming differ from those observed after priming with the native protein.

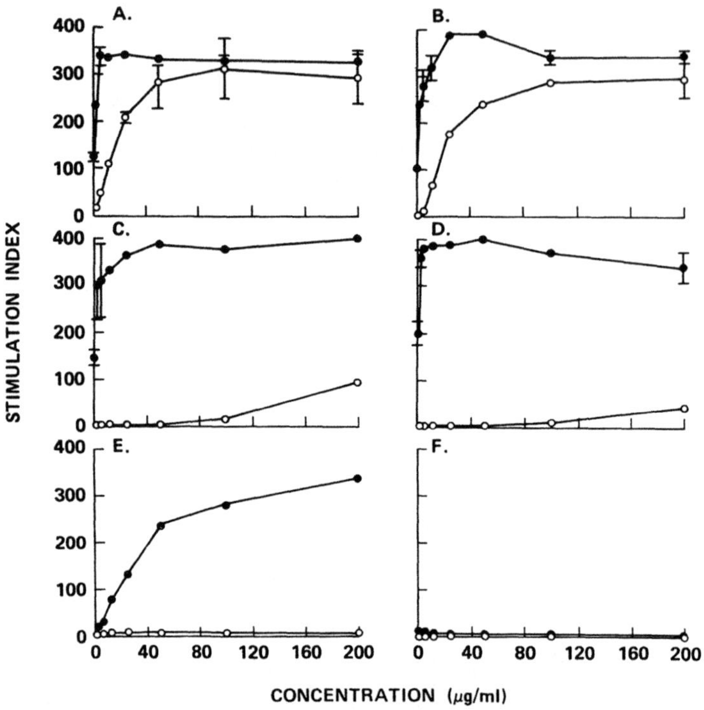

Fig. 8. Representative dose response curves to peptides of the natural sequence (o) or peptides extended by 'non-sense' sequence to a uniform size (•) of a site-specific DBA/2 T cell clone (clone No. E4.15.15). The responses, which were examined over a broad dose range, are shown in the panels as follows: (A) peptides 108-120 and N (108-120), (B) peptides 109-120 and N (109-120), (C) peptides 110-120 and N (110-120), (D) peptides 111-120 and N (111-120), (E) peptides 112-120 and N (112-120), (F) peptides 113-120 and N (113-120). Stimulation index is defined in the legend to Fig. 3. The background response of unstimulated cells was 535 cpm. (From Atassi et al., 1987).

If antigen fragmentation is a prerequisite to its presentation then those peptides containing T sites would be expected to be presented and prime for both an anti-peptide and an anti-protein response. Results obtained (Bixler and Atassi, 1985) with several peptides (Table 3) were consistent with this expectation (in Balb/c, peptides 61-77 and 109-125; in DBA/2, peptides 61-77; 73-89, 109-125 and 133-149; in SJL, peptides 37-53, 109-125, 133-149 and 141-153) and appeared to support the concept of fragmentation prior to antigen presentation. However, the majority of the patterns of recognition observed, were not satisfactorily explained by antigen processing prior to its presentation. Several regions (Table 3), in all three strains, previously shown (Bixler and Atassi, 1983, 1984) to contain T sites in Mb, were found (Bixler and Atassi, 1985) to be ineffective in priming for anti-protein response (in

Balb/c, peptides 49-65 and 133-149; in DBA/2, peptides 13-29, 37-53, 49-65 and 141-153; in SJL, peptides 49-65, 73-89 and 121-137). In addition, several regions (in DBA/2, peptide 49-65; in SJL, peptides 49-65 and 121-137) were not effective in priming for anti-peptide or anti-protein responses despite the fact that the peptides were recognized by Mb primed T cells. If fragmentation is an integral part of presentation, then the T-site containing peptides should be effective in priming T cells that will recognize not only the immunizing peptide but also the intact protein. Clearly, these results (Bixler and Atassi, 1985) do not confirm this expectation. Similar findings were obtained in our recent analysis of the presentation of lysozyme (Bixler et al., 1985; see Chapter in this volume).

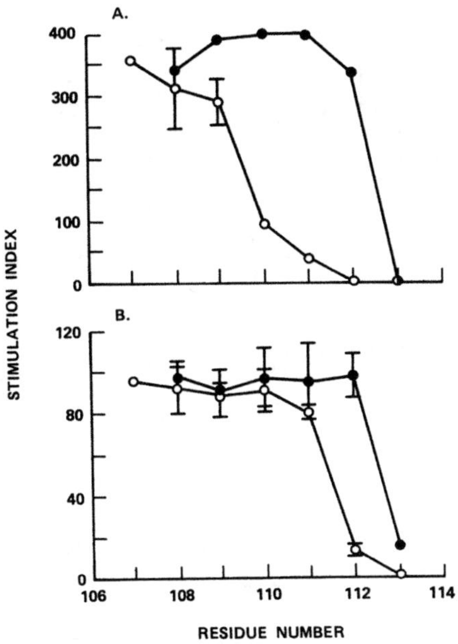

Fig. 9. Summary of proliferative responses of two site-specific DBA/2 T cell clones to in vitro challenge with peptides of the natural sequence (o) or peptides extended by 'non-sense' sequence to a uniform size (•). The maximum proliferative responses obtained are plotted against the corresponding Mb residue added. The clones correspond to (A) T cell clone No. E4.8.19 and (B) T cell clone No. E4.15.15. Stimulation index is defined in legend to Fig. 3. Background responses for the unstimulated cells were 557 and 535 cpm, respectively. (From Atassi et al., 1987).

Conversely, other peptides (Table 3) were very effective in priming for both an anti-peptide and anti-protein response, but these peptides did not contain T sites, i.e. did not stimulate T cells from Mb-primed mice (in Balb/c mice, peptide 37-53; in SJL mice, peptide 61-77). In several cases, peptides elicited a response only to the priming peptide (in Balb/c, peptides 1-17, 13-29, 25-41, 73-89, 85-101 and 133-149; in DBA/2, peptides 1-17, 25-41, 85-101, 97-113 and 121-137; in SJL, peptides 13-29, 25-41, and 97-113).

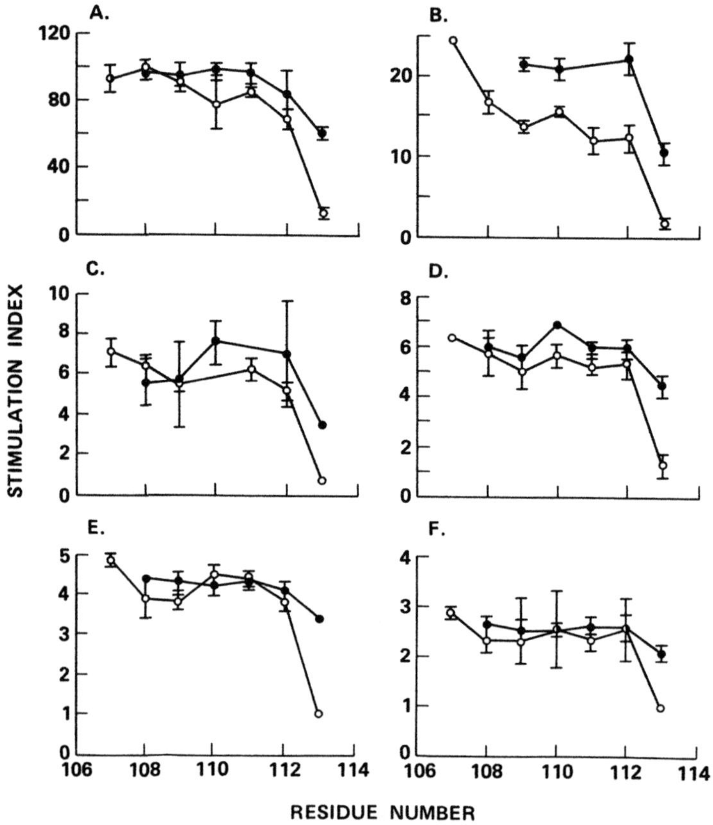

Fig. 10. Summary of proliferative responses of six site-specific SJL T cell clones to in vitro challenge with peptides of the natural sequence (o) or peptides extended by 'non-sense' sequence to a uniform size (•). The maximum proliferative responses obtained are plotted against the corresponding Mb residue added. The clones correspond to: T-cell clone No. L4.5.4 and (B) T-cell clone No. E4.5.1 (C) T cell clone No. VII 2.2 (D) T cell clone No. E4.4.8 (E) T cell clone No. E4.5.6 and (F) T cell clone No. E4.5.10. Stimulation index is defined in the legend to Fig. 3. Background responses for the unstimulated cells were 329, 474, 2392, 2915, 4817 and 5708 cpm, respectively. (From Atassi et al., 1987).

The possibility that these differences may have been caused by regulatory inter-site influences (Atassi et al., 1981, Krco et al., 1981) was examined with a mixture containing equimolar quantities of all the peptides (Bixler and Atassi, 1985). Mixture-primed mice responded (Table 3) to the majority of the peptides with three exceptions (in Balb/c, peptides 1-17 and 49-65; in SJL, peptide 61-77). By screening with the individual peptides, it was found that the T-cell recognition profile obtained after immunization with the protein was different from that obtained after immunization with the peptide mixture. These

Table 3: Summary of the proliferative responses of T cells primed with Mb, individual peptides or mixture primed to in vitro challenge with peptide or native protein.

	BALB/c				DBA/2				SJL			
Priming:	Protein	Peptide		Mixt.	Protein	Peptide		Mixt.	Protein	Peptide		Mixt.
Challenge:	Pept.	Mb	Pept.	Pept.	Pept.	Mb	Pept	Pept.	Pept.	Mb	Pept.	Pept.
Overlapping peptides												
1–17	–	–	++	–	–	–	+++	+++	–	–	–	+
13–29	–	–	++	++	+	–	+++	+++	–	–	++	+++
25–41	–	–	+++	+	–	–	++++	++	–	–	+++	+
37–53	–	+	++++	++	++	–	++	+++	+	+	++	++
49–65	+	–	–	–	++	–	–	+	+	–	–	++
61–77	+	+	+++	++	++	+++	++++	+++	–	++	++	–
73–89	–	–	+++	++	+	+	++++	+++	+	–	+++	++++
85–101	–	–	+++	+++	–	–	++++	++++	+	–	++	+++
97–113	–	–	–	+	–	–	++++	+++	–	–	+	++++
109–125	++	+	++++	++++	+++	++	++++	++++	+++	++++	++++	++++
121–137	–	–	–	+++	–	–	+	+++	+	–	–	++++
133–149	+	–	++++	++++	++	++	++++	++++	+	+++	++++	++++
141–153	–	–	–	+++	+	–	+++	++	+	++	+	++++

Mice were primed with Mb, peptide or an equimolar mixture (Mixt.) of all of the peptides and challenged in vitro with Mb or with each of the synthetic peptides. Assignments of positive and negative responses for the purpose of this table were based on considerations of both stimulation index and net cpm values. Proliferative responses with stimulation indicates less than 2.0 and which correspond to Δ cpm less than 2000 cpm, the response was denoted (–). For the positive responses the symbols are used to denote the following Δ cpm values: (+) 2000–10 000 cpm; (++) 10 000–25 000 cpm; (+++) 25 000–50 000 cpm; (++++) >50 000 cpm. For actual values see Tables 1 and 2 and the previous report [24] on the localization of sites of T cell recognition. Table is from Bixler and Atassi (1985). For details of the data, see that reference.

differences could not be attributed to inter-site regulation because all the regions of the molecule were present in both immunogens, the protein and the peptide mixture.

The finding that the pattern of peptide recognition obtained by *in vivo* priming with native protein was different from that obtained following priming with individual peptides or with a peptide mixture indicated that the regions recognized by priming with peptides, either individually or in mixture, bears little or no relationship to the T sites on the protein. All of the peptides were immunogenic in at least one of the strains examined and several of these peptides induced a response reactive to native protein, but only a few of the active peptides corresponded to the actual T sites of the native protein. Thus, fragmentation as a prerequisite to presentation could not satisfactorily explain why these regions are not recognized by protein primed T cells (Bixler and Atassi, 1985).

The concept of antigen presentation being dependent on processing has evolved from several lines of circumstantial evidence. These include experiments showing that during the lag period paraformaldhyde fixation interferred with presentation (Ziegler and Unanue, 1981; Chestnut et al, 1982). Prefixed antigen presenting cells, however, were able to present protein fragments but not the whole protein (Shimonkewitz et al., 1983; Allen and Unanue, 1984). Lysosomotropic

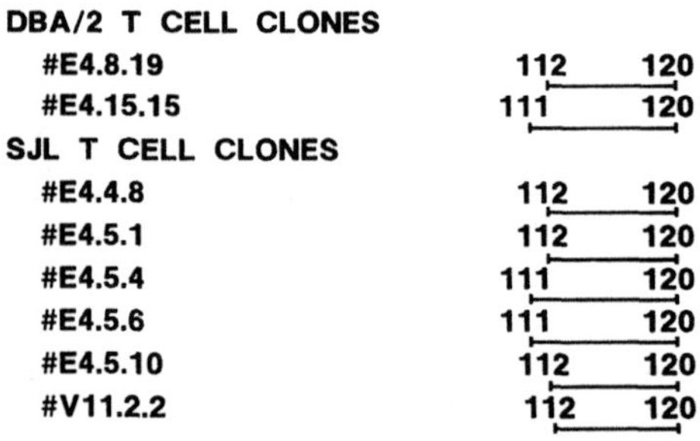

Fig. 11. Boundary shifts of T site recognition by several T-cell clones The site specific T-cell clones were isolated from peptide region 107-120) or myoglobin-driven long-term T-cell cultures of T cells obtained from mice that were immunized with intact Mb. (From Atassi et al., 1987).

agents, which were presumed to alter the pH of lysozomes, or monovalent carboxylic ionophores such as monensin also interferred with antigen presentation (Ziegler and Unanue, 1982; Chestnut et al., 1982; Lee et al., 1984; Allen et al., 1984; Allen and Unanue, 1984). Studies of enzymatic degradation of membrane-bound antigen suggested that the antigen may be sequestered in an enzymatically resistant compartment (Chestnut *et al.*, 1982; Allen et al., 1984). Collectively, these results have been interpreted as demonstrating the internalization, degradation of the antigen in the lysosomes to immunogenic fragments and the subsequent cycling of the processed fragments to the cell membrane for presentation. These approaches have serious shortcomings and the interpretation of the data derived from them is highly equivocal (for recent discussions, see Bixler and Atassi, 1985; Bixler et al., 1985).

The failure of peptide priming to produce a pattern of recognition similar to that observed after protein priming suggests to us that the event of antigen presentation in immune recognition may not be too different in principle from other biological membrane-mediated cellular activities. Such activities are triggered by the binding event to receptor and lead to elaboration by the cell of chemical signals or some other yet unknown mechanisms. Subsequent internalization of receptor-protein complexes would rescue some receptor molecules and these are recycled to the membrane and protein and complexes are degraded. Whether antigen presentation involves the recycling of a membrane receptor as has been demonstrated in several receptor-ligand models (Fan et al;, 1982; Anderson et al., 1977; Tolleshaug and Berg, 1979; Gonzalez-Noriega et al., 1980; Kaplan, 1980; Steer and Ashwell, 1980; Van Leuven et al., 1980; Basu et al., 1981) is not yet determined.

ACKNOWLEDGEMENTS

This work was supported by grant AI-21336 from the National Institutes of Health, U.S. Public Health Service and in part by the Robert A. Welch Foundation from grant Q994 and the award to M.Z. Atassi of the Robert A. Welch Chair of Chemistry.

REFERENCES

Allen, P.M. and Unanue, E.R. (1984) J. Immunol. 132, 1077.

Allen, P.M., Beller, D.I., Braun, J. and Unanue, E.R. (1984) J. Immunol. 132, 323.

Allen, M.E., Abramoff, P., Fink, J.N. and Calvanico, N.J. (1985) Immunol. Invest. 14, 329.

Anderson, R.G.W., Goldstein, J.L. and Brown, M.Z. (1977) Nature, 270, 695.

Atassi, M.Z. (1964) Nature, 202, 496.

Atassi, M.Z. (1975) Immunochemistry 12, 423.

Atassi, M.Z. (1978) Immunochemistry 15, 909.

Atassi, M.Z. (1980) Mol. Cell Biochem. 32, 21.

Atassi, M.Z. (1982) BBA 704, 552.

Atassi, M.Z. (1984) Eur. J. Biochem. 145, 1.

Atassi, M.Z. and Saplin, B.J. (1968) Biochemistry 7, 688.

Atassi, M.Z. and Singhal, R.P. (1970) J. Biol. Chem. 245, 5122.

Atassi, M.Z. and Pai, R.C. (1975) Immunochemistry 12, 735.

Atassi, M.Z. and Smith, J.A. (1978) Immunochemistry 15, 609.

Atassi, M.Z. and Kurisaki, J.I. (1984) Immunol. Commun. 13, 539.

Atassi, and Young, C.R. (1985) Crit. Revs. Immunol. 5, 387.

Atassi, H. and Atassi, M.Z. (1986) Europ. J. Immunol. 16, 229.

Atassi, M.Z. and Kurisaki, J.I. (1986) Proteides Biol. Fluids 34, 165.

Atassi, M.Z. and Bixler, G.S. (1987) in "Antigen Specific T-Cell Receptors and Factors" (Marchalonis, J.J., Ed.), Vol. 1, pp. 7-63, CRC Press, Boca Raton, Fl.

Atassi, M.Z., Sakata, S. and Kazim, A.L. (1979) Biochem. J. 179, 327.

Atassi, M.Z., Yokota, S., Twining, S.S, Lehmann, H. and David, C.S. (1981) Mol. Immunol. 18, 945.

Basu, S.K., Goldstein, J.L., Anderson, R.G.W. and Brown, M.S. (1981) Cell 24, 493.

Benjamin, D.C., Berzofsky, J.A., East, I.J., Gurd, F.R.N., Hannum, C., Leach, S.J., Margoliash, E., Michael, J.G., Mille, A., Prager, E.M., Reichlin, M., Sercarz, E.E., Smith-Gill, S.J., Todd, P.E. and Wilson, A.C. (1984) Ann. Rev. Immunol. 2, 67.

Berkower, I., Buckenmeyer, G.K., Gurd, F.R.N. and Berzofsky, J.A. (1982). Proc. Natl. Acad. Sci. USA 79, 4723.

Berkower, I., Matis, L.A., Buckenmeyer, G.K., Gurd, F.R.N., Longo, D.L. and Berzofsky, J.A. (1984) J. Immunol. 132, 1370.
Bixler, G.S. and Atassi, M.Z. (1983) Immunol. Comm. 12, 593.
Bixler, G.S. and Atassi, M.Z. (1984) J. Immunogenet. 11, 339.
Bixler, G.S. and Atassi, M.Z. (1985) Europ. J. Immunol. 15, 917.
Bixler, G.S., Bean, M. and Atassi, M.Z. (1986) Biochem. J., (in press).
Bixler, G.S., Yoshida, T. and Atassi, M.Z. (1984a) Expl. Clin. Immunogen. 1, 99.
Bixler, G.S., Yoshida, T. and Atassi, M.Z. (1984b) J. Immunogen. 11, 327.
Bixler, G.S., Yoshida, T. and Atassi, M.Z. (1985) Immunology 56, 103.
Cease, K.B., Berkower, I., York-Jolley, J. and Berzofsky, J.A. (1986), 6th International Congress of Immunology Abstract No. 2.71.5.
Chestnut, R.W., Colon, S.M. and Grey, H.M. (1982) J. Immunol. 129, 2382.
David, C.S. and Atassi, M.Z. (1982) in "Immunobiology of Proteins and Peptides (Atassi, M.Z., Ed.), Vol. 2, pp. 97-125, Plenum Press, New York.
Epand, R.M. and Scherga, H.A. (1968) Biochem. 7, 2864.
Fan, J.Y., Carpentier, J.L., Gordon, P., Van Obberghen, E., Blackett, N.M., Grunfeld, C. and Orei, L. (1982) Proc. Natl. Acad. Sci. 79, 7788.
Gonzalez-Noriega, A., Grubb, J.H., Talkad, V. and Sly, W.S., J Cell Biol. 1980, 85, 839.
Kaplan, J. (1980) Cell 19, 197.
Kazim, A.L. and Atassi, M.Z. (1980a) Biochem. J. 191, 261.
Keck, K., (1975) Nature 254, 78.
Koketsu, J. and Atassi, M.Z. (1973) BBA 328, 289.
Koketsu, J. and Atassi, M.Z. (1974) Immunochemistry 11, 1.
Krco, C.J., Kazim, A.L., Atassi, M.Z. and David, C.S. (1981) J. Immunogen. 8, 395.
Kurisaki, J., Atassi, H. and Atassi, M.Z. (1986) Eur. J. Immunol. 16, 236.
Lee, K.-C., Wong, M. and Spitzer, D. (1982) Transportation 34, 150.
Lozner, E.C., Sachs, D.H. and Shearer, G.M. (1974) J. Exp. Med. 139, 1204.
Melchers, I., Rajewsky, K. and Shreffler, D.C. (1973) Eur. J. Immunol. 3, 754.
Moller, G. (Ed.), (1978) Immuno. Rev. 40, 1.
Okuda, K., Christadoss, P.R., Twining, S.S., Atassi, M.Z. and David, C.S. (1978) J. Immunol. 121, 866.
Okuda, K., Twining, S.S., David, C.S. and Atassi, M.Z. (1979) J. Immunol. 123, 182.
Okuda, K., Twining, S.S., David, C.S. and Atassi, M.Z. (1979) J. Immunol. 123, 182-188.
Rosenthal, A.S.N., (1980) Engl. J. Med. 303, 1153.
Schmitz, H.E., Atassi, H. and Atassi, M.Z. (1983) Immunol. Comm. 12, 161.
Shimonkevitz, R., Kappler, J., Marrack, P. and Grey, H.M. (1983) J. Exp. Med. 158, 303.
Simpson, E. (1986) Immunol. Letters 12, 185.
Singhal, R.P. and Atassi, M.Z. (1970) Biochemistry 9, 4252.
Steer, C.J. and Ashwell, G. (1980) J. Biol. Chem. 225, 3008.
Tolleshaug, H. and Berg, T. (1979) Biochem. Pharmacol. 28, 2912.
Twining, S.S. and Atassi, M.Z. (1979) J. Immunol. Methods 30, 139.
Twining, S.S., David, C.S. and Atassi, M.Z. (1981) Mol. Immunol. 18, 7.
Unanue, E.L. and Allen, P.M. (1987) Science 236, 551.
Van Leuven, F., Cassiman, J.-J. and Van den Berghe, H. (1980) Cell 20, 37.
Yoshioka, M., Bixler, G.S. and Atassi, M.Z. (1983) Mol. Immunol. 20, 1133.
Yoshioka, M., Yoshioka, N. and Atassi, M.Z. (1986) Biochem. J. 234, 449.
Young, C.R. and Atassi, M.Z. (1982) Adv. Exp. Med. Biol. 150, 79.

Young, C.R. and Atassi, M.Z. (1983) J. Immunogenet. 10, 139.
Yoshioka, N. and Atassi, M.Z. (1986) Biochem. J. 234, 441.
Yokoi, T., Mulac-Jericevic, B. and Atassi, M.Z. (1987) Adv. Exptl. Med. Biol., in press.
Ziegler, K. and Unanue, E.R. (1981) J. Immunol. 127, 1869.
Ziegler, K. and Unanue, E.R. (1982) Proc. Natl. Acad. Sci. USA 79, 175.

T-CELL RECOGNITION AND ANTIGEN PRESENTATION OF LYSOZYME

Garvin S. Bixler, Jr. and M. Zouhair Atassi

Verna and Marrs McLean Department of Biochemistry
Baylor College of Medicine
Houston, Texas, 77030

ABSTRACT

Several years ago, this laboratory introduced a comprehensive strategy for the systematic localization of all the continuous sites on a protein that are involved in B- and T-cell recognition. The strategy depends on the synthesis of consecutive overlapping peptides that together account for the entire protein chain. Using this approach, the full submolecular profile of continuous regions on hen egg lysozyme recognized by T cells (T sites) were localized. Four major T-cell recognition sites, three of which were subject to individual genetic control, were localized in the six mouse strains examined. In addition to these four continuous T sites, T-cell recognition of lysozyme also involved the three previously defined discontinuous antibody binding sites as demonstrated with lysozyme-specific long-term T cell cultures. Contrary to a long held impression, T-cell recognition, therefore, is not restricted only to sequence features, but can also be directed to protein discontinuous surface areas of high conformational dependency. More recently, we have examined in two mouse strains the proliferative response to peptides and to native protein of lymph node cells from mice primed with synthetic overlapping peptides either individually or as a mixture. It was found that the pattern of T-cell recognition observed after priming with peptides differs from that obtained when the native protein is used as the immunogen. If antigen processing proceeds via fragmentation, then only those regions containing T sites would be expected to be effective in priming for a T-cell response to the intact protein. Since this was not found to be the case, it is unlikely that fragmentation of lysozyme is a prerequisite for antigen presentation. Rather, we suggest that the critical aspects in the presentation of a protein antigen involve predominantly recognition of an intact protein.

INTRODUCTION

In recent years, the full profile of antigenic sites involved in B-cell recognition (antibody binding) of several proteins [myoglobin (Atassi, 1975), lysozyme (Atassi, 1978), serum albumin (Atassi et al., 1979; Sakata and Atassi, 1980; Atassi, 1982), ragweed allergen Ra3 (Atassi and Atassi, 1985, 1986), hemoglobin (Kazim and Atassi, 1980; Yoshioka and Atassi, 1986), acetylcholine receptor α chain (Mulac-Jericevic et al., 1987) and human DR2β chain (Atassi et al., 1987)] have been elucidated. In contrast, only within the last four years has the fine specificity of T-cell recognition of proteins been studied in similar detail with rigorous synthetic peptide strategies. Hen egg lysozyme and myoglobin were the first two proteins for which full profiles of their T-and B-cell recognition became known (Bixler et al., 1984a,b; Bixler and Atassi, 1983, 1984a,b).

The complete antigenic (antibody binding) structure of lysozyme has been determined (Atassi, 1978). Three major sites accounting for over 98% of anti-lysozyme antibodies have been precisely defined and synthetically confirmed by the concept of surface-simulation synthesis (Atassi, et al., 1976; Lee and Atassi, 1976, 1977a,b; Atassi and Lee, 1978a,b). These sites comprise amino acid residues that are spatially adjacent but distant in sequence (termed discontinuous antigenic sites; Atassi and Smith, 1978) and thus are different in architecture from the antigenic sites of myoglobin (Atassi, 1975) which comprise conformationally sensitive continuous portions of the polypeptide chain (termed continuous antigenic sites; Atassi and Smith, 1978).

Several reports have suggested that, in lysozyme, T and B cells recognize different structural features (Thompson et al., 1972; Sugimoto et al., 1975; Scibienski et al., 1978). B cells were thought to recognize the native conformation whereas T cells recognize the unfolded protein. Studies with large lysozyme fragment produced by cyanogen bromide cleavage apparently identified a broad area (encompassing 93 residues) of T-cell recognition (Maizels et al., 1980). The large size of the fragments did not permit resolution of the number and the location of T-cell recognition site(s) within this large area. Recent studies from this laboratory using synthetic uniform overlapping peptides representing the entire lysozyme chain have permitted localization of four continuous regions of T-cell recognition in six high responder mouse strains (Bixler et al., 1984b). Additional studies have demonstrated that T cells also recognize discontinuous features of a molecule (Bixler and Atassi, 1984b).

In presentation, an antigen is recognized in association with Ia molecules on the cell surface (Keck, 1975, Melchers et al., 1973, Lozner et al., 1974; Okuda et al., 1978, 1979b), and each antigenic site of a multi-determinant protein is under separate Ir gene control (Okuda et al., 1979a). It is widely believed that the antigen must be fragmented prior to its presentation to T cells (Ziegler and Unanue, 1981, 1982; Chesnut et al., 1982; Shimonkevitz, 1983; Lee et al., 1982; Allen and Unanue, 1984,; Allen et al., 1984). This "processing" event, however, has not been clearly resolved because of the antigenic complexity of the models used. In contrast, protein antigens whose full profiles of T- and B-cell recognition are known, such as lysozyme (Atassi, 1978, Bixler et al., 1984a,b; Bixler and Atassi, 1984b) offer distinct advantages for the unravelling of antigen processing. From the T-cell proliferative responses obtained after priming with synthetic peptides which encompass the entire protein, we have found (Bixler et al., 1985) that the pattern of recognition observed after peptide-priming differs from that obtained after priming with the native protein. These findings have presented strong evidence against processing of the antigen into fragments as a prerequisite to its presentation.

MATERIALS AND METHODS

Materials

A/J ($H\text{-}2^a$), Balb/c and DBA/2 ($H\text{-}2^d$), B10.BR ($H\text{-}2^k$), DBA/1 ($H\text{-}2^q$) and SJL ($H\text{-}2^s$) mice, 6-10 weeks of age, were purchased from Jackson Laboratories, Bar Harbor, ME. Native hen's egg white lysozyme (three times crystallized) and concanavalin A (Con A) were obtained from Sigma Chemical

Co., St. Louis, MO. Purified protein derivative (PPD) was purchased from Connaught Laboratories Ltd., Swiftwater, PA.

Synthetic Peptide

The primary structure, synthesis, purification and characterization of the overlapping peptides (Figure 1) which encompass the entire poly-peptide chain of lysozyme (Bixler et al., 1984b) and the surface-simulation sites of lysozyme (For review see Atassi, 1978) have been previously described. The structures of the surface-simulation synthetic sites are:

Site 1: ARG-GLY-GLY-ARG-GLY-GLU-GLY-GLY-ARG-LYS
Site 2: PHE-GLY-LYS-LYS-ASN-THR-ASP
Site 3: LYS-ASN-ARG-GLY-PHE-LYS

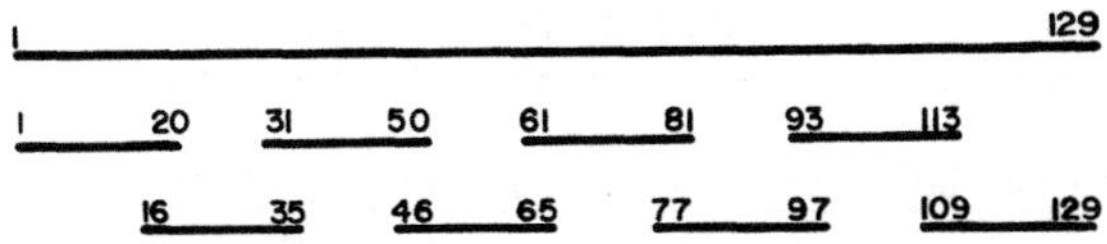

Fig. 1. Schematic diagram illustrating the overlapping peptide strategy used to localize the continuous sites of T-cell recognition in lysozyme. The identity of the overlapping synthetic peptides is indicated by the numbers which refer to the first and last residues in the covalent structure. Figure is from Bixler et al (1984b).

Immunization of Mice

Mice were immunized subcutaneously at the base of the tail with 100 µg of a lysozyme, 25 µg of peptide or 100 µg of an equimolar mixture of the overlapping peptides emulsified in Freund's complete adjuvant containing Mycobacterium tuberculosis, strain H37Ra (Difco, Detroit, MI) as previously described (Bixler and Atassi, 1983). Seven days after immunization, inguinal and periaortic lymph node were removed for proliferative assay or preparation of long-term T-cell cultures.

Preparation of long-term T cell cultures

Long-term cultures of T cells were prepared as previously described (Yoshioka et al., 1983; Bixler, et al., 1984b). The T cells were maintained without exogenous growth factors in 25 cm^2 tissue culture flasks by reculturing, at approximately two week intervals, 6 x 10^5 viable T cells with 40 x 10^6 syngeneic, x-irradiated (3,300 R) normal spleen cells and an optimal concentration of antigen (50 µg/ml).

Proliferative assay

Viable lymph node cells (5 - 7.5 x 10^5 cells/well) in RPMI containing 1% normal mouse serum or T cells (0.5 - 1 x 10^4 cells/well) and syngeneic, X-irradiated spleen cells (0.5 - 1 x 10^6 cells/well) in RPMI containing 10% fetal bovine serum were cocultured in triplicate with various concentrations of antigen, mitogen or peptide. Human adult hemoglobin and several control peptides (from our library of synthetic peptides) that are unrelated to lysozyme were used as negative control antigens. After three days of incubation at 37°C in a humidified 5% CO_2 atmosphere, the lymphocytes were pulsed for 18 hr with 2 µCi/well [^{3}H]-thymidine (Research Products International Corp., Mount Prospect, IL) and then harvested onto glass microtiter filters (Whatman, Clinton, NJ) for counting by liquid scintillation.

RESULTS

Proliferative response to overlapping synthetic peptides

The proliferative response to synthetic peptides of lymph node cells from six lysozyme-responding mouse strains were examined (Table 1). In each strain, cultures were challenged with 50 ug/ml of lysozyme, 1 μg/ml Con A or 100 μg/ml PPD responded. No responses to myoglobin or unrelated peptides were observed. All of the mouse strains examined responded to peptides 16-35 and 46-65. Peptide 93-113 elicited a response in T cell from all the mouse strains, except B10.BR. Positive responses to peptides 31-50 were only observed with lymph node cells from DBA/1 and A/J strains while SJL was the only strain responsive to peptide 109-129. The remaining peptides did not provoke responses in any of the mouse strains examined.

Proliferative response to surface-simulation peptides

The proliferative responses of lysozyme-primed T cells, maintained *in vitro* by several (seven) passages with lysozyme, to the surface-simulation synthetic sites were determined (Table 2). These cells gave substantial responses when challenged with sites 1 or 3. However, the cells were only moderately responsive to site 2. The T cells responded appropriately to lysozyme or Con A, but were unresponsive to PPD, LPS, or unrelated proteins or peptides.

Proliferative response of peptide-primed lymph node cells to synthetic peptides and to native lysozyme

Lymph node cells from DBA/1 and B10.BR mice immunized with the individual peptides were examined for proliferative activity to the immunizing peptide as well as to the intact protein. Representative experiments are shown in Figures 2 and 3. When either of the peptides 16-35 or 31-50 was used as the priming antigen in DBA/1 mice, the cells gave high responses to the priming peptide and intermediate or high responses, respectively, to native lysozyme. Cells from mice primed with peptide 93-113 or 46-65 responded to challenge with their respective peptides but were unresponsive to native lysozyme. The remaining groups of peptide-primed cells responded weakly or not at all to challenge with either peptide or whole protein. Cells from B10.BR mice primed with peptide 109-129 had the highest *in vitro* responses to both peptide and the native protein while cells primed with peptide 93-113 also responded strongly to peptide and mounted an intermediate response to whole protein. In contrast, although intermediate peptide responses were observed in cells primed with peptides 46-65, 77-97 or 16-35, the cells had either weak or no responses to intact protein. Cells from mice that had been primed with peptides 61-81 and 31-50 were also weakly responsive only to the peptide whereas cells primed with peptide 1-20 were unresponsive to challenge with either peptide or whole protein. As a positive control, cells from protein-primed mice were challenged *in vitro* with each of the overlapping peptides, the responses observed agreed with the profile previously reported (Bixler *et al.*, 1984a,b). All of the groups responded to Con A and PPD, but were unresponsive to myoglobin or synthetic myoglobin peptides (unrelated negative controls). Unstimulated cells had a range of background responses from 1,455 to 4,988 cpm.

Table 1. The proliferative response of lysozyme-primed lymph node cells to challenge with synthetic peptides.

	STIMULATION INDEX ± SD*					
Strain:	A/J	Balb/c	DBA/2	B10.BR	DBA/1	SJL
Haplotype:	a	b	d	k	q	s
Antigen						
Peptide+:						
1-19	1.32 ± 0.04	0.74 ± 0.08	0.53 ± 0.19	1.10 ± 0.06	1.10 ± 0.11	0.35 ± 0.10
16-35	4.79 ± 0.09	2.57 ± 0.04	2.08 ± 0.22	3.02 ± 0.07	3.40 ± 0.39	2.19 ± 0.14
31-50	3.05 ± 0.37	1.50 ± 0.06	0.83 ± 0.20	1.88 ± 0.14	5.20 ± 0.87	1.33 ± 0.27
46-65	8.55 ± 1.83	2.35 ± 0.12	2.30 ± 0.03	5.69 ± 0.23	2.95 ± 0.40	3.24 ± 0.72
61-81	0.99 ± 0.07	1.28 ± 0.01	1.03 ± 0.08	1.10 ± 0.05	1.10 ± 0.19	1.13 ± 0.30
77-97	1.77 ± 0.42	1.88 ± 0.29	1.56 ± 0.03	1.07 ± 0.08	1.18 ± 0.02	1.77 ± 0.53
93-113	2.11 ± 0.03	4.23 ± 0.14	2.85 ± 0.25	1.24 ± 0.08	9.09 ± 0.70	3.04 ± 0.14
109-129	1.80 ± 0.40	1.20 ± 0.11	0.90 ± 0.03	1.28 ± 0.16	1.14 ± 0.13	2.63 ± 0.64
Controls‡:						
Lysozyme	6.03 ± 0.55	18.60 ± 1.67	20.68 ± 0.41	10.14 ± 2.69	38.68 ± 4.92	11.47 ± 1.21
Con A	7.74 ± 0.70	15.01 ± 0.8	9.91 ± 0.61	28.26 ± 2.02	19.04 ± 0.58	22.78 ± 0.35
PPD	14.86 ± 1.15	40.78 ± 0.99	25.27 ± 0.88	12.31 ± 0.54	11.13 ± 0.18	19.93 ± 0.92
Unrelated Peptides	0.96 ± 0.08	1.00 ± 0.06	1.00 ± 0.04	1.29 ± 0.21	1.01 ± 0.01	1.00 ± 0.13

* Stimulation index is the ratio of label incorporated in stimulated cells/label incorporated in unstimulated cells. The amounts of label incorporated by unstimulated cells were: A/J, 9,029 cpm; Balb/c, 2,869 cpm; DBA/2, 6,220 cpm; B10.BR, 3,032 cpm; DBA/1, 3,122 cpm; SJL, 3,127 cpm.

+ The response at an optimum peptide concentration of 50 or 80 µg/ml is shown although a dose range of 12.5-100 µg/ml was examined.

‡ Lysozyme, Con A and PPD were used at doses of 50, 1 and 100 µg/ml, respectively. Several unrelated synthetic peptides were used as negative controls at a dose of 50 µg/ml.

Table is from Bixler et al., (1984b).

Table 2. Proliferative response to the surface-simulation synthetic sites of B10.BR T cells from lysozyme-driven long-term cultures*.

Challenge antigen	Opt. dose (μg/ml)	[^{3}H]-Thymidine incorporation (Δ CPM)
Site 1	6.25	10,821
Site 2	6.25	4,778
Site 3	1.56	8,564
Lysozyme	25	42,883
Con A		38,762
PPD		0
LPS		0
Myoglobin		0

* The T cells were harvested after seven in vitro passages with lysozyme. The Δ CPM is relative to the mean of the cell responses to unrelated proteins or peptides (3,048 ± 651 cpm). The cells were challenged with peptides or lysozyme in the dose range 50-0.78 μg/ml and the maximum response at the indicated optimum dose is given for each antigen. Note that the surface-simulation synthetic peptides are the sites to which the antibody response against native lysozyme is directed. Table is from Bixler and Atassi (1984b).

Table 3. Summary of the proliferative response of DBA/1 and B10.BR lymph node cells to peptides or whole protein*

Antigen:	DBA/1				B10.BR			
	Priming Peptide		Prot.	Mixt.	Peptide		Prot.	Mixt.
Challenge:	Pept.	Prot.	Pept.	Pept.	Pept.	Prot.	Pept.	Pept.
Peptide:								
1-20	-	-	-	-	-	-	-	-
16-35	+ + + +	+ +	+	+ + + +	+ + +	-	+	+ +
31-50	+ + + +	+ + + +	+ +	+ + +	+	-	-	-
46-65	+ +	-	+	+	+ + +	-	+ +	+ + +
61-81	-	-	-	-	+	-	-	-
77-97	-	-	-	+	+ + +	-	-	+
93-113	+ +	-	+ + +	+	+ + +	+ +	-	+
109-129	-	-	-	-	+ + + +	+ +	-	-

*The assignment of positive and negative responses for the purpose of this table was based on considerations of both stimulation index and net c.p.m. values. When the response was less than twice that of the background, and when the c.p.m. was less than 3000, the response was denoted (-). For the positive responses, the symbols are used to denote the following net c.p.m. values: (+) 3000-10,000 c.p.m.; (+ +) 10,000-25,000 c.p.m.; (+++) 25,000-50,000 c.p.m.; (++++) >50,000 c.p.m. For actual values, see Bixler et al (1985) and the previous reports on the localization of sites of T-cell recognition (Bixler et al., 1984a.b). Table is from Bixler et al., (1985).

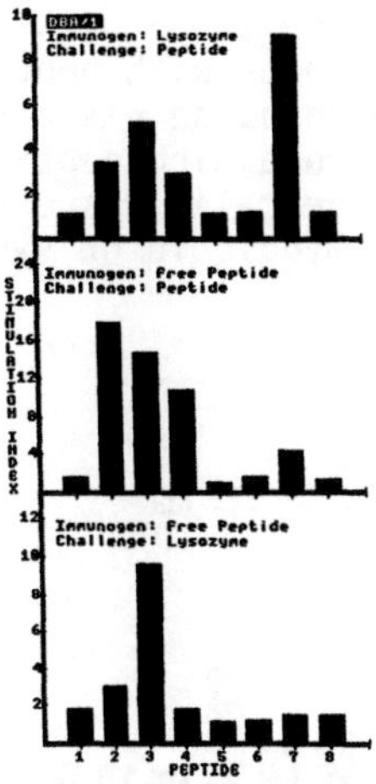

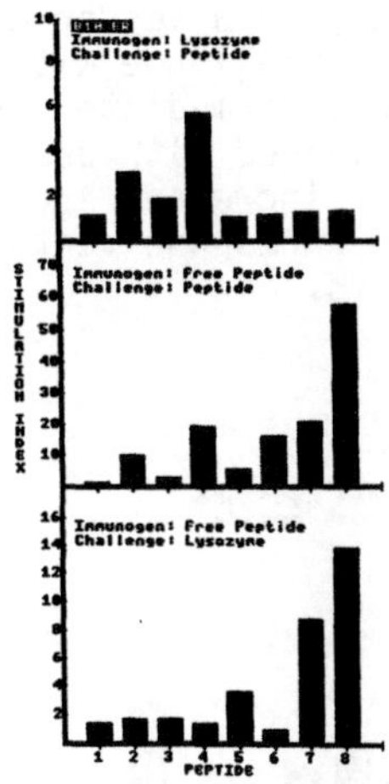

Fig. 2. (Left) The proliferative response of peptide-primed DBA/1 lymph node cells to in vitro challenge with peptide (center panel) or with the intact lysozyme molecule (bottom panel). For comparison, the proliferative response of protein primed lymph node cells which were challenged in vitro with peptides are also shown (top panel). Peptide numbers refer to: (1) peptide 1-20, (2) peptide 16-35, (3) peptide 31-50, (4) peptide 46-65, (5) peptide 61-81, (6) peptide 77-97, (7) peptide 93-113, (8) peptide 109-129. Figure is plotted from data reported by Bixler et al. (1985).

Fig. 3. (Right) The proliferative response of peptide-primed B10.BR lymph node cells to in vitro challenge with peptide (center panel) or the intact lysozyme molecule (bottom panel). For comparison, the proliferative response of protein primed lymph node cells which were challenged in vitro with peptides are also shown (top panel). Peptide numbers refer to the regions given in Figure 2. Figure is plotted from data reported by Bixler et al. (1985).

Proliferative response of lymph node cells primed with a mixture of the overlapping peptides

It is now known (Atassi et al., 1981; Krco et al., 1981) that recognition of various regions on a multi-determinant complex antigen is subject to inter-site regulatory effects. Therefore, it was necessary to rule-out the possibility that differences in the patterns of peptide recognition between protein-primed and peptide-primed mice could be due to some inter-site regulatory effects among various regions of the whole protein which would not play a role when each peptide individually is used for priming. A peptide mixture consisting of equimolar quantities of all of the peptides was used to prime both DBA/1 and B10.BR mice. Representative experiments showing the proliferative responses of these mice to challenge with individual peptides, a peptide mixture, or native protein are presented in Figure 4.

Lymph node cells from DBA/1 mice responded strongly to peptides 16-35 and 31-50 as well as to the peptide mixture. The response to the whole protein was intermediate. Several peptides, 46-65, 77-97, and 93-113, evoked only low proliferative responses. No response was obtained on challenge with the remaining peptides. Unrelated molecules evoked no response. The cells also responded appropriately to both Con A and PPD.

In lymph node cells from peptide mixture-primed B10.BR mice (Figure 5), the strongest responses to in vitro peptide challenge were obtained with peptide 46-65 and, to a lesser extent, with peptide 16-35 or with the peptide mixture. Challenge with the whole protein or with peptide 93-113 generated low-to-intermediate responses. A low response was also observed in cultures challenged with peptide 77-97. The remaining peptides elicited very little or no increases in proliferation. The cells responded to Con A and PPD but were unresponsive to challenge with myoglobin or synthetic myoglobin peptides.

4
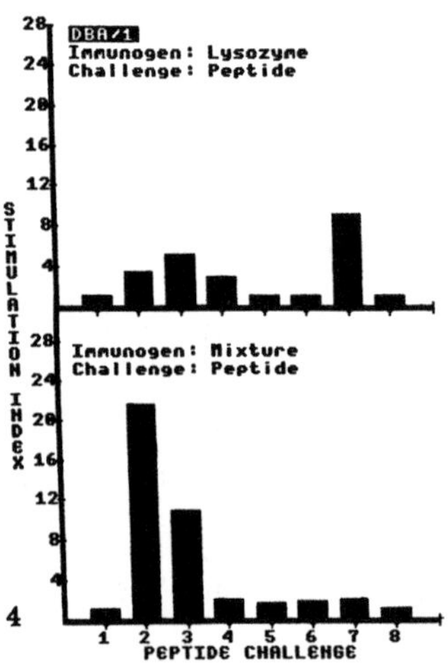

5
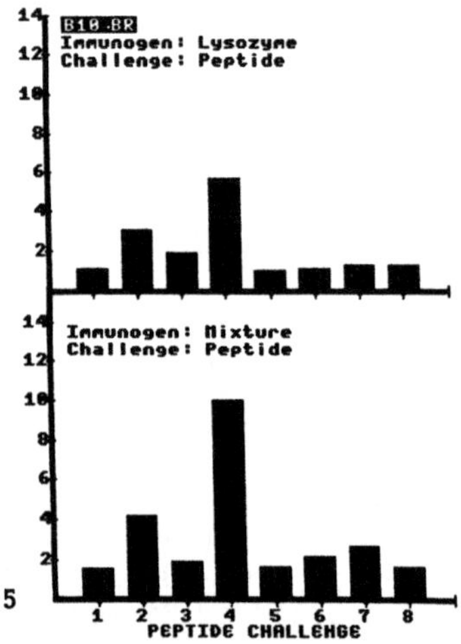

Fig. 4. (Left) The proliferative response of peptide mixture-primed DBA/1 lymph node cells (lower panel) and, for comparison, the proliferative response of protein primed lymph node cells (upper panel) to challenge *in vitro* with peptides. Peptide numbers are defined in Figure 2. This figure is plotted from data reported by Bixler *et al* (1985).

Fig. 5. (Right) The proliferative response of peptide mixture-primed B10.BR lymph node cells (lower panel) and, for comparison, the proliferative response of protein primed lymph node cells (upper panel) to challenge *in vitro* with peptides. Peptide numbers are defined in Figure 2. This figure is plotted from data required by Bixler *et al* (1985).

DISCUSSION

In order to localize the continuous regions of T cell recognition a comprehensive synthetic strategy introduced earlier by this laboratory (Kazim and Atassi, 1980) was adopted. This strategy consists of systematically synthesizing a series of consecutive overlapping peptides of uniform size which together account for the entire protein chain (Kazim and Atassi, 1980). The advantages of this approach have been discussed in detail (Kazim and Atassi, 1980, 1982). We have determined that a 5-residue overlap at each end of the consecutive peptides is optimal for avoiding scission of antigenic sites and in terms of synthetic load. In recent studies (Young and Atassi, 1982, 1983) on the effect of peptide size on T cell proliferation to a myoglobin antigenic site, it was found that peptides greater than 14 residues gave an optimal response. Accordingly, we decided to employ 20 or 21-residue peptides.

Examination of the proliferative responses of lymph node cells to the peptides enabled the localization of 'continuous' regions of T-cell recognition (Figure 6) on the polypeptide chain (Bixler et al., 1984a,b). Taking into account the absence of reactivity of adjacent overlapping peptides and applying rationale previously discussed (Kazim and Atassi, 1982), it was possible to conclude that lysozyme has four continuous T sites residing within the regions shown in Figure 6. In SJL mice, a shift in the boundaries of T site 4 was exhibited which is reminiscent of that previously found for protein sites recognized by antibodies (Koketsu and Atassi, 1973, 1974; Atassi, 1975; Kazim and Atassi, 1982). A similar shift in the recognition of T site 1 in SJL and B10. BR mice was also observed. The H-2^d, H-2^k and H-2^s haplotypes did not recognize site 2 because of Ir gene control. It should be noted that these localized regions (For summary, see Figure 6) were made intentionally larger than the expected size of T sites (Young and Atassi, 1982) to avoid errors in assignments at this stage. Accurate narrowing down of the boundaries of these regions will require synthesis of apprporiate overlapping peptides around these indicated sites (Atassi, 1975; Bixler et al., 1986).

As seen here, it is not unexpected that individual antigenic sites of proteins are each under separate control since it was previously shown that the T-lymphocyte and antibody responses to the five synthetic antigenic sites of myoglobin are each under separate genetic control (Okuda et al., 1979a; Twining et al, 1981). Furthermore, the immune responses to the individual antigenic sites of a multideterminant protein antigen are complicated by the regulatory effects of intersite influences which can be of either help or suppression in nature (Atassi et al., 1981; Krco et al., 1981). In fact a region in lysozyme has been postulated, from comparison of T-cell response to lysozyme from various species, to induce suppressor T cells (Semma et al., 1981). However, this still lacks confirmation by independent studies with synthetic peptides.

Several years ago, the antigenic (antibody binding) sites of lysozyme were localized, defined and confirmed by 'surface-simulation' synthesis (Atassi et al., 1976; Lee and Atassi, 1976; Atassi, 1978). The sites were found to consist of surface residues from distant portions of the sequence which were brought into close spatial proximity by the folding of the polypeptide chain (Atassi, 1978). The three discontinuous lysozyme sites account for greater than 98 of anti-lysozyme antibodies raised in several host species (Atassi, 1978, 1979). Their participation in T-cell recognition, however, required investigation.

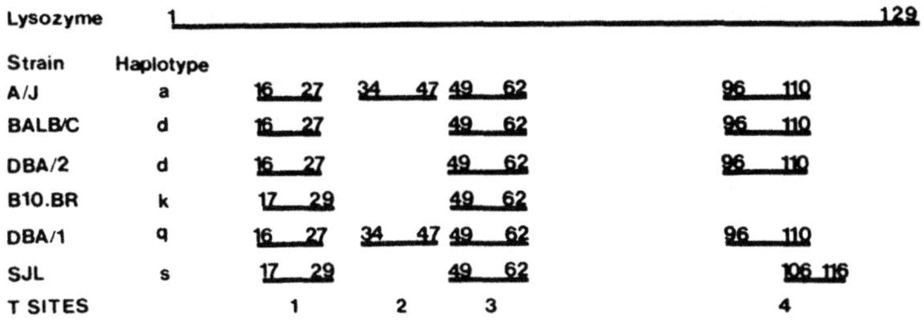

Fig. 6. Schematic diagram summarizing the sites localized within the polypeptide chain of lysozyme in several mouse strains. Note that each T site falls within but may not necessarily include all of the regions indicated. Only those regions which generated a proliferative response exceeding a stimulation index of 2.0 are shown here. In addition to these continuous sites to which no antibody responses are detected, lysozyme-specific T-cell long-term cultures have been shown to respond to the three discontinuous surface- simulation synthetic sites that are the target of antibody (B-cell) recognition. Figures is from Bixler et al (1984b).

In our studies of the T-cell recognition sites of myoglobin, it was found that the sites recognized by antibody (i.e. B cells) are also recognized by T cells (Okuda et al., 1979a; Bixler and Atassi, 1983; Yoshioka et al., 1983; Young and Atassi, 1982, 1983). Initial attempts to detect T-cell proliferative activity to the surface-simulation peptides in lysozyme-primed lymph node cells gave erratic but yet tantalizing results. In order to increase the probability of detecting T-cell proliferative activity to the surface-simulation sites, T-cell long-term cultures derived from lysozyme primed mice were examined for T-cell responses to the surface-simulation synthetic sites. It was fascinating, yet somewhat unexpected by present dogma, that each of the three surface-simulation synthetic sites provoked a response, with site 1 being the most immunogenic in this mouse strain.

The demonstration of T cell responses to discontinuous (surface-simulation) sites is very significant. From studies with native lysozyme and its S-carboxymethyl derivatives it was suggested (Thompson et al., 1972; Sugimoto et al., 1975) that the structures recognized by T and B cells were different since the native protein and its unfolded derivative cross-reacted at the T-cell level but not at the antibody (B-cell) level. Subsequent studies with cyanogen bromide cleavage fragments gave a fragment that was recognized by T cells but not by antibodies (Maizels et al., 1980), further supporting this view. However, our results clearly show that T cells are not restricted to recognition of continuous features of the protein but that they do recognize discontinuous sites (Bixler and Atassi, 1984b) whose existence is entirely dependent on the integrity of the native three-dimensional structure (Atassi, 1978). In light of this data, the previously perceived dichotomy thought to exist (Maizels et al., 1980) between T-and B-cell reactivities, i.e. that T and B cells recognize fundamentally different structural features, has been resolved. Similar findings have been demonstrated with sperm whale myoglobin where the sites recognized by antibody (B cells) (Atassi, 1975) are also recognized by T cells (Okuda et al., 1979a; Bixler and Atassi, 1983, 1984a; Yoshioka et al., 1983), but there are also regions recognized by T cells for which no detectable antibody response can be found (Bixler and Atassi, 1983, 1984a).

The finding that T cells recognize the surface-simulation synthetic peptides (Bixler and Atassi, 1984b) which mimic the discontinuous sites that bind to antibody (Atassi, 1978) is of basic consequence to our understanding of antigen presentation. The integrity of discontinuous sites is entirely dependent on the retention of the three-dimensional structure of the protein and would be destroyed by its fragmentation (Atassi, 1978) during processing. Clearly, the synthetic peptides which simulate surface regions of lysozyme and which, after all, do not exist in the protein, could not be generated by a fragmentation process. Consistent with this conclusion, is the finding that populations of T-cell clones following priming with native cytochrome c were reported to be different from those obtained after priming with the denatured protein (Buchmuller and Corradin, 1982). The dependence of immune recognition on the conformation of the protein is not easily explained by the current dogma of antigen presentation as being that of 'processed' fragments.

From more recent studies using individual peptides for priming, it was found (Bixler et al., 1985) that some peptides, which carry T sites, prime T cells to respond to the respective peptide as well as to the protein (e.g. peptides 16-35 and 31-50 in DBA/1). However, it should be noted that the levels of in vitro responses to these peptides were much higher after peptide priming than after protein priming (for summary, see Table 3). Also, some peptides that are not associated with T sites, (i.e. were not recognized after protein priming), did not prime for either anti-peptide or anti-protein in vitro responses (in DBA/1, peptides 1-20, 61-81, 77-97 and 109-129; in B10.BR, peptide 1-20). If, as indicated by current dogma, antigen presentation proceeds via antigen fragmentation, then it would be expected that those peptides that are associated with protein T sites should prime for in vitro responses to both the priming peptide and the protein. Conversely, regions that are not associated with T sites on the protein should not prime for an in vitro response to the priming peptide or to the protein. Thus, the results discussed in this paragraph, are consistent with the idea (at least qualitatively) that peptide fragments are the species presented after priming with native protein.

The fragmentation of antigen prior to its presentation, however, is not supported by the rest of the results. Several regions that coincide with protein T sites were effective in priming for an in vitro anti-peptide response, but these cells did not respond to native protein (in DBA/1, peptides 46-65 and 93-113; in B10.BR, peptides 16-35 and 46-65). Some peptides which are not associated with protein T sites primed T cells for in vitro response only to the immunizing peptide but not to the protein (in B10.BR, peptides 31-50, 61-81 and 77-97). Further, some peptides, though not associated with the protein T sites, primed T cells for in vitro response to the immunizing peptide and to the protein (e.g. in B10.BR, peptides 93-113 and 109-129). These findings do not support, and indeed pose serious problems for the current dogma.

Inter-site regulatory influences have been shown (Atassi et al., 1981; Krco et al., 1981) to play an important role in the immune response to a protein antigen. Therefore, we examined the possibility that the above differences may be due to absence of these regulatory influences when individual peptides are used as the priming antigens (Bixler et al., 1985). A mixture containing equimolar quantities of all the overlapping peptides was employed for priming at the same dose that was used in priming with lysozyme. Indeed, differences were found in the pattern of recognition of various peptides after priming with individual peptides as compared to that obtained after priming with the mixture (Bixler et al., 1985). These differences may well reflect inter-site regulatory effects operating in the case of priming with the peptide mixture. However, this point needs more study. At any rate, priming with peptide mixture generated T cells that responded in vitro to peptides which carry protein T sites (in DBA/1, peptides 16-35, 31-50, 46-65 and 93-113; in B10.BR, peptides 16-35 and 46-65). There were, however, large quantitative differences in the levels of the in vitro responses to the peptides that are recognized both after mixture priming or after protein priming (for summary, see Table 3). In addition, it should be noted that some peptides were recognized in vitro after in vivo priming with the peptide mixture but not after protein priming (peptides 93-113 in B10.BR and 77-97 in both DBA/1 and B10.BR). Since all the regions present in the peptide mixture are presumably present in the native protein (if it were processed), then the differences in patterns of recognition cannot entirely be attributed to the absence of inter-site regulatory effects.

In conclusion, the T-cell recognition and antigen presentation of lysozyme have been investigated. Using synthetic overlapping peptides encompassing the entire lysozyme chain to challenge lysozyme-primed lymph node cells, four continuous regions of T-cell recognition have been identified. These regions were mapped to small, discrete regions of the protein. Significantly, in addition to these regions, the surface-simulation peptides, representing the discontinuous antigenic (antibody-binding) sites which are known to bind greater than 98% of anti-lysozyme antibodies, also stimulated T cells obtained from long term lysozyme specific T-cell lines. Clearly, therefore, T and B cells can recognize the same regions of a protein. With the advantage of knowing the full profile of the T-cell recognition regions, a comparison of the patterns of recognition following protein priming as opposed to peptide priming was undertaken. Significant differences in the patterns were revealed. As seen here, the T-cell response to a free peptide often has little or no relationship to the recognition by T cells of the same region on the protein. Thus, although protein fragments can be presented and induce an immune response and can be sequestered in the interior of the cell, their significance to immune recognition of the native protein cannot be assessed unless the full profiles of T- and B-cell recognition of the protein are known. These findings afford strong evidence against a mechanism of antigen presentation which is dependent on the generation of peptide fragments with the latter being the 'presented' species. Rather, the protein molecule must be presented in its intact form.

ACKNOWLEDGEMENTS

This work was supported by the Welch Foundation due to grant Q-994 and by the award to MZA of the Robert A. Welch Chair of Chemistry.

REFERENCES

Allen, P.M. and Unanue, E.R. (1984) J. Immunol. 132, 1077-1079.
Allen, P.M., Strydom, D.J. and Unanue, E.R. (1984a) Proc. Natl. Acad. Sci. USA 81, 2489-2493.
Allen, P.M., Beller, D.I., Braun, J. and Unanue, E.R. (1984b) J. Immunol. 132, 323-331.
Atassi, M.Z. (1975) Immunochemistry 12, 423-438.
Atassi, M.Z. (1978) Immunochemistry 15, 909-936.
Atassi, M.Z. (1979) CRC Reviews in Biochemistry 6, 371-400.
Atassi, M.Z. (1982) Biochim. Biophys. Acta 704, 552-555.
Atassi, M.Z. and Lee, C.-L. (1978a) Biochem. J. 171, 419-427.
Atassi, M.Z. and Lee, C.-L. (1978b) Biochem. J. 171, 429-434.
Atassi, M.Z. and Smith, J.A. (1978) Immunochemistry 15, 609-610.
Atassi, M.Z., Lee, C.-L. and Pai, R.-C. (1976) Biochem. Biophys. Acta 427, 745-751.
Atassi, M.Z., Sakata, S. and Kazim, A.L. (1979) Biochem. J. 179, 327-331.
Atassi, M.Z., Yokota, S., Twining, S.S., Lehmann, H. and David, C.S. (1981) Mol. Immunol. 18, 945-948.
Atassi, H., Ulrich, R.G. and Atassi, M.Z. (1987) Europ. J. Immunol., in press.
Bixler, G.S. and Atassi, M.Z. (1983) Immunol. Comm. 12, 593-603.
Bixler, G.S. and Atassi, M.Z. (1984a) J. Immunogen. 11, 339-353).
Bixler, G.S. and Atassi, M.Z. (1984b) J. Immunogen. 11, 245-250.
Bixler, G.S., Yoshida, T. and Atassi, M.Z. (1984a) Expl. Clin. Immunogen. 1, 99-111.
Bixler, G.S., Yoshida, T. and Atassi, M.Z. (1984b) J. Immunogen. 11, 327-337.
Bixler, G.S., Yoshida, T. and Atassi, M.Z. (1985) Immunology 56, 103-112.
Bixler, G.S. Bean, M. and Atassi, M.Z. (1986) Biochem. J. 240, 139-146.
Buchmuller, and Corradin, G. (1982) Eur. J. Immunol. 12, 412-416.
Chesnut, R.W., Colon, S.M. and Grey, H.M. (1982) 129, 2382-2388.
Kazim, A.L. and Atassi, M.Z. (1980) 191, 261-264.
Kazim, A.L. and Atassi, M.Z. (1982) Biochem. J. 203, 201-208.
Keck, K. (1975) Nature 254, 78.
Koketsu, J. and Atassi, M.Z. (1973) Biochim. Biophys. Acta 328, 289-302.
Koketsu, J. and Atassi, M.Z. (1974) Immunochemistry 11, 1-8.
Krco, C.J., Kazim, A.L., Atassi, M.Z. and David, C.S. (1981) J. Immunogenet. 8, 315-322.
Lee, C.-L. and Atassi, M.Z. (1976) Biochem. J. 159, 89-93.
Lee, C.-L. and Atassi, M.Z. (1977a) Biochim. Biophys. Acta 495, 354-368.
Lee, C.-L. and Atassi, M.Z. (1977b) Biochem. J. 167, 571-582.
Lee, K.-C., Wong, M. and Spitzer, D. (1982) Transplantation 34, 150-152.

Lozner, E.C., Sachs, D.H. and Shearer, G.M. (1974) J. Exp. Med. 139. 1204.
Maizels, R.M., Clarke, J.A., Harvey, M.A., Miller, A. and Sercarz, E.E. (1980) Eur. J. Immunol. 10, 509-515.
Melchers, I., Rajewsry, K. and Shreffler, D.C. (1973) Eur. J. Immunol. 3, 754.
Mulac-Jericevic, B., Kurisaki, J. and Atassi, M.Z. (1987) Proc. Nat. Acad. Sci. USA, in press.
Okuda, K., Christadoss, P.R., Twining, S., Atassi, M.Z. and David, C.S. 1978) J. Immunol. 121, 866-868.
Okuda, K., Twining, S.S., David, C.S. and Atassi, M.Z. (1979a) J. Immunol. 123, 182-188.
Okuda, K., Sakata, S., Atassi, M.Z. and David, C.S. (1979b) J. Immunogen. 6, 447-452.
Sakata, S. and Atassi, M.Z. (1980) Mol. Immunol. 17, 139-142.
Scibienski, R.J., Klingmann, V., Leung, C., Thompson, K. and Benjamini, E. (1978) (Atassi, M.Z. and Stavitsky, A.B., Eds.), Vol. 1, pp. 305-317. Plenum Press, New York.
Semma, M., Sakata, N., Fujio, H. and Amano, T. (1981) Immunol. Letters 3, 57-61.
Shimonkevitz, R., Kappler, J., Marrack, P. and Grey, H. (1983) J. Exp. Med. 158, 303-316.
Sugimoto, M., Kohima, A., Yaginuma, K. and Egashira, Y. (1975) Japan J. Med. Sci. Biol. 28, 23-25.
Thompson, K., Harris, M., Benjamini, E., Mitchell, G. and Noble, M. (1972) Nature N.B. 238, 20-21.
Twining, S.S., David, C.S. and Atassi, M.Z. (1981) Mol. Immunol. 18, 447-450.
Yoshioka, M., Bixler, G.S. and Atassi, M.Z. (1983) Mol. Immunol. 20, 1133-1137.
Yoshioka, N. and Atassi, M.Z. (1986) Biochem. J. 234, 441-447.
Young, C.R. and Atassi, M.Z. (1982) Adv. Exp. Med. 150, 79-93.
Young, C.R. and Atassi, M.Z. (1983) J. Immunogen. 10, 151-160.
Ziegler, K. and Unanue, E.R. (1981) J. Immunol. 127, 1869-1875.
Ziegler, K. and Unanue, E.R. (1982) Proc. Natl. Acad. Sci. USA 79, 175-178.

THE REGIONS OF T-CELL RECOGNITION ON THE EXTRACELLULAR PART OF THE α CHAIN OF *TORPEDO CALIFORNICA* ACETYLCHOLINE RECEPTOR

Tsuyoshi Yokoi, Biserka Mulac-Jericevic and M. Zouhair Atassi[+]

Marrs McLean Department of Biochemistry
Baylor College of Medicine
Houston, Texas, 77030, U.S.A.

ABSTRACT

A comprehensive synthetic approach was employed to identify the continuous regions of T-cell recognition on the α-chain of *Torpedo californica* acetylcholine receptor (AChR). Eighteen synthetic consecutive overlapping peptides, of uniform size and overlaps, that spanned the entire extracellular part (residues 1-210) of the α chain were examined for their *in vitro* stimulation of lymph node cells from AChR-primed C57BL/6 (H-2^b), C3H/He (H-2^k), SWR(H-2^q) and SJL (H-2^s) mice. The T-cell recognition sites (T sites) in the AChR-primed mouse strains resided within six regions on the extracellular part of the α-chain. Three of the regions recognized by T cells coincided with regions recognized by antibodies (i.e. B cells) and one of these three regions also coincided with an α-neurotoxin binding region. It is noteworthy that, in addition to sites recognized by both T and B cells, the protein has at least two sites which are recognized exclusively by T cells and to which no detectable antibody responses are directed.

INTRODUCTION

The nicotinic acetylcholine receptor (AChR) plays a central role in postsynaptic neuromuscular transmission by mediating ion flux across the cell membrane in response to binding of acetylcholine (McCarthy et al., 1986; Changeux et al., 1984). This regulatory activity is inhibited by binding to an α-neurotoxin (Lee, 1979) or by some anti-receptor antibodies. The receptor is a pentamer composed of four subunits ($\alpha_2\beta\gamma\delta$). The primary structures of all four AChR subunits of *Torpedo californica* have been deduced from the respective cDNA sequence (Noda et al., 1982, 1983a,b). Functional studies have focussed mostly on the α subunit because it has been shown to be responsible for binding acetylcholine (Sobel et al., 1977; Moore and Raftery, 1979, Tzartos and Changeux, 1983) and α-neurotoxins (Lee, 1979). From the primary structure of each subunit, it was possbile to identify transmembrane hydrophobic regions and the extracellular part of the chain (Noda et al., 1983b; Claudio et al., 1983; Devillers-Thiery et a;., 1983).

Previous immunological studies on acetylcholine receptor (AChR) have focussed, almost exclusively, on the antibody response to the molecule, probably because of the association of the autoantibody response with the neurological disease, myasthenia gravis (Appel et al., 1975). However, autoimmune recognition of a protein has been shown (Yokota et al., 1980) to involve autoimmune T-cell responses. Recently, the role of the T cells in autoimmune myasthenia gravis was demonstrated (Lennon et al., 1985; Lisak et al., 1986; Sinigaglia et al., 1984). Similar emphasis has also been shown in studies of other proteins. In fact, it was only very recently, that the complete T-cell recognition profiles of proteins were determined [sperm whale myoglobin (Bixler and Atassi, 1983, 1984a), hen lysozyme (Bixler and Atassi, 1984b; Bixler et al., 1984a, 1984b), the β chain of human hemoglobin A (Yoshioka et al., 1986) and ragweed allergen Ra3 (Kurisaki et al., 1986)]. These profiles were mapped by application of a comprehensive synthetic peptide strategy (Kazim and Atassi, 1980). In the case of lysozyme, the surface-simulation synthetic sites (Atassi, 1978) were also recognized by T-cells (Bixler and Atassi, 1984b).

Recently we derived (Mulac-Jericevic et al., 1987), by a set of consecutive overlapping synthetic peptides which spanned the entire extracellular part (residues 1-210) of the α chain of AChR, the full profile of the continuous antigenic regions recognized by anti-AChR antibodies. These synthetic overlapping peptides were then employed (Yokoi et al., 1987) to localize the T-cell recognition profile of this part of the α chain in mouse strains that had been immunized (primed) with native AChR.

MATERIALS AND METHODS

Preparation of receptor and synthetic peptides

The AChR was prepared from the electric organ of *Torpedo californica* as described elsewhere (Mulac-Jericevic et al., 1987). The primary structures, of the eighteen overlapping peptides encompassing the entire extracelluar part (residues 1-210) of the α chain of AChR (Mulac-Jericevic and Atassi, 1987) are shown in Figure 1.

Immunization of mice

C57BL/6(H-2^b), C3H/He (H-2^k), SWR (H-2^q), RIIIS (H-2^r) and SJL (H-2^s) mice between 6 and 10 weeks of age were obtained from Jackson Laboratories (Bar Harbor, ME). To determine the optimum priming dose for each mouse strain, the mice were immunized subcutaneously at the base of the tail with varying doses of AChR in the range 5-50 μg per mouse. The antigen, in PBS (50 μl), was emulsified with Freund's complete adjuvant (50 μl) containing *Mycobacterium tuberculosis*, strain H37Ra (Difco, Detroit, MI) as described by Corradin et al. (1977).
1987) are shown in Figure 1.

Proliferative assay

Seven days after priming with AChR, lymph node cells were harvested from the mice and suspended in RPMI 1640 containing 1% fresh, autologous normal mouse serum. The number of viable cells was determined by vital staining with flourescein diacetate (Rotman and Papermaster, 1966). Viable lymph node cells (3.0 x 10^5 cells/well) were cocultured in triplicates with various concentrations of AChR (from 2.5-20 μg/ml), peptides (from 10-40 μg/ ml), mitogen or control unrelated proteins and peptides [lysozyme synthetic peptide 31-50 (Bixler et al., 1984b), hen egg lysozyme and ovalbumin]. The cultures were incubated five days at 37°C in a humidified 5% CO_2 atmosphere, pulsed (18 hrs) with 2 μCi/well [^{3}H]-thymidine (Research Products International Corp., Mount Prospect, IL) and then harvested onto glass microfiber filters (Whatman, Clinton, NJ) and counted by liquid scintillation.

Peptide	Structure
1-16	S-E-H-E-T-R-L-V-A-N-L-L-E-N-Y-N
12-27	L-E-N-Y-N-K-V-I-R-P-V-E-H-H-T-H
23-38	E-H-H-T-H-F-V-D-I-T-V-G-L-Q-L-I
34-49	G-L-Q-L-I-Q-L-I-S-V-D-E-V-N-Q-I
45-60	E-V-N-Q-I-V-E-T-N-V-R-L-R-Q-Q-W
56-71	L-R-Q-Q-W-I-D-V-R-L-R-W-N-P-A-D
67-82	W-N-P-A-D-Y-G-G-I-K-K-I-R-L-P-S
78-93	I-R-L-P-S-D-D-V-W-L-P-D-L-V-L-Y
89-104	D-L-V-L-Y-N-N-A-D-G-D-F-A-I-V-H
100-115	F-A-I-V-H-M-T-K-L-L-L-D-Y-T-G-K
111-126	D-Y-T-G-K-I-M-W-T-P-P-A-I-F-K-S
122-138	A-I-F-K-S-Y-C-E-I-I-V-T-H-F-P-F-D
134-150	H-F-P-F-D-Q-Q-N-C-T-M-K-L-G-I-W-T
146-162	L-G-I-W-T-Y-D-G-T-K-V-S-I-S-P-E-S
158-174	I-S-P-E-S-D-R-P-D-L-S-T-F-M-E-S-G
170-186	F-M-E-S-G-E-W-V-M-K-D-Y-R-G-W-K-H
182-198	R-G-W-K-H-W-V-Y-Y-T-C-C-P-D-T-P-Y
194-210	P-D-T-P-Y-L-D-I-T-Y-H-F-I-M-Q-R-I

Fig. 1 Structure of the synthetic overlapping peptides representing the extracellular part (residues 1-210) of the α chain of the *Torpedo californica* AChR. The regions of overlaps between consecutive peptides are underlined. The single letter notations of the amino acids are: A, alanine; C, cysteine; D, aspartic acid; E, glutamic acid; F, phenylalanine; G, glycine; H, histidine; I, isoleucine; K, lysine; L, leucine; M, metionine; N, asparagine; P, proline; Q, glutamine, R, arginine; S, serine, T, threonine; V, valine; W, tryptophan; Y,tyrosine.

RESULTS

Determination of optimum dose conditions for various mouse strains

Several mouse strains were studied so that some potentially recognizable T sites will not be overlooked due to genetic exclusion of their recognition. We examined the responses of five mouse strains to AChR. These were: C57BL/6 ($H-2^b$), C3H/He ($H-2^k$), SWR ($H-2^q$), RIIIS ($H-2^r$) and SJL ($H-2^s$).

In each of these mouse strains, we determined the optimum *in vivo* priming (from 5.0 to 50μg/mouse) and the *in vitro* challenge (from 2.5 to 20 μg/ml) doses of AChR. Figure 2 shows the challenge dose response curves in two mouse strains at different priming doses of AChR. Figure 3 shows, for the five mouse strains immunized with optimum priming doses, the response curves as a function of challenge dose. The SJL strain mice responded very strongly to AChR. In this strain, the optimum priming dose was 5 μg AChR per mouse giving a maximum proliferative response at the challenge dose of 5.0 μg AChR/ml. The SWR strain, also responded very strongly to AChR. The optimum priming and challenge doses of AChR in the SWR strain were 5 μg per mouse and 5 μg/ml, respectively. C57BL/6 mice gave an intermediate response at optimum AChR priming and challenge doses of 5 μg per mouse and 5 μg/ml, respectively. RIIIS mice responded very weakly with optimum priming and challenge AChR doses of 5 μg/mouse and 2.5 μg/ml, respectively. Finally, C3H/He gave no response to AChR at any of the priming and challenge doses tested. In all subsequent work, the optimum priming dose appropriate for each strain was used and the cultures were routinely challenged with three doses of 2.5, 5 and 10 μg per ml of AChR and with peptide doses of 10, 20 and 40 μg per ml of culture. The strains, SJL, SWR (high responders to AChR), C57BL/6 (an intermediate responder to AChR) and C3H/He (a non-responder to AChR) were selected for screening by the peptides.

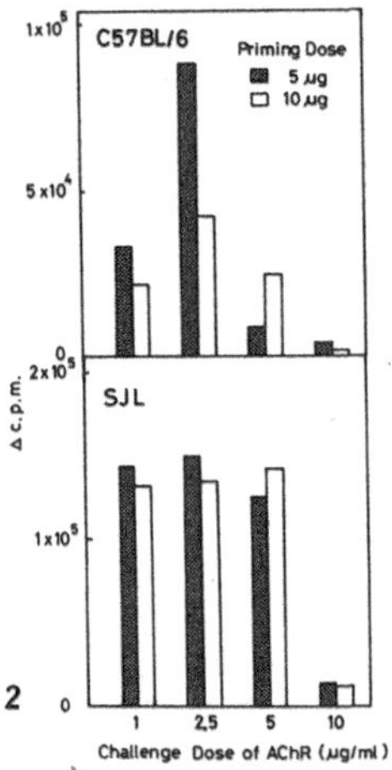

2

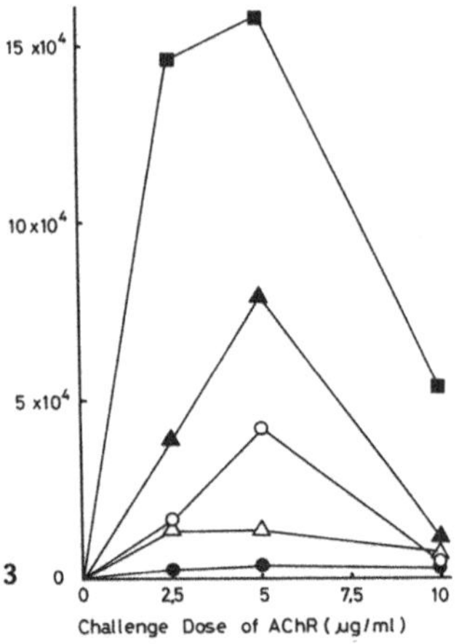

3

Fig. 2 (Left) A schematic diagram showing examples in two mouse strains of the dependence of the T-cell responses on the priming and challenge doses of AChR. Upper panel shows the responses of C57BL/6 ($H\text{-}2^b$) and the lower panel gives the responses of SJL ($H\text{-}2^s$) mice. The results at two AChR priming doses used (5 µg and 10 mg per mouse) and four challenge doses (1 to 10 µg/ml) are shown. Cultures containing unstimulated lymph node cell had the following background radioactivities; C57BL/6: 5 µg prime, 1,386 c.p.m.; 10 µg prime, 3,203 c.p.m.; SJL: 5 µg prime, 5,059 c.p.m.; 10 µg prime, 9,688 c.p.m.

Fig. 3 (Right) Dose response curves of AChR-primed lymph node cells from (o) C3H/He ($H\text{-}2^k$); (Δ) RIIIS ($H\text{-}2^r$); (o) C57BL/6 ($H\text{-}2^b$); (Δ) SWR ($H\text{-}2^q$) and ( ) SJL ($H\text{-}2^s$) mice. Cultures containing unstimulated lymph node cells had the following background radioactivities: C57BL/6, 1,386 c.p.m.; C3H/He, 1,571 c.p.m.; RIIIS, 6,701 c.p.m.; SWR, 2,849 c.p.m.; SJL, 1,172 c.p.m.

Proliferative responses of AChR-primed T-cells to the synthetic peptides

Typical peptide dose response curves are shown in Figure 4. The results with the four mouse strains are summarized in Table 1 and are given in a convenient diagramatic presentation in Figure 5. AChR-primed T cells from SJL mice responded very strongly to AChR and, in decreasing levels of responses, to the following synthetic overlapping peptides: 111-126, 67-82, 146-162, 23-38, 12-27, 100-115 and 78-93 (Table 1). The remaining peptides caused very little or no significant responses. AChR-primed T cells from SWR mice responded very strongly to AChR and, in decreasing order of activity, to the following peptides: 67-82, 1-16, 146-162, 12-27 and 34-49 (Table 1). The remaining peptides did not stimulate significant responses. AChR-primed T cells from C57BL/6 mice gave a moderate *in vitro* response to AChR and, in decreasing order of activity, to the following peptides: 182-198, 146-162 and 111-126. The remaining peptides did not stimulated significant responses. Finally, in C3H/He mice, priming with AChR induced cells which, although did not respond to AChR, they did mount, in decreasing order of activity, responses to *in vitro* challenge with the following α-chain peptides: 67-82, 146-162, 170-186 and very weakly to 12-27. The remaining peptides had little, or no, proliferative responses.

The specificity of the responses to the peptides was confirmed by absence of *in vitro* responses, by AChR-primed cells, to unrelated proteins and peptides. Conversely, AChR or its peptides did not stimulate any proliferative activity in cells from unimmunized mice or from mice that had been primed with unrelated proteins (data not shown). The viability of the cells in all the present studies was indicated from their responses to Con A, PPD and LPS.

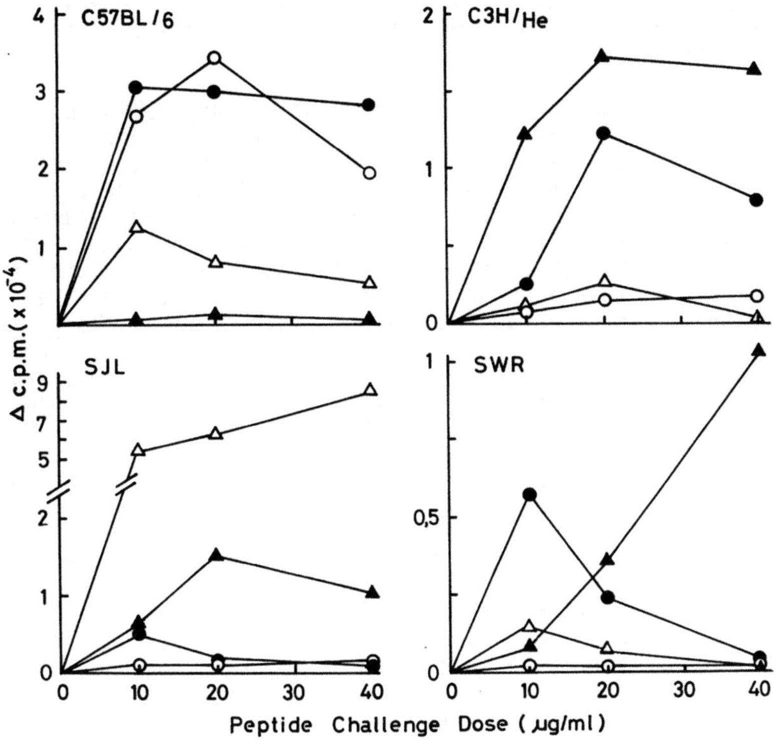

Fig. 4 Examples of dose response curves to the synthetic peptides of AChR-primed lymph node cells from C57BL/6, C3H/He, SJL and SWR mice. (Δ) peptide 67-82, (Δ) peptide 111-126, (o) peptide 146-162 and (o) peptide 182-198. Cultures containing unstimulated lymph node cells had the following background radioactivities; C57BL/6, 2,538 c.p.m.; C3H/He, 3,841 c.p.m.; SJL, 1,172 c.p.m.; SWR, 2,849 c.p.m.

DISCUSSION

The immune responses to protein antigens are under Ir gene control (David and Atassi, 1982; Keck, 1975; Lozner *et al.*, 1974; Melchers *et al.*, 1973; Okuda *et al.*, 1978, 1979a). More importantly, the responses to each of the antigenic sites are under separate genetic control (Bixler and Atassi, 1983, 1984a, 1985, Bixler *et al.*, 1984a, 1984b; David and Atassi, 1982; Kurisaki *et al.*, 1986; Okuda *et al.*, 1979b; Twining *et al.*, 1981). Thus, the genetic diversity and response levels of the mouse strains were selected so that most, or all, of the potential T sites on the protein will be identified.

The mouse strains selected represented four independent haplotypes ($H\text{-}2^b$, $H\text{-}2^k$, $H\text{-}2^q$ and $H\text{-}2^s$) of different genetic backgrounds. Two strains ($H\text{-}2^q$ and $H\text{-}2^s$) were high responders to AChR, one strain ($H\text{-}2^b$) was a moderate responder, while the fourth strain ($H\text{-}2^k$) was essentially a nonresponder. The findings that the $H\text{-}2^k$ (C3H/He) and the $H\text{-}2^r$ (RIIIS) haplotypes are low responders and that the $H\text{-}2^b$ (C57BL/6) haplotype is an intermediate-to-high responder to Torpedo AChR are in agreement with other reports (Christadoss et al., 1979, 1982; Gorzynski et al., 1985) using these three haplotypes, but different mouse strains than those used here. On the other hand, $H\text{-}2^s$ (ASW and B10.S) and $H\text{-}2^q$ (B10.Q) haplotypes were reported to be low and intermediate responders, respectively, while our results show that $H\text{-}2^s$ (SJL) and $H\text{-}2^q$ (SWR) are both high responders. However, since the mouse strains were not the same, the differences are most probably due to non-H-2 gene influences.

The rationale and design of the comprehensive overlapping peptide strategy have been discussed previously in detail (Kazim and Atassi, 1980, 1982; Bixler and Atassi, 1984a). The size of the peptides was selected to be in the optimal range for in vitro stimulation of T cells and to take into account the synthetic load and the protein size (210 residues) being screened. Earlier studies from this laboratory have shown that, although synthetic antigenic sites of myoglobin (6-7 amino acid residues) can stimulate in vitro T-cell proliferation (Okuda et al., 1979b), this activity improved greatly on extention of the sites by an additional 5-6 residues (Yoshioka et al., 1983; Young and Atassi, 1982, 1983). In fact, these extended sites were used (Yoshioka et al., 1983) to drive the culture into a T-cell population (i.e. T-cell lines) of a single desired specificity and, from these T-cell lines, T-cell clones possessing the same pre-determined specificity are prepared.

Localization of the sites takes into consideration activities of individual peptides as well as activities residing in the overlap regions of adjacent peptides (Kazim and Atassi, 1980, 1982). Six major T sites were found to reside within the regions shown in Figure 6. It should be stressed that the strategy applied here is not designed to define the precise boundaries of the T sites. The boundary frame shifts observed for the T sites from strain to strain are not unexpected and have been reported for the boundaries of the protein sites recognized by antibodies (Atassi, 1975; Koketsu and Atassi, 1973, 1974; Yoshioka and Atassi, 1986) as well as the sites of T-cell recognition (Bixler et al., 1984a,b; Bixler and Atassi, 1984a; Kurisaki et al., 1986).

The magnitude of the responses to the various sites varied with the haplotype. For example, the T-site within residues 113-124 was inactive in the $H\text{-}2^k$ and $H\text{-}2^q$ haplotypes but provoked strong and moderate responses in the $H\text{-}2^s$ and $H\text{-}2^b$ haplotypes, respectively. Similarly, the T site within residues 67-82 stimulated T cells of the $H\text{-}2^s$, $H\text{-}2^k$ and $H\text{-}2^q$ haplotypes but evoked little or no response in the $H\text{-}2^b$ mice. Other examples can be seen in Table 1 and Figures 5 and 6. These results are consistent with genetic control operating at the antigenic site level (Okuda et al., 1979b) (i.e. each site is under separate genetic control).

It is significant to note that even though T cells of AChR-immunized C3H/He ($H\text{-}2^k$) mice did not give an in vitro response to AChR, they did give significant responses to at least three different peptides. The immune response is regulated, in addition to Ir gene control, by inter-site cellular influences (Atassi et al., 1981a; Krco et al., 1981a,b,c, 1984). The cellular response to a T site in a protein exerts regulatory effects (help or suppression) upon the responses to other T sites of the same protein. It would appear therefore, that the cellular responses of the $H\text{-}2^k$ haplotype to some AChR site(s) have the effect of turning off the responses to other sites. The networks of these site-directed cell-cell interactions are now being studied.

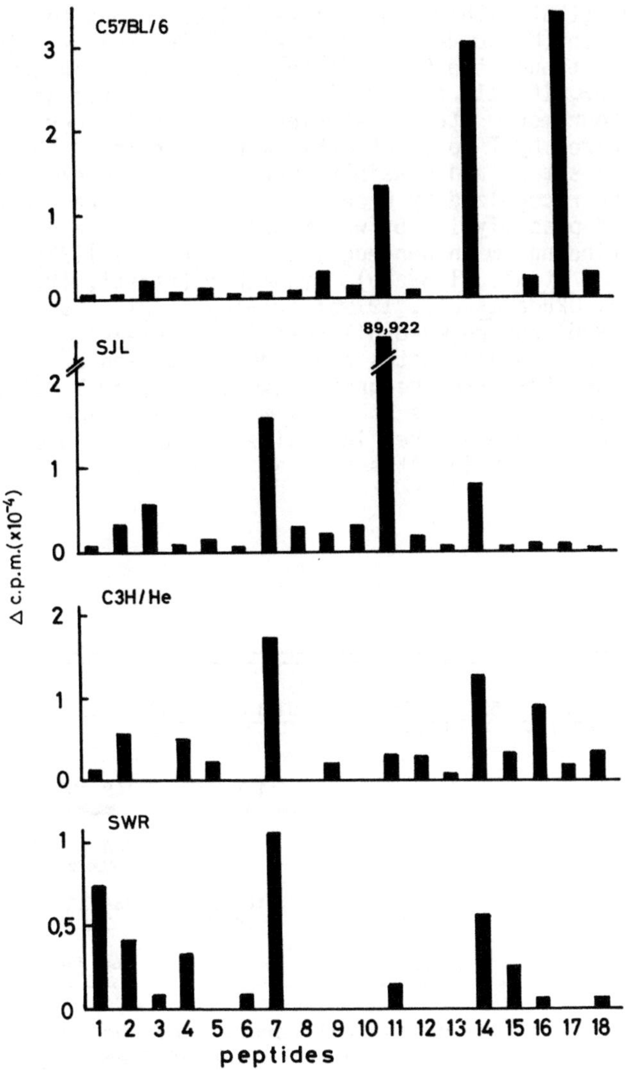

Fig. 5 Schematic presentation of the *in vitro* stimulating activity by the synthetic AChR peptides. The diagram shows the net c.p.m. at the optimum challenge dose of each peptide: (1) peptide 1-16; (2) peptide 12-27; (3) peptide 23-38; (4) peptide 34-49; (5) peptide 45-60; (6) peptide 56-71; (7) peptide 67-82; (8) peptide 78-93; (9) peptide 89-104; (10) peptide 100-115; (11) peptide 111-126; (12) peptide 122-138; (13) peptide 134-150; (14) peptide 146-162; (15) peptide 158-174; (16) peptide 170-186; (17) peptide 182-198; (18) 194-210.

The determination of the full profile of the continuous T-cell recognition regions on the extracellular part (residues 1-210) of the α chain of AChR provides a unique opportunity for comparison of the T-cell recognition profile with the full profile of recognition by antibodies (Mulac-Jericevic *et al.*, 1987). Three (and possibly four) of the T sites on the α chain coincide with the antigenic (antibody binding) sites that are recognized by outbred mouse antibodies (Mulac-Jericevic *et al.*, 1987) (Figure 6). One of these three T sites (that within region 184-196) coincides (or overlaps) with a toxin binding region (Mulac-Jericevic et al., 1986; Mulac-Jericevic and Atassi, 1987). Even though the B-cell recognition sites (in outbred mice) within residues 41-53, 102-114 and 128-138 are not significantly recognized by T cells of the four mouse strains studied here, it is very likely that, they will be recognized by T cells of other mouse strains. There are, however, at least two T sites (and possibly three) which are exclusively T cell specific and are not recognized by B cells. These sites reside within regions 113-124, 148-160 and possibly 14-25 (which shifts in $H-2^s$ and $H-2^q$). This is similar to our findings with hen egg lysozyme (Atassi 1978; Bixler and Atassi, 1984b; Bixler et al., 1984a,b), myoglobin (Atassi, 1975; Bixler and Atassi, 1983, 1984a; Okuda et al., 1979b; Twining et al., 1981), hemoglobin (Yoshioka et al., 1986) and ragweed allergen Ra3 (Kurisaki et al., 1986). Each of these proteins contains sites that are recognized by both B and T cells as well as sites that are recognized exclusively by T cells. The functions of these various T sites in the immune recognition of a protein may be concerned with the aforementioned intersite influences which regulate the immune responses to the protein (Atassi et al., 1981; Krco et al., 1981a-c).

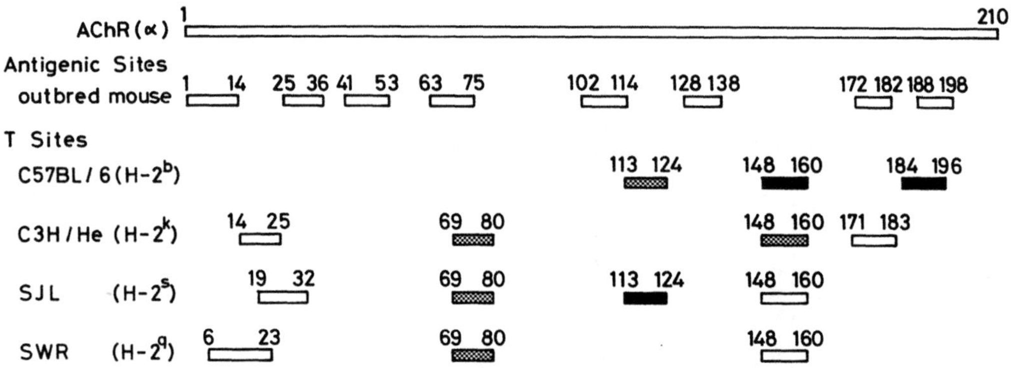

Fig. 6 Schematic diagram showing the full profile of the regions on the AChR α subunit that carry the continuous sites of T-cell recognition (T-sites) in four mouse strains. The T-cell recognition sites are compared with the sites of antibody (B-cell) recognition (i.e. antigenic sites) in outbred mouse which were localized in the preceding article (14). The T sites notations are as follows: (solid bars) regions stimulating high T-cell responses (Δ cpm > 20,000); (stippled bars) regions stimulating intermediate responses (Δ cpm, 10,000-20,000); (open bars) region stimulating low responses (Δ cpm, 5,000-10,000). It is not implied that the entire regions shown comprise the T sites, rather that the sites reside within these regions. Indeed, the T sites are localized within intentionally larger regions than their expected size.

The regions localized here reflect the responses of numerous T-cell clones, each of which perceives the T site somewhat differently (i.e. showing frame shifts to the right or to the left). The maximal effective response detected here (i.e. the T site) is the average of all of these activities (Bixler and Atassi, 1983; Atassi et al., 1987). This would be consistent with a heterogenous nature of the T-cell response at the clonal level as has previously been found to occur during B-cell recognition of other proteins (Atassi, 1975, 1980, 1984). In view of this heterogeneity, it is possible that T-cell clones with specificity for a region that is shifted with respect to a known T site (Atassi *et al*., 1987) or to other regions (outside the six T sites) which are present *in* traces would not be detected in proliferative assays of bulk cultures but could be isolated by appropriate cloning methods. Long-term T-cell cultures passaged *in vitro* with a protein have been shown (Bixler *et al*., 1984c) to exhibit drifts with time leading to dramatic alterations in the relative proportions of T-cell populations having various specificities. Therefore, T-cell populations that may initially be present in very low amounts in lymph node cell cultures can proliferate and expand so rapidly so as to overtake the entire culture (Bixler *et al*., 1984c). In the case of B-cell recognition, monoclonal antibodies have been prepared against regions to which trace or no detectable antibody responses are present in anti-protein antisera (Atassi, 1984; Schmitz *et al*., 1983). It remains uncertain whether such trace amounts of T- and B-cell clones whose specificity is directed toward non-dominant regions, termed "background responses" (Atassi, 1980) have any biological significance.

It was postulated recently (Benjamini *et al*., 1984) that the sites recognized by T cells may be different from, and more limited in number than, the sites recognized by antibodies. These views have no experimental basis and they overlooked the fact that the sites of myoglobin that are recognized by B cells had previously already been shown to be recognized by T cells as well (Bixler and Atassi, 1983; Okuda *et al*., 1979b; Yoshioka *et al*., 1983; Young and Atassi, 1982, 1983). Similarly, the aforementioned postulate (Benjamin *et al*., 1984) is not supported by the present findings nor by recent studies of other proteins (Bixler and Atassi, 1983, 1984a, 1984b; Bixler *et al*., 1984a, 1984b; Yoshioka *et al*., 1986; Kurisaki *et al*., 1986; Atassi and Kurisaki, 1984, 1986) which clearly show that T cells can indeed recognize the same sites as B cells and they can also recognize other regions to which no antibody responses are detectable.

The hypothesis that immunodominant T sites coincide with amphipathic helices in proteins (DeLisi and Berzofsky, 1985) is not supported by the present findings and the above referenced studies. Also, these findings do not support the postulates (Spouge *et al*., 1987) that lysine residues occur frequently at the *C*-terminal end of the T sites and that immunodominant helper T sites belong to one particular conformational feature. It should be stressed that, as already discussed here and in all the studies referenced in the above paragraph, the immuodominance of a T site is not an absolute property of the T site, but is a function of the genetic restriction of the host (see Figures 4 and 5). Clearly, immune recognition is not only dependent on the shape of the protein, but is a complex biological phenomenon subject to control and regulation by the host cellular immune system by mechanisms that are still largely unknown.

ACKNOWLEDGEMENTS

The work was supported in part by grant (AI 21336) from the National Institutes of Health and a grant (Q994) from the Welch Foundation and the award to M.Z. Atassi of the Robert A. Welch Chair of Chemistry.

REFERENCES

Appel, S.H., Almon, R.R. and Levy, N. (1975) N. Engl. J. Med. 293, 760-761.
Atassi, M.Z. (1975) Immunochemistry 12, 423-438.
Atassi, M.Z. (1978) Immunochemistry 15, 909-936.

Atassi, M.Z.(1980) Mol. Cell. Biochem. 32, 21-44.
Atassi, M.Z. (1984) Europ. J. Biochem. 145, 1-20.
Atassi, M.Z. and Kurisaki, J.I. (1984) Immunol. Commun. 13, 539-551.
Atassi, M.Z. and Kurisaki, J.I. (1986) Proteides of the Biol. Fluids 34, 157-160.
Atassi, M.Z., Yokota, S., Twining, S.S., Lehmann, H. and David, C.S. (1981) Mol. Immunol. 18, 945-948.
Atassi, M.Z., Yoshioka, M., Bean, M. and Bixler, G.S. (1987) Biochem. J., in press.
Benjamin, D.C., Berzofsky, J.A., East, E.J., Gurd, F.R.N., Hannum, C., Leach, S.J., Margoliash, E., Michael, J.G., Miller, A., Prager, E.M., Reichlin, M., Sercarz, E.E., Smith-Gill, S.J., Todd, P.E. and Wilson, A.C. (1984) Ann. Rev. Immunol. 2, 67-101.
Bixler, G.S. and Atassi, M.Z. (1983) Immunol. Comm. 12, 593-603.
Bixler, G.S. and Atassi, M.Z. (1984a) J. Immunogen. 11, 339-353.
Bixler, G.S. and Atassi, M.Z. (1984b) J. Immunogen. 11, 245-250.
Bixler, G.S. and Atassi, M.Z. (1985) Europ. J. Immunol. 15, 917-922.
Bixler, G.S., Yoshida, T. and Atassi, M.Z. (1984a) Exptl. Clin. Immunogen. 1, 99-111.
Bixler, G.S., Yoshida, T. and Atassi, M.Z. (1984b) Immunol. Commun. 13, 161-172.
Bixler, G.S., Yoshida, T. and Atassi, M.Z. (1984c) J. Immunogen. 11, 327-337.
Changeux, J.-P., Devillers-Thiery, A. and Chemouilli, P. (1984) Science 225 1335-1345.
Christadoss, P., Lennon, V.A. and David, C.S. (1979) J. Immunol. 123, 2540-2543.
Christadoss, P., Lennon, V.A., Krco, C.J. and David, C.S. (1982) J. Immunol. 128, 1141-1144.
Claudio, T., Ballivet, M., Patrick, J. and Heinemann, S. (1983) Proc. Natl. Acad. Sci. USA 80, 1111-1115.
Corradin, G., Etlinger, H.M. and Chiller, J.M. (1977) J. Immunol. 119, 1048-1053.
DeLisi, C. and Berzofsky, J. (1985) Proc. Natl. Acad. Sci. USA 82, 7048-7052.
David, C.S. and Atassi, M.Z. (1982) Adv. Exp. Med. Biol. 150, 97-126.
Devillers-Thiery, A., Giraudat, J., Bentaboulet, M. and Changeux, J.P. (1983) Proc. Natl. Acad. Sci. USA 80, 2067-2071.
Gorzynski, T.J., Lennon, V.A., Nathanson, R.M.. and David, C.S. (1985) J. Immunol. 134, 2079-2083.
Kazim, A.L. and Atassi, M.Z. (1980) Biochem. J. 191, 261-264.
Kazim, A.L. and Atassi, M.Z. (1982) Biochem. J. 203, 201-208.
Keck, K. Nature (London) (1975) 254, 78-79.
Koketsu, J. and Atassi, M.Z. (1973) Biochim. Biophys. Acta 328, 289-302.
Koketsu, J. and Atassi, M.Z. (1974) Immunochemistry 11, 1-8.
Krco, C.J., Kazim, A.L., Atassi, M.Z. and David, C.S. (1981a) J. Immunogen. 8, 315-322.
Krco, C.J., Kazim, A.L., Atassi, M.Z. and David, C.S. (1981b) J. Immunogen. 8, 395-404.
Krco, C.J., Kazim, A.L., Atassi, M.Z. and David, C.S. (1981c) J. Immunogen. 8, 471-476.
Krco, C.J., Abramson, F.J., Yoshioka, N., Atassi, M.Z. and David, C.S. (1984) J. Immunogen. 11, 33-43.
Kurisaki, J., Atassi, H. and Atassi, M.Z. (1986) Europ. J. Immunol. 16, 236-240.
Lee, C.Y. (1979) Adv. Cytopharmacol. 3, 1-16.
Lennon, V.A., McCormick, D.J., Lambert, E.H., Griesmann, G.E. and Atassi, M.Z. (1985) Proc. Natl. Acad. Sci. (U.S.A.) 82, 8805-8809.
Lisak, R.P., Laramore, C., Levinson, A.I., Zweiman, B. and Moskocitz, A.R. (1986) Ann. Neurol. 19, 87-89.
Lozner, E.C., Sachs, D.H. and Shearer, G.M. (1974) J. Exp. Med. 139, 1204-1214.

McCarthy, M.P., Earnest, J.P., Young, E.T., Choe, S. and Stroud, R.M. (1986) Annu. Rev. Neurosci. 9, 383-413.
Melchers, I., Rajewsky, K. and Shreffler, D.C. (1973) Eur. J. Immunol. 3, 754-761.
Moore, H. and Raftery, M.A. (1979) Biochemistry 18, 1862-1867.
Mulac-Jericevic, B. and Atassi, M.Z. (1986) FEBS Lett. 199, 68-74.
Mulac-Jericevic, B. and Atassi, M.Z. (1987) Biochem. J., in press.
Mulac-Jericevic, B., Kurisaki, J. and Atassi, M.Z. (1987) Proc. Natl. Acad. Sci. USA., in press.
Noda, M., Takahashi, H., Tanabe, T., Toyosato, M., Furutani, Y., Hirose, T., Asai, M., Inayama, S., Miyata, T. and Numa, S. (1982) Nature London 299, 793-797.
Noda, M., Takahashi, H., Tanabe, T., Toyosato, M., Kikyotani, S., Furutani, Y., Hirose, T., Takashima, H., Inayama, S., Miyata, T. and Numa, S. (1983) Nature London 302, 528-532.
Okuda, K., Christadoss, P., Twining, S.S., Atassi, M.Z. and David, C.S. (1978) J. Immunol. 121, 866-868.
Okuda, K., Sakata, S., Atassi, M.Z. and David, C.S. (1979a) J. Immunogen. 6, 447-452.
Okuda, K., Twining, S.S., David, C.S. and Atassi, M.Z. (1979b) J. Immunol 123, 182-188.
Rotman, B. and Papermaster, B.W. (1966) Proc. Natl. Acad. Sci. (U.S.A.) 55, 134-141.
Schmitz, H.E., Atassi, H. and Atassi, M.Z. (1983) Mol. Immunol. 20, 719-726.
Sinigaglia, F., Gotti, C., Castagnoki, R. and Clementi, F., (1984) Proc. Natl. Acad. Sci. (U.S.A.) 81, 7569-7573.
Sobel, A., Weber, M. and Changeux, J.P. (1977) Eur. J. Biochem. 80, 215-224.
Spouge, J.L., Guy, H.R., Cornette, J.L., Margalit, H., Cease, K., Berzofsky, J. and DeLisi, C. (1987) J. Immunol. 138, 204-212.
Twining, S.S., David, C S. and Atassi, M.Z. (1981) Mol. Immunol. 18, 447-450.
Tzartos, S.J., Changeux, J.-P. (1983) EMBO J. 2, 281-387.
Yokota, S., David, C.S. and Atassi, M.Z. (1980) Mol. Immunol. 17, 1079-1082.
Yoshioka, M., Bixler, G.S. and Atassi, M.Z. (1983) Mol. Immunol. 20, 1133-1137.
Yoshioka, M. and Atassi, M.Z. (1986) Biochem. J. 234, 441-447.
Yoshioka, M., Yoshioka, N. and Atassi, M.Z. (1986) Biochem. J. 234, 449-452.
Young, C.R. and Atassi, M.Z. (1982) Adv. Exp. Med. Biol. 150, 73-93.
Young, C.R. and Atassi, M.Z. (1983) J. Immunogen. 10, 161-169.

STRUCTURAL CONSIDERATIONS OF T-CELL COGNIZANCE OF ANTIGEN

Eli Benjamini, Beatrice C. Langton and Carl E. Mackewicz

Department of Medical Microbiology and Immunology

School of Medicine, University of Calif. Davis, CA 95616

ABSTRACT

Work summarized herein describes two congenic strains of mice, C57BL/10 and B10.BR, which differ at the I-A region of the MHC where C57BL/10 and B10.BR are $I\text{-}A^b$ and $I\text{-}A^k$ respectively. Using various antigens to stimulate, in vitro, primed T lymphocytes, studies on the responsiveness of these two strains to immunization with TMVP and with its tryptic peptide number 8 representing residues 93-112 of the protein are described. These studies revealed that in the C57BL/10 strain TMVP and peptide 8 exhibit cross reactivity on the T-cell level, whereas in the B10.BR strain these two antigens do not exhibit such cross reactivity. Further studies revealed that the cross reactivity is mapped to the I-A region of the MHC with cross reactivity between TMVP and peptide 8 exhibited in mice with $I\text{-}A^b$ (referred to as cross reactive-CR) but not with $I\text{-}A^k$ (referred to as non cross reactive-NCR). Cell depletion and reconstitution experiments revealed that cross reactivity (or the lack thereof) could be attributed to antigen presenting cells (APC). A profound difference between the strains was also expressed on the level at which their immune T-cells reacted in vitro to stimulation by various derivatives of peptide 8. The studies suggest that the strains differ in their responsiveness to the various orientations in which the T-cell epitope(s) are presented. Assuming that TMVP, but not peptide 8, is altered during processing by APC and assuming that antigen processing by APC of CR and NCR is similar, the difference which the strains exhibit in recognizing different orientations of the epitope may account for the difference in the cross reactivity between TMVP and peptide 8 exhibited by these strains. Further investigations revealed that the strains also differ in their response to pre-immunization with TMVP prior to immunization with peptide 8. Whereas preimmunization of the C57BL/10 (CR) mice with TMVP did not affect subsequent response to immunization with peptide 8, preimmunization of B10.BR (NCR) mice with TMVP suppressed the response to subsequent immunization with peptide 8. It is suggested that the presentation of the T-cell epitope(s) in the correct orientation by the appropriate Ia is crucial for the activation of T helper cells but that such presentation does not play a decisive role in the activation of T suppressor cells.

INTRODUCTION

It is well established that Ia molecules on antigen presenting cells (APC) play an important role in the interaction of antigen with T-lymphocytes (Shevach and Rosenthal, 1973; Kappler and Marrack, 1978; Geha et al., 1979). The ability of the antigen presenting cell to process and present antigen to the T-cell constitutes one level on which the genetic control of the immune response is expressed (Rosenthal and Shevach, 1973). In a series of elegant experiments, Rosenthal and Shevach have shown that the difference between "responder" and "non-responder" strains of animals to a given antigen could be contributed to the APC: APC from responder strains could present antigen to T-cells of F_1 (responder x non-responder) offspring, while the APC of non-responders could not, thus indicating that antigen processing and presentation by the APC is crucial in determining whether or not T-cells of a certain individual would respond to a given antigen. The molecular events which are governed by the genetic control of the immune response associated with antigen processing and presentation are still not clear. It appears that at least in some cases which involve high molecular weight antigens the antigen is internalized by the APC and "processed" by mechanisms which include enzymatic cleavage (reviewed by Unanue, 1984). Small immunogenic peptides apparently do not require such processing and cleavage (Shimonkevitz et al., 1984). It is possible that such small peptide portions of a protein represents entities similar to cleaved fragments of the larger protein. After internalization and cleavage, the "processed" antigen emerges on the surface of the APC where, in some form of association with the Ia of the APC,it is presented to the T lymphocyte antigen receptor, leading to the activation of the T-cell (reviewed by Unanue, 1984).

It has been shown that "processing" of antigen by APC of responders and non-responders can be similar (Friedman et al, 1983). If so, non-responsiveness, expressed on the level of APC, must be attributed to the inability of the APC to properly present antigen. Because presentation involves some form of association of antigen with Ia it may be postulated that non-responsiveness is a result of the lack of proper interaction between antigen and Ia in a manner which leads to T-cell interaction and activation. Indeed, in support of this possibility, direct binding between antigen and Ia of responder strain has been demonstrated while no such binding could be demonstrated between antigen and Ia of the non-responder strain (Babbit et al., 1985).

Several models have been proposed for the interaction between antigen, Ia, and the T-cell antigen receptor leading to T-cell activation (reviewed by Schwartz, 1985). Nevertheless, this interaction is still poorly understood. In the work described herein we have utilized the immune response of different strains of mice to a well-defined epitope of a protein antigen. This was performed in an attempt to elucidate, on a molecular level, some parameters involved in the differential responsiveness of these strains to the epitope and to correlate the findings with the role of APC in T-cell activation. As antigen we have utilized the tobacco mosaic virus protein (TMVP) which has been used in our laboratory for many years as a model protein antigen.

TMVP is a single polypeptide chain consisting of 158 amino acids of a known sequence (Anderer et al., 1960; Tsugita et al., 1960). TMVP is immunogenic in many animal species inducing both T-cells and antibodies to several portions of the protein (Benjamini, 1977;

Benjamini et al., 1985). One important antigenic area of the protein consists of its tryptic peptide number 8. This tryptic peptide represents residues 93-112 of the protein and has the amino acid sequence Ile-Ile-Glu-Val-Glu-Asn-Gln-Ala-Asn-Pro-Thr-Thr-Ala-Glu-Thr-Leu-Asp-Ala-Thr-Arg (Woody and Knight, 1959). The peptide has been demonstrated to constitute an area of the protein recognized by both T-cells and B-cells of many animal species (Benjamini, 1977; Benjamini et al., 1985; Morrow, Rennick and Benjamini, 1983). Experiments on the immunogenicity of tryptic peptide 8 demonstrated that the peptide is immunogenic in many strains of mice leading to the production of antibodies capable of binding with peptide 8 as well as with the whole protein TMVP (reviewed by Benjamini et al., 1985).

Recent work from our laboratory has indicated that immunization of some strains of mice with TMVP leads to the induction of T-cells which can be stimulated in vitro by TMVP as well as by peptide 8. Similarly, immunization of these strains with peptide 8 induces T cells capable of being stimulated in vitro by peptide 8 as well as by TMVP. Thus, these strains exhibit cross reactivity, on the T-cell level, between TMVP and peptide 8; these strains are referred to as cross reactive (CR) strains. In contrast, immunization of other strains with TMVP induces T-cells which react in vitro with TMVP, but not with peptide 8. Similarly, immunization of these strains with peptide 8 induces T cells which are stimulated in vitro by peptide 8 but not by TMVP. These strains do not exhibit cross reactivity on the T-cell level between TMVP and peptide 8 and are referred to as non-cross reactive (NCR) strains. Interestingly while mice of the NCR strain do not exhibit cross reactivity between TMVP and peptide 8 on the T-cell level they do exhibit cross reactivity between these antigens on the B cell level (Benjamini et al., 1985).

In the studies described below we have focused our attention on T-cell activation and on differences in T-cell cross reactivity between the CR and NCR strains. The in vitro proliferative response of lymph node cells to antigen, as described by Wan et al., 1986, served as a measure of antigen-specific T-cell activation. That the proliferative response is due to stimulated T-cells has been previously shown in our laboratory (Wan et al., 1986). Moreover, it has been shown that the proliferating cells are mainly T helper cells (Schreir et al., 1979). The studies described herein have been conducted with the aim of elucidating underlying mechanisms responsible for the differences exhibited by the strains in the cross reactivity between TMVP and peptide 8. These studies have been conducted on the genetic, cellular and molecular levels. Some parts of these studies have been recently reported (Benjamini et al., 1986; Benjamini, Langton and Wan, 1986).

GENETIC ASPECTS OF THE DIFFERENCES BETWEEN CROSS REACTIVE (CR) AND NON-CROSS REACTIVE (NCR) STRAINS

Preliminary studies showed that immunization of some strains of mice with TMVP induces T-cells which respond in vitro to TMVP as well as to peptide 8, and that immunization with peptide 8 induces cells which respond in vitro to peptide 8 and to TMVP. Strains which exhibit such cross reactivity on the T-cell level between TMVP and peptide 8 include C3H.SW, C3H.WB, and C57BL/10. Strains which do not exhibit this cross reactivity include A/J, and B10.BR. In an attempt to identify the genetic locus involved in this differential cross reactivity, we have utilized congenic and recombinant strains of mice. In these experiments the animals were immunized in the base of tail with 10-50 μg TMVP in Freund's Complete Adjuvant (FCA). Fourteen days

Table 1. The Responsiveness, in vitro, to TMVP and to Peptide 8 of Congenic and Recombinant Strains of Mice Immunized with TMVP

Strain	MHC							Response* to	
	H-2	K	I-A	I-J	I-E	S	D	TMVP	Peptide 8
C57BL/10	b	b	b	b	b	b	b	++	++
B10.BR	k	k	k	k	k	k	k	++	-
B10.S	s	s	s	s	s	s	s	++	++
B10.D_2	d	d	d	d	d	d	d	++	++
B10.A	a	k	k	k	k	d	d	++	-
B10.A(2R)	h2	k	k	k	k	d	b	++	-
B10.A(3R)	i3	b	b	b	k	d	b	++	++
B10.A(4R)	h4	k	k	b	b	b	b	++	-
B10.A(5R)	i5	b	b	k	k	d	d	++	++
B10.A(18R)	i18	b	b	b	b	b	d	++	++

*(-) Stimulation index (S.I.) less than 1.5; (±) S.I. 1.5 - 1.9; (+) S.I. 2.0 - 2.4, (++) S.I. above 2.5

later lymph node cells were harvested and cultured, in vitro, in the presence of various concentrations of TMVP (0.05-5 μM) or of peptide 8 (0.3-30 μM) as described (Wan et al., 1986). A strain is considered responsive (+) to an antigen when the stimulation index, in the presence of antigen at the optimal concentration, is greater than 1.5 (a value derived statistically from virtually hundreds of experiments).

Results in Table 1 clearly indicate that the difference in responsiveness between the strains is mapped to the I-A locus of the MHC, where cross reactivity on the T-cell level, between TMVP and peptide 8, is exhibited by strains with I-A^b while no such cross reactivity is exhibited by strains with I-A^k. These results, linking non-cross reactivity with I-A^k help explain the previously mentioned non-cross reactivity exhibited by A/J mice which are of H-2^a haplotype but with I-A^k, and the cross reactivity exhibited by C3H.SW which are I-A^b.

It is important to reiterate at this point that the above difference which is mapped to the I-A of the MHC is with respect to the cross reactivity on the T-cell level between TMVP and peptide 8. It does not involve the lack of T cells capable of recognizing and reacting to peptide 8. In fact, as has been mentioned earlier, immunization of these NCR strains with peptide 8 induces T-cells which respond, in vitro, to stimulation by peptide 8 but not by TMVP.

CELLULAR ASPECTS OF THE DIFFERENCES BETWEEN CROSS-REACTIVE (CR) AND NON-CROSS- REACTIVE (NCR) STRAINS

Because the difference in the cross reactivity between TMVP and peptide 8 exhibited by the various strains of mice was mapped to the I-A of the MHC it was reasonable to assume the involvement of antigen processing and presentation by antigen presenting cells (APC) in the difference. To ascertain the possible role of APC in the difference we have resorted to depletion and reconstitution experiments. In order to avoid problems arising from non-histocompatibility we have utilized F_1

Table 2. The Responsiveness of C57BL/10 x B10.BR F_1 (CRxNCR) TMVP Immune T-cells to TMVP and to Peptide 8 in the presence of Adherent Peritoneal Exudate Cells (PEC) of CR or NCR Strains

Responding Cells	Response* to TMVP	Response* to Peptide 8
Lysozyme - immune F_1 lymph node (LN) cells	-	-
TMVP - immune F_1 (LN) cells	++	++
TMVP - immune purified T-cells only	-	-
TMVP - immune purified F_1 T-cells in the presence of F_1 adherent PEC	++	++
TMVP - immune purified F_1 T-cells in the presence of CR adherent PEC	++	++
TMVP - immune purified F_1 T-cells in the presence of NCR adherent PEC	++	-

* (-) Stimulation index (S.I.) less than 1.5; (±) S.I. 1.5 - 1.9; (+) S.I. 2.0 - 2.4; (++) S.I. above 2.5

mice which constitute offsprings of CR x NCR (C57BL/10 x B10.BR) mice. The experiments consisted of testing the *in vitro* stimulation by TMVP and by peptide 8 of T-cells obtained from TMVP-immunized F_1 mice, in the presence of APC obtained from CR or from NCR mice. APC were depleted from lymph node cells of F_1 mice by passage through sephadex and subsequent pannings on rabbit anti mouse Ig. APC were isolated by first adhering peritoneal exudate cells (PEC) on plastic plates and recovering the adherent cells by a cold shock. For reconstitution, APC-depleted T-cells were mixed with PEC at a ratio of 1 PEC per 30 T cells.

Results of the reconstitution experiments summarized in Table 2 clearly demonstrate that the ability of a strain to exhibit cross reactivity between TMVP and peptide 8 (which, as described above, was mapped to the I-A) is dominant. This is concluded from the finding (Table 2) that TMVP-immune lymph node T-cells from F_1 mice respond *in vitro* to both TMVP and to peptide 8. The depletion and reconstitution experiments summarized in Table 2 indicate that TMVP-immune T-cells respond *in vitro* to both TMVP and to peptide 8 in the presence of adherent PEC of the CR strain but not of the NCR strains. The results suggest that a difference in the antigen presentation capacity by APC is involved in the difference in cross reactivity on the T-cell level exhibited by the CR and NCR strains. It is interesting to note that the involvement of Ia of the APC in the difference between the cross reacting and non-cross reacting strains is similar to the involvement of Ia of APC in the difference in the total responsiveness (or non-responsiveness) to an antigen exhibited between different strains of mice. The latter has been demonstrated by the classical experiments of

Rosenthal, Shevach and others (Rosenthal and Shevach, 1973; Shevach and Rosenthal, 1973; Thomas and Shevach 1977; Yano, Schwartz and Paul, 1978) where the non-responsiveness has been attributed to the inability of APC to either process or present antigen and has been mapped to the I-A region of the MHC of the APC (Paul et al., 1977).

The participation of APC in the activation of antigen-specific T-cells could be expressed on the level of antigen processing, on the level of antigen presentation, or both. Since experiments have indicated that APC from responder and non-responder animals "process" antigen in a very similar manner (Friedman et al., 1983) it is logical to assume that the difference between responder and non-responder strains associated with APC is due to differences in presentation rather than processing. Only recently have some advances been made towards the understanding of the association between antigen and Ia. It has been shown that antigen binds to Ia of a responder strain but not of a non-responder strain (Babbit et al., 1985). With respect to an antigen capable of activating specific T-cells it has been proposed that a portion of the antigen to which the term agretope has been coined, binds with the Ia of APC (Heber-Katz, Hansburg and Schwartz, 1983, reviewed by Schwartz, 1985). Thus, the antigen-Ia complex interacts with the T-cell receptor which recognizes some portion of the Ia molecule and the T-cell recognizable epitope. It is conceivable that there are instances where the antigen indeed binds to Ia, as has been demonstrated, but where the Ia-antigen complex does not present the T-cell recognizable epitope to the T-cell receptor in the proper manner. Put differently, the Ia-agretope interaction is such that it "selects" the determinant to be presented to the T-cell (reviewed by Paul, 1984). This selection would result in the activation of T-cells with the appropriate specificity. However, should there be a "hole" in the T-cell repertoire where a T-cell with such specificity is absent from the total T-cell population of the individual, that individual would obviously not mount a response to this epitope (reviewed by Paul, 1984). We have utilized the system described in the present studies (i.e. cross reactivity versus non-cross reactivity) to investigate some aspects of the structural features of the antigen as they may pertain to interaction with Ia and the T-cell, and to correlate these structural features with the differences in cross reactivity between TMVP and peptide 8 exhibited by the CR and NCR strains.

STRUCTURAL ASPECTS OF THE ANTIGEN ASSOCIATED WITH DIFFERENCES BETWEEN CROSS REACTING AND NON-CROSS REACTING STRAINS

Having ascertained some of the genetic and cellular aspects associated with the ability (or inability) of the different strains of mice to exhibit cross reactivity, on the T-cell level, between TMVP and peptide 8 we proceeded to ascertain whether we could detect differences between the strains in their reactivity with various portions and derivatives of peptide 8. This was peformed with the hope of defining structural aspects of the antigen which may participate in antigen presentation and T-cell activation. To this end, CR (C57BL/10) and NCR (B10.BR) mice were immunized with either TMVP or with peptide 8 and the reactivity of their immune T-cells with various synthetic portions and derivatives of peptide 8 was tested.

Results presented in Table 3 indicate differences in the responsiveness of immune T-cells to the test antigens. TMVP-immune and peptide 8-immune T-cells of the CR strain respond <u>in vitro</u> to stimulation by the C-terminal hexadecapeptide portion of peptide 8. In contrast, peptide 8-immune T-cells of the NCR strain do not respond to this peptide. (Since TMVP-immune T-cells of the NCR strain do not

Table 3. The Stimulation of TMVP-Immune or Peptide 8-Immune T-Cells from C57BL/10 or B10.BR Mice by Peptide 8 and its Derivatives

Test Peptide (88 Asp, 89 Thr, 90 Arg, 91 Asn, 92 Arg, 93 Ile, 94 Ile, 95 Glu, 96 Val, 97 Glu, 98 Asn, 99 Gln, 100 Ala, 101 Asn, 102 Pro, 103 Thr, 104 Thr, 105 Ala, 106 Glu, 107 Thr, 108 Leu, 109 Asp, 110 Ala, 111 Thr, 112 Arg)	CR C57BL/10 Stimulation* *in vitro* after immunization with TMVP	CR C57BL/10 Pept.8	NCR B10.BR TMVP	NCR B10.BR Pept.8
(Peptide 8) (93-112)	++	++	-	++
(C-decapeptide) (103-112)	-	-	-	-
(C-dodecapeptide) (101-112)	-	-	-	-
(C-tetradecapeptide) (99-112)	-	-	-	-
(C-hexadecapeptide) (97-112)	++	++	-	-
("middle" peptide) (97-107)	-	-	-	-
(N-pentadecapeptide) (93-107)	±	+	-	±
[N-(4D) pentadecapeptide] (93-107) (D-residues 93-96)	-	-	-	-
(N-undecapeptide) (93-103)	-	-	-	-
(N5N-undecapeptide) (88-103)	-	-	-	-

* (-) Stimulation index (S.I.) less than 1.5; (±) S.I. 1.5 - 1.9; (+) S.I. 2.0 -2.4; (++) S.I. above 2.5

respond _in vitro_ to peptide 8 it is not surprising that these cells did not respond to the test peptide nor to any of the test peptides shown in Table 3).

Another difference between the two strains is expressed by the finding that peptide 8-immune T-cells of the CR strain respond to the N-pentadecapeptide portion of peptide 8. Peptide 8-immune T-cells of the NCR strain exhibit only a marginal response to this peptide.

The findings that the C-hexadecapeptide portion of peptide 8 is stimulatory to peptide 8-immune cells of the CR strain and that peptide 8 immune cells of both strains exhibit a response (albeit weak) to the N-pentadecapeptide portion of peptide 8 suggest that peptide 8-immune T-cells of both strains recognize a portion of peptide 8 which consists of the overlapping portion of the C-hexadecapeptide and the N-pentadecapeptide portions of peptide 8. Since peptide 8-immune T-cells of both strains respond _in vitro_ to peptide 8 but not to many of the tested peptides, the possibility that some of the latter peptides do not contain a T-cell recognizable epitope, an agretope, or both was investigated. To this end we tested the stimulatory capacity of conjugates consisting of proteins and the C-decapeptide or the N-undecapeptide portions of peptide 8. These peptides were conjugated to BSA, to transferrin or to the succinylated forms of the proteins as described recently (Wan et al., 1985).

The Data in Table 4 indicate that while none of the C-terminal decapeptide conjugates were stimulatory, the N-undecapeptide conjugated to BSA or to transferrin stimulated, _in vitro_, T-cells derived from TMVP- or from peptide 8-immunized C57BL/10 (CR) but not B10.BR (NCR) mice. These findings again demonstrate differences between the strains. Interestingly the results presented in Table 4 show that immunization of both strains with peptide 8 (but not with TMVP) induced T-cells capable of being stimulated _in vitro_ by the N-undecapeptide conjugated to succinylated BSA or to succinylated transferrin (with conjugation taking place exclusively through the N-terminal portion of the peptide). The results further indicate that immunization with peptide 8 induces, in both strains, T-cells which recognize the N-undecapeptide as a T-cell epitope. The inability of this free peptide to stimulate these cells but its capacity to do so when conjugated to a carrier may be due to the stabilization of a certain conformation of the peptide, even if the free peptide itself contains an appropriate agretope. On the other hand, the finding that the free peptide is not stimulatory but when conjugated to a protein carrier is stimulatory suggests that the latter provides appropriate features necessary for an effective agretope for this peptide, as has been suggested by Wan et al., (1986). An agretope is also provided by the C-terminal portion of peptide 8 since the entire peptide or even only its N-pentadecapeptide portion is stimulatory to peptide 8-immune T-cells. The ability of the protein carriers to provide for an agretope for the N-undecapeptide indicates that, at least in some instances, the agretope-Ia interaction may not be highly specific. This is not surprising in view of the limited polymorphism of the Ia molecule.

Results in Tables 3 and 4 suggest that immunization of mice of the CR as well as of the NCR strains with peptide 8 induces T-cell population(s) with specificity towards an area which overlaps the N-terminal undecapeptide and the C-terminal hexadecapeptide portions of peptide 8. The N-undecapeptide portion of peptide 8 by itself, is unable to stimulate these T-cells unless additional areas are added to it. These areas may consist of portions of peptide 8, such as amino acid residues C-terminally to the peptide, or of areas provided by

Table 4. The Stimulation of TMVP-Immune or Peptide 8-Immune T-Cells From C57BL/10 or B10.BR Mice by the C-Decapeptide or N-Undecapeptide Portions of Peptide 8 and their Conjugates to BSA, Transferrin or to the Succinylated Forms of the Proteins

Test Antigens: 93 Ileu, 94 Ileu, 95 Glu, 96 Val, 97 Glu, 98 Asn, 99 Gln, 100 Ala, 101 Asn, 102 Pro, 103 Thr, 104 Thr, 105 Ala, 106 Glu, 107 Thr, 108 Leu, 109 Asp, 110 Ala, 111 Thr, 112 Arg

Test Antigens	CR C57/BL10 Stimulation* in vitro following immunization with TMVP	CR C57/BL10 Pept. 8	NCR B10.BR TMVP	NCR B10.BR Pept. 8
(103-112) (C-decapeptide) ← 103–112 →	-	-	-	-
Conjugated to BSA ← 103–112 →	-	-	-	-
Conjugated to Transferrin ← 103–112 →	-	-	-	-
Conjugated to succinyl-BSA ← 103–112 →	-	-	-	-
Conjugated to succinyl-Transferrin ← 103–112 →	-	-	-	-
(93-103) (N-undecapeptide) ← 93–103 →	-	-	-	-
Conjugated to BSA ← 93–103 →	++	++	-	-
Conjugated to Transferrin ← 93–103 →	++	++	-	-
Conjugated to succinyl-BSA ← 93–103 →	-	++	-	++
Conjugated to succinyl-Transferrin ← 93–103 →	-	++	-	++

*(-) Stimulation index (S.I.) less than 1.5; (±) S.I. 1.5 - 1.9; (+) S.I. 2.0 - 2.4; (++) S.I. above 2.5

protein carriers such as BSA and transferrin. Because of the exquisite specificity towards an epitope expected from T lymphocytes and because the N-undecapeptide which by itself is non stimulatory becomes stimulatory upon the addition of various areas which exhibit only limited specificty, we postulate that such areas serve as or provide for an agretope. These agretopes are necessary for interaction with Ia and presentation of the N-undecapeptide to T-cells leading to their activation.

Data presented in Tables 3 and 4 indicate that peptide 8-immune T-cells of the CR strain are stimulated by the N-undecapeptide conjugated to BSA, transferrin or to their succinylated forms whereas peptide 8-immune T-cells of the NCR strain are stimulated by the N-undecapeptide only when conjugated to the succinylated forms of the proteins. It thus appears that the orientation in which the T-cell recognizable epitope (N-undecapeptide or a portion thereof) is presented can play a crucial role in the activation of the T-cell. Working with the protein antigen lysozyme, a recent report suggests that the orientation in which an epitope of lysozyme is presented to the T-cell is important for T-cell activation (Shastri et al., 1986).

Regarding the differences between the strains in their capacity to exhibit cross reactivity on the T-cell level between TMVP and peptide 8, the data in Tables 3 and 4 indicate that during immunization of either strain with peptide 8, T-cells are induced which recognize the N-undecapeptide when presented through its N-terminal orientation (as is the case when it is conjugated to the succinylated carriers). Immunization of the CR strain with peptide 8 also induces T-cells which recognize the N-undecapeptide in a different orientation (such as when conjugated to the non-succinylated carriers). However, T-cells of this latter specificity are not induced in the NCR strain since T-cells of the NCR strain recognize the peptide only when presented through the N-terminal orientation.

Although definitive proof is lacking, it is possible that because the protein TMVP constitutes an immunogen of high molecular weight it is "processed" by APC with an alteration taking place at an area consisting of several N-terminal residues of peptide 8. Thus, immunization with TMVP would induce T-cells which recognize the T-cell epitope within the N-undecapeptide only when this putative epitope is presented through its carboxyl groups but not through the N-terminal orientation. These cells would be stimulated by the N-undecapeptide conjugated to the non-succinylated forms of the protein; they would not be stimulated by the N-undecapeptide conjugated through its N-terminal to the succinylated forms of the carriers. The same type of alteration in the N-terminal portion of the immunogen TMVP is expected to occur following immunization of the NCR strain with TMVP. However, this strain recognizes the epitope within the N-undecapeptide only when presented conjugated through its N-terminal orientation. Thus, like in the CR strain, immunization with TMVP will fail to induce T-cells which recognize the epitope presented through its N-terminal orientation. Since the NCR strain does not recognize the epitope unless it is presented through its N-terminal orientation, immunization with TMVP would fail to induce T-cells which react with this epitope presented via its carboxyl groups even if the test peptide is the entire peptide 8. Hence, TMVP and peptide 8 exhibit cross reactivity, on the T-cell level, in the CR strains but not in the NCR strain. Work is in progress to ascertain possible alterations in the N-terminal area of peptide 8 during immunization with TMVP.

Table 5. The Effect of Preimmunization with TMVP or Lysozyme Upon the Induction of Peptide 8-Reactive Lymph Node Cells by Immunization with Peptide 8

In Vivo Treatment	Ag used for In Vitro Stimulation	Suppression (CR)* C57BL/10	Suppression (NCR)** B10.BR
TMVP ⟶ Peptide 8 (I.P.) (B.O.T.)	Peptide 8	9.5 ± 5.7	72 + 4.2
Lysozyme ⟶ Peptide 8 (I.P.) (B.O.T.)	Peptide 8	0	0

*Average ± S.E.M. of four experiments
**Average ± S.E.M. of three experiments

DIFFERENCES BETWEEN THE CROSS REACTING AND NON-CROSS-REACTING STRAIN IN SUPPRESSION OF IMMUNOGENICITY.

So far we have dealt with the phenomenon of a differential cross reactivity on the T-cell level between TMVP and peptide 8. This differential cross reactivity has been attributed to the Ia of APC. The CR and NCR strains also differ in their T-cell recognition and reactivity with various derivatives of peptide 8. As suggested above these differences reflect differences in the recognition of different orientations or the context in which a T-cell epitope is presented. Since immunization of the NCR strain with TMVP does not induce T-cells capable of being stimulated in vitro by peptide 8 it was of interest to assess what effect, if any, immunization with TMVP would have upon subsequent immunization with peptide 8. To this end CR and NCR mice were first immunized intraperitoneally with 50 μg TMVP in FCA. This was followed 1 week later by immunization in the base of tail with 50 μg of peptide 8 in FCA. Immunization with the unrelated protein lysozyme in FCA prior to immunization with peptide 8 served as control. Two weeks thereafter the mice were sacrificed and the stimulatory capacity of peptide 8 on the lymph node cells was assessed.

Results in Table 5 clearly demonstrate that immunization of the CR strain with TMVP prior to immunization with peptide 8 had no effect on the induction of peptide 8-responsive cells. In contrast, immunization of the NCR strain with TMVP prior to immunization with peptide 8 greatly suppressed the induction of peptide 8-reactive cells.

The finding of the differential suppressive effect of TMVP on subsequent induction of peptide 8-reactive cells adds another functional difference to the differences between the CR and NCR strains described so far.

Although the mechanism(s) for the suppression are still unknown it may be postulated that suppressor T-cells would be involved. If so, the following explanation is suggested to account for the differences in suppression observed between the CR and NCR strain: It is well accepted that in general, immunization with a given antigen triggers the induction of different functional T-cells specific for given epitopes. These include T-helper cells as well as T suppressor cells. In a normal immune response to an antigen, the T helper cell population with specificity to a given epitope undergoes a more vigorous amplification than does the T suppressor cell population to that epitope. This competition in favor of the T helper cells leads to a discernable immune response to the epitope and can be detected by specific in vitro proliferation to antigen. As has been mentioned earlier, the proliferating cells, in vitro, are primarily T helper cells (Schrier et al., 1979). If, however, for some reason the T suppressor cells undergo expansion while T helper cells to the same epitope do not the immune response will be suppressed to that epitope.

In the case of the CR strain, pre-immunization with TMVP apparently induces more peptide 8-reactive T helper cells than T suppressor cells. Thus, subsequent immunization with peptide 8 would result in the continuation of the induction of peptide 8-specific T helper cells which respond in vitro to peptide 8. On the other hand, immunization of the NCR strains with TMVP induces T helper cells with specificity to various areas of TMVP but not with specificity to peptide 8. This failure of TMVP to induce in the NCR strain peptide 8-specific T helper cells is I-A related and may be due to the improper presentation of this epitope to the T-cells. However, it is conceivable that TMVP and peptide 8 do cross react on the level of the T suppressor cell for which the activation requirements are distinct from the activation requirements for T helper cells and have been implicated as not being significantly dependent on I-A (reviewed by Dorf and Benacerraf, 1985). Thus, pre-immunization of the NCR strain with TMVP could induce peptide 8-specific T suppressor cells. These cells would suppress the subsequent induction of peptide 8-specific T-helper cells upon immunization with peptide 8. The presence of peptide 8-specific T suppressor cells in animals of the NCR strain pre-immunized with TMVP awaits experimental demonstration.

ADKNOWLEDGMENTS

This work was supported in part by grants number PCM 8103264 and PCM 8411235 from the National Science Foundation, and by the Ann B. Ashworth Memorial Grant for Cancer Research number IM 291 and grant number IM 401 from the American Cancer Society.

REFERENCES

1. Anderer, F.A., Uhlig, H., Weber, E., and Schramm, G., 1960, Nature, 186:922.
2. Babbit, B.P., Allen, P.H., Matsueda, G., Haber, E., and Unanue, E.R., 1985, Nature (London) 317:359.
3. Benjamini, E., 1977, in: Immunochemistry of Proteins, Vol. 2, M.Z. Atassi, ed., Plenum Press, New York.
4. Benjamini, E., Wan, A.M., Langton, B.C., and Andria, M.L., 1985, in: High Technology Route to Virus Vaccines, G.R. Dreesman, J.G. Bronson, and R. Kennedy, eds., Am. Soc. Microbiol., Pub., Washington, D.C.

5. Benjamini, E., Langton, B.C., Wan, A.M., Andria, M.L., and Leung, C.Y. 1986, in: Immunomodulation, G. Torrigiani, ed., W.H.O. Pub., Geneva (in press).
6. Benjamini, E., Langton, B.C., and Wan, A.M., 1986, Fed. Proc., 45:726.
7. Champness, J.N., Bloomer, A.C., Bricogne, G., Butler, P.J.G., and Klug, A., 1976, Nature, 259:20.
8. Dorf, E.M., and Benecerraf, B., 1985, Immunol. Rev., 83:23.
9. Friedman, A., Zerubavel, R., Gitler, C., and Cohen, I.R., 1983, Immunogenetics, 18:277.
10. Geha, R.S., Milgrom, H., Broff, M., Alpert, S., and Yunis, E.J., 1979, Proc. Natl. Acad. Sci. (U.S.), 76:4038.
11. Heber-Katz, E., Hansburg, D., and Schwartz, R.H., 1983, J. Mol. Cell. Immunol., 1:3.
12. Kappler, J.W., and Marrack, P., 1978, J. Exp. Med., 148:1510.
13. Morrow, P.R., Rennick, D.M., and Benjamini, E., 1983, J. Immunol., 131:2875.
14. Paul, W.E., Shevach, E.M., Pickeral, S., Thomas, D.W., and Rosenthal, A.S., 1977, J. Exp. Med., 145:618.
15. Paul, W.E., 1984, in: Fundamental Immunology, W.E. Paul, ed., Raven Press, New York.
16. Rosenthal, A.S., and Shevach, E.M., 1973, J. Exp. Med., 138:1194.
17. Schrier, R.D., Skidmore, B.J., Kurnick, J.T., Goldstine, S.N., and Chiller, J.M., 1979, J. Immunol., 123:2525.
18. Schwartz, R.H., 1985, Ann. Rev. Immunol., 3:237.
19. Shastri, N., Gammon, G., Miller, A., and Sercarz, E.E., 1986. J. Exp. Med., 164:882.
20. Shevach, E.M., and Rosenthal, A.S., 1973, J. Exp. Med., 138:1213.
21. Shimonkevitz, R., Colon, S., Kappler, J.W., Marrack, P., and Grey, H.M., 1984, J. Immunol., 133:2067.
22. Thomas, D.W., and Shevach, E.M., 1977, Proc. Natl. Acad. Sci. (U.S.A.), 74:2104.
23. Tsugita, A.D., Gish, D., Young, J.D., Fraenkel-Conrat, H., Knight, C.A., and Stanley, W.M., 1960, Proc. Natl. Acad. Sci. (U.S.A.), 46:1463.
24. Unanue, E.R., 1984. Ann. Rev. Immunol., 2:395.
25. Wan, A.M., Langton, B.C., Andria, L., and Benjamini, E., 1986, Mol. Immunol., 23:467.
26. Woody, B.R., and Knight, C.A., 1959, Virology, 9:359.
27. Yano, A., Schwart, R.H., and Paul, W.E., 1978, Eur. J. Immunol., 8:344.

ANTIGEN PRESENTING CELLS: DETECTION AND QUANTIFICATION OF A CYTOCHROME c DETERMINANT IMPORTANT FOR ACTIVATION OF T-CELLS ON BONE MARROW DERIVED MACROPHAGES BY USING SPECIFIC ANTI CYTOCHROME c MONOCLONAL ANTIBODY

Stéphane Demotz*, Claudio Vita+ and Giampietro Corradin*

*Institut de Biochimie, Université de Lausanne, Epalinges, Switzerland; +Istituto di Chimica Organica, Universita di Padova, Padova, Italy.

SUMMARY

The region of the horse cytochrome c molecule recognized by Mab SJL2-4 specific for the denatured form of the protein was located around residues 22-28. Binding studies on antigen pulsed macrophages were also performed.Surprisingly, heme peptide 1-65 was not recognised by Mab when bound on macrophages. This correlates with the incapacity of the same peptide to activate the T-cell clone 2-16. Binding sites on antigen pulsed macrophages varied between $0.5\text{-}2\times10^6$ per cell depending on the conditions used. The expression of the antigenic determinant as detected by Mab was also followed under different conditions (chloroquine, trypsin treatment) and time. Kinetics parameters of the antigen-antibody reaction in solution and on antigen bound macrophages were also determined and are dramatically different. This is correlated with a different structure of the peptide in solution and on macrophage cell surface.

INTRODUCTION

The structural feature of an antigenic peptide(s) present on the cell surface of an antigen presenting has not yet been characterized. Furthermore, the number of antigenic molecules present per cell has not been determined as well as the influence of various chemical modification of the antigen presenting cells (fixation, treatment with lysomotropic reagents) on the display on the cell surface of the antigenic moiety. In addition, no data are available at this moment whether the conformation of antigenic peptide in solution and that eventual recognized by T-cell differ from one another as suggested by several authors (Pincus et al., 1983; De Lisi and Berzofsky, 1985). Recently, data have appeared on the interaction of peptide antigen with purified class II molecules which can eventually represent a first step in the interaction with the antigen T-cell receptor (Babbitt et al., 1985; Babbitt et al., 1986; Buus et al., 1986). On the other hand, interaction of an antigenic peptide with the cell surface may be a general phenomenon which precedes the interaction with class II molecule and thus independent of the H-2 haplotype as seen for ovalbumin peptide 323-337 (Shimonkevitz et al., 1984).

In the last few years, we have been able to show that a monoclonal antibody specific for denatured cytochrome *c* (apo cytochrome *c*) is capable of inhibiting proliferation of apo cytochrome *c* specific T-cell clones and that the cytochrome *c* segment recognized by the Mab and T cell clones was similar (Corradin and Engers, 1984; Corradin et al., 1984). In this paper, we compare kinetics and equilibrium parameters of the antigen antibody reaction in solution and on macrophage bound antigen. In addition, we followed the appearence and disappearence of the antigenic determinant on the cell surface of the APC under different experimental conditions. We used mainly as antigen apo horse peptide 1-65 which is in denatured form in solution and which can be presented to different clones recognizing epitope 11-25 by fixed macrophages.

MATERIALS AND METHODS

Animals

BALB/c, C57BL/6 and SJL mice were raised at the Swiss Institute for Experimental Cancer Research, Epalinges, with breeding pairs which originated from Jackson Labs, Bar Harbor, ME (Balb/c) or Bomholtgard, Ry, Denmark (SJL).

Antigens

All cytochrome *c* species used were purchased from Sigma Chemical Co., St. Louis, MO and further purified either by ion exchange or gel filtration chromatography. Apo-cyt *c* or peptides were obtained according to Fisher et al. (1973). The synthetic peptides 11-25 to which a tyrosine residue was attached at the N-terminus and 13-25 was obtained according to the Merrifield method modified by Atherton et al. (1979). They were purified by gel filtration, ion exchange and high performance liquid chromatography (HPLC). Horse heme peptides 1-38 was obtained according to Fanger and Harbury (1965), respectively. Horse, beef and tuna heme peptides 1-65, *yeast* and *Candida Krusei* heme peptides 1-69 and 1-70 were obtained by cyanogen bromide cleavage according to Corradin and Harbury (1970).

Heme peptide 5-21 was obtained by treating 18 mg of horse heme peptide 1-38 with 1.5 mg of *staphylococcus Aureus* V8 protease (Miles Laboratories, Elkart, IN) in 2.6 ml of 0.1 M sodium citrate buffer at pH 4.0 for 41 h at 39°. Purification of the material was performed by gel filtration on a Sephadex G-50 superfine (1 x 220 cm column) followed by reverse phase HPLC on a microbondapak C-18 (Waters, Milford, MA) using a linear gradient of 0.05 % trifluoroacetic acid and 0.025 % triethylamine and acetonitrile (0 to 60 % acetonitrile in 80 min). The amino acid composition of heme fragment obtained 5-21 corresponded to the expected values.

The concentration of the various peptide preparations was determined by weight from lyophilized samples. The concentration of cytochrome *c* was determined spectrophotometrically (Margoliash et al., 1967).

Determination of the association constant and binding specificity

Association constant (Ka) of the three Mab was determined in sodium phosphate buffer saline (PBS) at pH 7.2 supplemented with 10% normal rabbit serum by using a constant amount of ^{125}I-labeled horse apopeptide 1-65 and horse cyt *c* and increasing amount of affinity purified

Mab. The antigen-antibody complex was precipitated by addition of polyethylenglycol (PEG 6000) at 13% final concentration. The concentration of bound Mab is equal to the concentration of radiolabeled antigen precipitated minus the background value (no Mab added). thus, the concentration of free Mab can be easily determined from the equation $Mab_{free} = Mab_{o} - Mab_{bound}$.

The association rate constants (k_1) were calculated using the second order kinetic equation k_1 = initial rate/ $ab_0 \cdot antigen\ bound_0$, where Ab_0 and $antigen\ bound_0$ are the initial antibody and antigen bound concentrations, respectively. Antigen bound was determined from the Scatchard plot.

Dissociation rates were determined by binding radiolabeled Mab antibody to antigen bound macrophages. At time zero, 100 ul of a medium containing 1000-10000 excess of antigen was added to each well. The antibody-bound vs free was then determined at different time. The data were expressed as a percentage of maximum antibody bound vs time and the dissociation rate constants (K_{-1}) were determined from the slope of the natural log plots of the data.

The dissociation rate constant in solution could not be determined because it is to fast. The dissociation rate constant was determined by preforming antigen-antibody complex in which the antigen was radiolabeled. At time zero, the immunocomplexes were dissolved in 200 ul of PBS containing 1000 fold excess of unlabeled antigen. At different time, bound vs unbound labeled antigen was separated by precipitation of the immunocomplexes with polyethylenglycol (13% final concentration). Data were then analysed as described above.

Inhibition assays were performed in PBS by adding increasing amount of unlabeled antigens to the radiolabeled preparation prior to addition of Mab. The reaction mixture was incubated for 2 hr at room temperature prior to addition of PEG 6000 at 13% final concentration. All the dilutions were done in 10% normal rabbit serum.

Cross-reactivity among different cyt <u>c</u> preparations was also determined by solid phase binding using a ^{125}I-rabbit anti-mouse $F(ab)'_2$ fragment antibody or by ELISA. . Hundred ul of 100 ug/ml of various preparations in PBS were used for coating the polyvinyl plates for 1 hr. After three repetitive washings, 0.2% bovine serum albumin (BSA) or gelatin was used to saturate the plates for 1 hr. Plates were again washed (3x) and monoclonal antibodies were added for one additional hour. After washing (3 times) ^{125}I-rabbit anti-mouse $F(ab)'_2$ fragment antibodies (50.000 to 100.000 cpm) was added for 1 hr. Wells were then washed (3x), cut and counted. For ELISA, sheep anti-mouse immunoglobulines coupled to phosphatase (Sigma Chemical Co) was added at 1:1000 dilution. Washing was done 1 hr later (3 times) and p-nitrophenolphosphate was added and optical density was usually determined after 1 hr. All the washings and dilution of Mab and antisera were done in 0.2% gelatin or BSA.

Monoclonal antibodies

SJL 2-4 Mab was obtained by fusing inguinal and periaortic lymph nodes from SJL mice.

Mice were first immunized with apo-cyt c in complete Freund's adjuvant (50 ug/50 ul) at the base of the tail (Corradin et al. 1977) and boosted 3 weeks later and 3 days before fusion with 50 ug of the homologous antigen in 50 ul of incomplete Freund's adjuvant. Cell fusion was performed according to Koehler and Milstein (1975) using the myeloma cell line P3/653. To screen the resulting hybridoma cultures, a solid phase radioimmunoassay was used as described previously. Horse apo cyt c at 100 ug/ml in PBS (100 ul per well) were used to coat the polyvinyl plates. The Mab was purified from liquid supernatants or ascites fluids by affinity chromatography using a Sepharose 4B column to which the cyt c heme peptide 1-65 was coupled by the CNBr method (Parikh et al, 1974).

Mab concentration was determined spectrophotometrically (1 mg = 1.4 O.D.at 280 nm) and its purity was determined by SDS-PAGE in 5% acrylamide.

Pulse of macrophages with peptides and binding analysis with Mab

Two x 10^6 macrophages (Mø) in 2 ml DMEM were incubated with variable concentrations of different peptide preparations at different temperatures for 0 to 1 hr. Mø were then washed twice in Hank's medium, resuspended in DMEM supplemented with 10% fetal calf serum (FCS) and plated in a 96 wells flat bottom plate at 5 x 10^4 cells per well. Binding experiments were performed after 0 to 6 h. Supernatant was removed and iodinated antibodies in DMEM + 10% FCS were added for 45 min. Supernatant was then harvested, cells were washed twice with Hank's medium and lysed with 200 ul of 2% sodium dodecylsulfate (SDS) in PBS. Supernatants and lysates were then counted.

Association constant (Ka) determination on pulsed Mø was performed by using increasing amounts of ^{125}I-Mab SJL 2-4 and the data were analysed by the Scatchard method. Similarly competition experiments were performed. A constant amount of ^{125}I-labeled Mab and increasing amounts of unlabeled Mab were mixed together prior to addition to pulsed Mø.

Fixation and trypsinization of BMMø

Mø were fixed as described by Shimonkevitz et al. (1983). Briefly, 5 µl of a 50% glutaraldehyde solution were added to 5 ml of Hank's medium. After 30 s, an equal volume of DMEM-10% FCS was added to block excess of free glutaraldehyde. Mø were then washed twice prior to use.

For trypsinization, Mø were resuspended in DMEM and treated with 50 ug/ml of enzyme (bovine pancreatic trypsin, Sigma chemical Co., St. Louis, MO) for 15 min at 37°C. Tryptic activity was quenched by addition of 10% final concentration of FCS. Mø were then washed twice prior to use. This treatment did not cause significant loss of viability as determined by trypan blue exclusion.

Cell culture

Mø were derived from bone marrow stem cells of C57BL/6 mice. Bone marrow of hind feet femurs was washed twice in Hank's medium and clumps of cells were gently dispersed. Six x 10^6 cells were plated in a Petri dish of 8 cm in diameter with 12 ml of the appropriate medium (50% Dulbecco's modified Eagle's medium, DMEM; 30% supernatant of L929 cells which were provided by Dr. M.L. Lohmann-Matthes; 20% horse serum) (Meerpohl et al., 1976). Mø were used after 6 to 9 days of culture. Cells were detached from Petri dishes by incubation with 10 ml phosphate buffer saline (PBS) 0.02% EDTA for 30 min at 4°. Cells were then centrifuged and resuspended in DMEM.

RESULTS

The fine specificity of Mab SJL 2-4 was determined either by solid phase binding or by inhibition assay in solution by using different cyt c preparations. In particular as shown in Table 1, SJL2-4 recognizes heme peptide 1-38 and peptide 1-25, synthetic apo-peptide Tyr-11-25 but not heme peptides 5-21. If one considers that an antigenic site is comprised of 4-6 amino acid residues (Sela, 1969)and that we are probably dealing with a sequential determinant, it follows that the sequence recognized by the Mab SJL2-4 should be located near residues 22-28 of the cyt c molecule.This region may be further defined when we consider that tuna cyt c heme peptide 1-65 is recognized by the Mab. In this fragment Candida krusei and yeast cyt c contain a proline instead of a lysine residue (Fig. 1). As expected, these two preparations are not recognized by the Mab.

The positive binding obtained when the wells were coated with native cyt c can be explained by a partial denaturation of the molecule upon binding to the solid phase. Since the solid phase binding gives only a qualitative indication of the capacity of the Mab to bind to a certain preparation, quantitative immunoprecipitation analysis and competitive inhibition assays were performed in solution by using a ^{125}I-radiolabeled preparation of horse apo-peptide 1-65. The association constant determined by Scatchard analysis was 9±1 x 10^{8} M.

Table I

Binding of SJL 2-4 and Mab to different cyt c preparations on solid phase[a]

Antigen	Bound CPM x 10^{-3}
Horse apo cyt c	11.2
Horse heme peptide 1-38	8.6
Horse synthetic peptide Tyr-11-25	3.0
Horse heme peptide 1-25	2.6
Horse heme peptide 5-21	0.2
Tuna heme peptide 1-65	8.8
Candida peptide 1-70	0.3
Yeast peptide 1-69	0.3
Horse cyt c	11.2
Bovine serum albumin	0.2

[a]Binding was performed as described in Material and Methods. Binding of SJL 2-4 were performed with 100 µl of 1:40 culture supernatant. This concentration of Mab is below the limit of saturation in our experimental condition. 100.000 cpm of ^{125}I-rabbit anti-mouse F(ab)'$_2$ fragment antibodies were added at each well.

```
          10                  20                  30
Horse     F V Q K C A Q C H T V E K G G K H K T G P N L H G L F G R
Tuna      ________________________N__________V_________W_________
Yeast     _ K T R _ L ________________P___V________________I_____
Candida   _ K T R ____________I _ A___A___V________________I _ S _
  krusei
```

Amino acid sequence of Horse, tuna, yeast and Candida k cytochrome c of segment 10-38.

Figure 1

When competitive inhibition assays were performed in solution with different cyt c preparations the following results were obtained (Table II). Homologous horse apo-cyt c, homologous horse apo-cyt c and homologous apo-peptide 1-65 and heme peptide 1-65 competed efficiently for the binding of ^{125}I-apo-peptide 1-65 at similar antigen concentration. On the contrary, tuna peptide 1-65, synthetic peptide Tyr-11-25 and native cytochrome c competed at much higher concentrations or not at all. This was in contrast with the results obtained by solid phase binding in which the response obtained for the three preparations was in general of the same order of magnitude as for the apo-protein. This might be due to the fact that on solid phase binding, an antibody can bind as a bivalent ligand and this can increase the overal affinity of the interaction. Support for this explanation is the capacity of peptide Tyr-11-25 coupled to ovalbumin (10 groups/ molecule) to effectively inhibit the antigen-antibody reaction in solution.

Tuna cyt c differs from horse cyt c in the region 22-28 at position 22 and 28 where two non conservative substitutions occur. Asparagine and alanine residues are substituted for a lysine and a threonine residue, respectively (Fig. 1). At present, uncertainty remains in the determination of which of the two residues of the horse cyt c molecule is part of the epitope recognized by Mab SJL2-4.

To test the specificity of the binding of SJL2-4 on Mø C57BL or Balb/c Mø were pulsed with various cyt c preparations. The antigen concentration used was 1 mg/ml since it was early found to be optimal for the activation of apo-cyt c specific T cells. Table 3 summarizes the results obtained when Mab SJL 2-4 was used.

Table II

Competitive inhibition of the binding of ^{125}I-radiolabeled horse apo-peptide 1-65 and Mab SJL 2-4[a]

Unlabeled antigen	Antigen concentration at 50% inhibition
Horse apo-cyt c	5.0×10^{-9} M
Horse apo-peptide 1-65	5.1×10^{-9} M
Horse heme peptide 1-65	5.1×10^{-9} M
Tuna heme peptide 1-65	3.5×10^{-6} M
Horse synthetic peptide Tyr-11-25 2/	2.5×10^{-5} M
Horse synthetic peptide Tyr-11-25-OVA	2.0×10^{-7} M
Horse cyt c[b]	10^{-5} M

[a]A constant amount of ^{125}I-radiolabeled horse apo-peptide 1-65 (30.000 cpm), Mab SJL 2-4 (50 ng) was selected to give approximately 50% binding of the radiolabeled antigen. Increasing amount of unlabeled preparations were added to the labeled peptide prior to addition of the Mab.The resulting mixture (200 ul total) was incubated for 2hr at room temperature and the antigen antibody complex was precipitated with PEG 6000 (13% final concentration).

[b]Horse synthetic peptide Tyr-11-25, horse peptide 81-104 and native horse cyt c did not compete at all at the concentrations indicated.

Table III

Comparison between the binding of Mab SJL 2-4 on macrophages pulsed with different peptide preparations and specificity of T-cell clone 2-16[a]

Peptides	cpm x 10^{-4b} Mø	T cell clone
Lysozyme	0.2 (–)[c]	–
Cyt c	0.4 (+)	–
Heme peptide 1-65	0.4 (+)	–
apo-cyt c	3.6 (+)	+
apo-peptide 1-65	4.4 (+)	+
synthetic peptide Tyr 11-25	0.7 (+)	+

[a]BM Mo were pulsed for 1h at 37° with 1 mg/ml of different peptide preparations, washed twice and then incubated 5 h at 37°.
[b]6 x 10^5 cpm of ^{125}I-Mab were added to 5 x 10^4 cells for 45 min at 37°. After two washings the radioactivity bound to Mo was determined by lysing the cells with 2% SDS in PBS. Standard deviation is less than 5%.
[c]The positive (+) or negative (-) binding obtained by solid phase assay is shown in parenthesis ( ).

These binding experiments showed that Mab SJL 2-4 could bind apo-cyt c,apo-peptide 1-65 and peptide Tyr-11-25. On the other hand, in contrast to solid phase binding, little binding was observed when cyt c or heme peptide 1-65 were used. Similar results were obtained with glutaraldehyde fixed Mo (data not shown). The binding data correlate well with the functional data obtained with the Balb/c clone 2-16 (Table III, Corradin et al., 1983) which were stimulated by apo protein and peptide 11-25 but not by heme peptide 1-65 and cyt c and were inhibited by the addition of Mab SJL 2-4 in the cultures (Corradin and Engers, 1984).

Time course of pulsing and effect of antigen concentration on the binding of ^{125}I-Mab SJL 2-4

Mo were pulsed for different lengths of time with apo-peptide 1-65 at 37° and were then washed twice. After 5hr incubation at 37°, ^{125}I-Mab SJL 2-4 was added. Results showed that the uptake of the cyt c peptide by Mo was a very rapid process, since 50 % of maximal binding occured already after 5 min of pulsing and a plateau was reached within 30 min (Fig. 2). Furthermore, the constant increase of ^{125}I-Mab SJL 2-4 binding as a function of increasing antigen concentration used for pulsing seemed to indicate that maximum uptake of apo-peptide 1-65 by Mo had not yet been reached, even at a concentration of 1 mg/ml (data not shown). On the other hand, at 4°, the amount of ^{125}I-Mab SJL 2-4 bound to Mo increased constantly over a period of 150 min. It should be pointed out also that little dissociation of bound ^{125}I-Mab SJL 2-4 to apo-peptide 1-65 pulsed Mo was observed at 4°. On the other hand, at 37°, about 50 % of bound ^{125}I-Mab SJL 2-4 could be displaced within 30 min with a 50 to 500 fold excess of cold Mab SJL 2-4 (data not shown). Due to these last observations, association constant was determined at 37° only.

Binding constant determination between Mab SJL 2-4 and apo-peptide 1-65

Association constant (Ka) of the interaction between Mab SJL 2-4 and apo-peptide 1-65 were determined at 37° by using increasing amounts of ^{125}I-Mab SJL 2-4.

Scatchard analysis of the binding was performed as shown in Fig. 3. It was determined that the Ka between Mab SJL 2-4 and apo-peptide 1-65 varied between 0.5 and 1.0 x 10^8 M^{-1}. It was also calculated that the number of antigenic sites varied between 1 to 2 x 10^6 per cell.

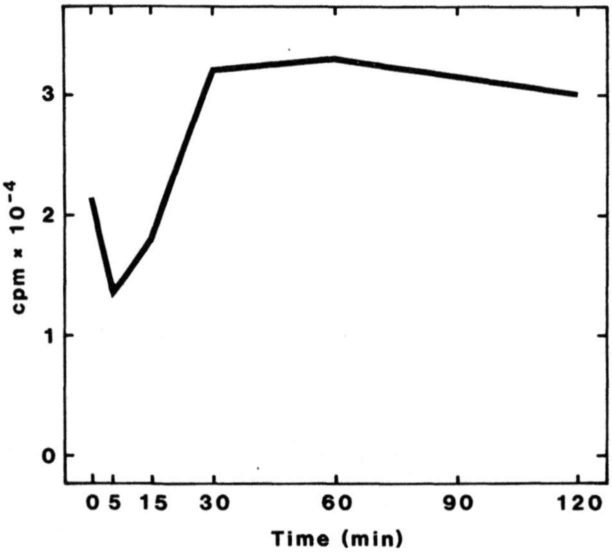

Figure 2

Kinetic of antigenic site appearance on antigen pulsed Mø.
BM Mø were pulsed with 1 mg/ml apo-peptide 1-65 for 0 to 120 min. and then washed twice. After 5 hr incubation at 37°, 5 x 10^5 cpm of ^{125}I-Mab SJL 2-4 were added to 5 x 10^4 cells for 45 min. at 37°. After two washings, the radioactivity bound to Mo was determined by lysing the cells with 2% SDS in PBS.

Mø were also fixed with glutaraldehyde before pulsing with apo-peptide 1-65. Also in this case no significant difference was observed between non treated and glutaraldehyde fixed Mø. In fact, Ka and the number of antigenic sites determined by Scatchard analysis were similar to the values obtained for not fixed Mø (Ka = 0.5 - 1 x 10^8 M^{-1}; 1-2 x 10^6 sites/Mø).

To determine if the structure of peptide was similar in solution or on Mø, kinetics parameters of the antigen-antibody reaction were determined. As shown in Table IV, the rate association constant for the reaction changed by a factor of 10^3 in the two experimental conditions used. The rate dissociation constant is also different in the two cases but one should consider the bivalency of the antibody when it reacts with the antigen on the Mø. This can decrease the rate dissociation constant by a factor or 10^2-10^3 (Karush, 1978). That the peptide 13-25 recognized by Mab SJL2-4 and the T cell clone is capable of undergoing a conformational change is provided by the circular dichroism data obtained in different solvent composition. As shown in Fig. 4 peptide 13-25 displays a higher -helical content by increasing the percentage of trifluoroethanol (TFE) as judged by the absorption at 222 and 207 nm. The percentage of -helix at 99% TFE calculated by taking the experimental value obtained at 222 nm varies from 37 to 50% depending on the value chosen as 100% heliplicity. This varies from -28.000 to 21.800 deg.cm^2dmol^{-1} for small peptides of 6-10 amino acids (Wu et al., 1981).

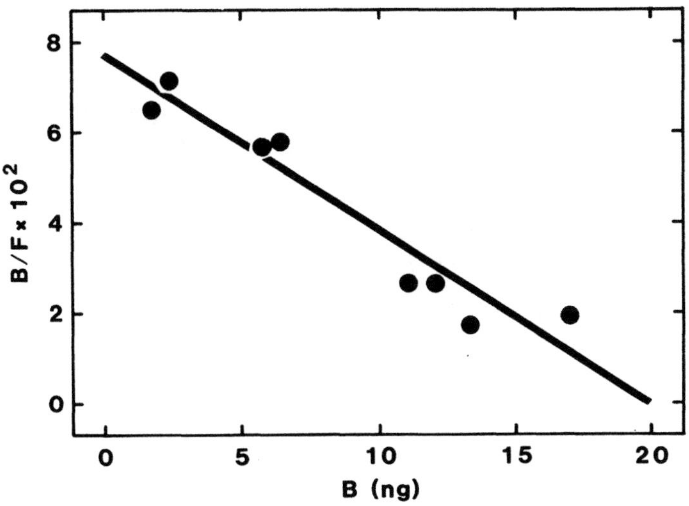

Figure 3

Association constant of the interaction between Mab SJL 2-4 antigen and pulsed Mø

BM Mø were pulsed for 1 hr at 37° with 1 mg/ml apo-peptide 1-65 and then washed twice. After 5 hr incubation at 37°, different amounts of ^{125}I-Mab SJL 2-4 in 100 ul were added to 5 x 10^4 cells for 45 min. at 37°. After two washings, the radioactivity bound to the Mø (B) and the radioactivity in supernatant (F) were determined for Scatchard analysis.

Ka = 0.6 x 10^8 M^{-1}

Number of antigenic sites/Mø = 1.8 x 10^6

Association constant and number of antigenic sites/Mø vary from 0.5 to 1.0 x 10^8 M^{-1} and 1 to 2 x 10^6 sites/Mø, respectively in the 4 experiments performed.

Table IV

Values of binding constants and K_{+1} and K_{-1} for apo-cyt c peptide 1-65 and Mab SJL2-4

Solution	$Ka(M^{-1})$	$K_{+1}(M^{-1}s^{-1})$	$K_{-1}(s^{-1})$
	$9x10^8$	$1.3x10^7$	$1.5x10^{-2}$
Macrophage	$0.7-3x10^8$	$3.5x10^3$	$10^{-4}-10^{-5}$

The association constant and on and off rate of the reaction between apo cytochrome c peptide 1-65 and Mab SJL2-4 were determined at 25°C.

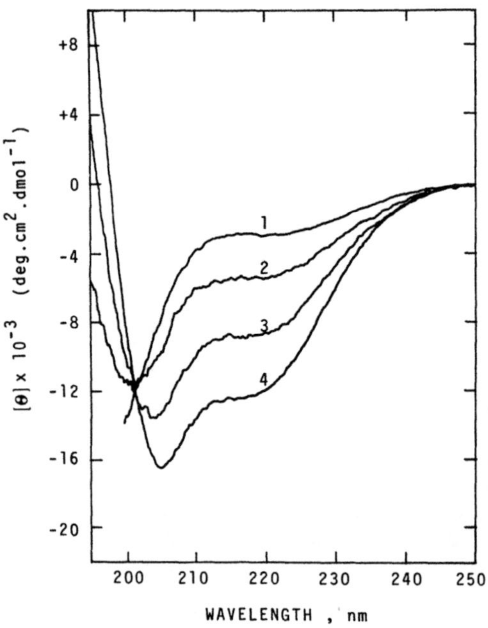

Figure 4

Far-ultraviolet circular dichroisim spectra of peptide 13-25 of horse cytochrome c.
Spectra were recordered at 25°C at the concentration of 50 ug/ml in 3 mM phosphate buffer, pH 7.0 and in the presence of 0.1 M NaCl (1), 60% (2), 80% (3), 99% (4) of trifluoroethanol.

Time course of expression of antigen on Mo cell surface

To test the possibility that antigen was taken up by Mo and reexpressed at a later time as seen in other experimental systems (Chesnut et al., 1982; Allen et al., 1984), the effect of trypsin after antigen pulsing was investigated at different times. As summarized in Fig. 5, binding of ^{125}I-Mab SJL 2-4 was detected over a period of 50 hr and the half-time of antigenic disappearance was about 15-20 hr. On the contrary, trypsinized Mo did not bind any ^{125}I-Mab SJL 2-4 over a period of 50 hr indicating that antigen determinants were not reexpressed in this

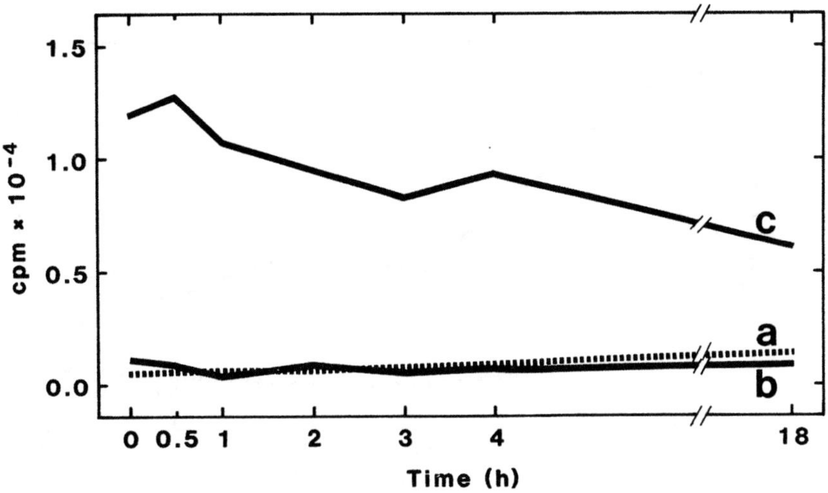

Figure 5

Kinetics of ^{125}I-Mab SJL 2-4 binding on Mo pulsed with different peptide preparations.
BM Mo were pulsed for 1 hr at 37° with 1 mg/ml of either lysozyme (a), cyt c (b) or apo-peptide 1-65 (c) and then washed twice. 2.5 x 10^5 cpm of ^{125}I-Mab SJL 2-4 were added to 5 x 10^4 cells for 45 min at 37° at different time as indicated in the figure. After two washings, radioactivity bound to Mo was determined by lysing the cells with 2% SDS in PBS.

period of time (Fig. 6). It is worth noting that trypsinization did not abolish the Mo capacity to bind apo-peptide 1-65. In fact, the degree of ^{125}I-Mab SJL 2-4 binding to Mo pulsed with antigen after trypsinization was similar to that observed for untreated Mo (data not shown).

Similarly, studies were performed on native cyt c pulsed MØ to determine whether or not the Mo could generate the antigenic site seen by Mab SJL 2-4. MØ pulsed with either lysozyme, cyt c or apo-peptide 1-65 were subjected to ^{125}I-Mab SJL 2-4 binding over a period of 18hr. In the case of cyt c, binding of Mab SJL 2-4 remained near the background level (lysozyme) while apo-peptide 1-65 pulsed Mo showed a slow decrease of ^{125}I-Mab SJL 2-4 binding with a halftime of antigen disappearance of about 15-20hr as previously shown in Fig. 5.

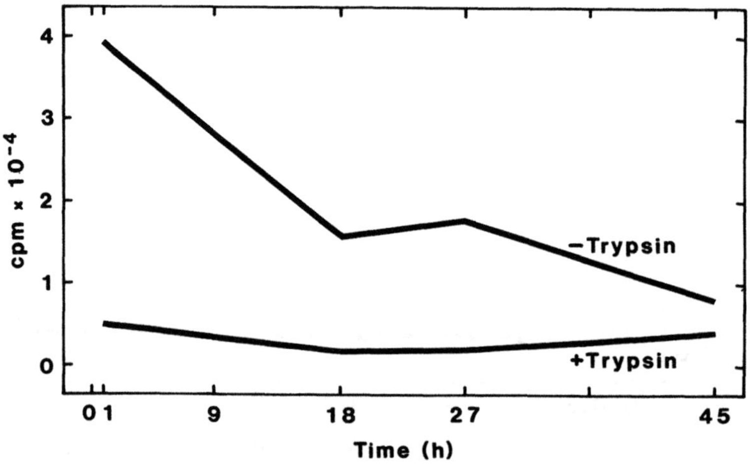

Figure 6

^{125}I-Mab SJL 2-4 binding on trypsinized-antigen pulsed MØ. BM MØ were pulsed for 1 hr at 37° with 1 mg/ml apo-peptide 1-65. After two washings, cells were treated with 50 ug/ml trypsin for 15 min. at 37°. Tryptic activity was quenched by adding FCS to final concentration of 10%. 5 x 10^5 cpm of ^{125}I-Mab SJL 2-4 were added to 5 x 10^4 cells for 45 min. at 37° at different time as indicated in the figure. After two washings, the radioactivity bound to the MØ was determined by lysing the cells with 2% SDS in PBS.

These negative results obtained with native cyt c were not due to a low uptake of native protein since cyt c was taken up by MØ to the same extent as apo-cyt c as judged by using radiolabeled preparations of the two forms.

The effect of chloroquine treatment before and after antigen pulsing was also determined. As shown in Table V, no difference in the bound cpm was found between the two experimented procedures.

Table V

Effect of chloroquine on the binding of ^{125}I-Mab SJL 2-4 to apo-peptide 1-65 pulsed Mø

Pretreatment[a] and pulse	Incubation[b]	cpm x 10^{-4}[c]
−	−	1.7 ± 0.1
−	+	2.2 ± 0.1
+	−	2.2 ± 0.1
+	+	2.3 ± 0.2

[a]BMMø were treated for 1hr either with (+) or without (-) 0.1 mM chloroquine prior to 1hr pulsing with 1 mg/ml of apo-peptide 1-65.
[b]Mø were washed twice and then incubated 1.5 hr in the presence (+) of the drug.
[c]5 x 10^5 cpm of ^{125}I-Mab SJL 2-4 were added to 5 x 10^4 Mø for 45 min at 37°. After two washings, the radioactivity bound to Mø was determined by lysing the cells with 2% SDS in PBS. Control cpm (no antigen) was 0.1 x 10^4 cpm/5 x 10^4 Mø.

All these experiments indicated that very little if any internalization of the antigen was needed under our experimental conditions either during or after pulsing for the expression of the antigenic determinant 23-28.

DISCUSSION

The results presented here indicate that the Mab SJL 2-4 recognizes the denatured horse cyt c molecule with an association constants of 9 x 10^8 M^{-1}. In particular, it recognizes heme or apo peptide 1-65, heme peptide 1-25, apo-peptides Tyr-11-25 but not heme peptides 5-21. This suggests that the sequence recognized by the Mab is located in the C-terminal segment of peptide 11-25. Yeast and Candida krusei cyt c peptide 1-69 and 1-70 in which a proline residue is substituted for a lysine in position 25 do not bind to the Mab. If we consider that an antigen determinant is comprised of 4 to 6 amino acid residues (Sela, 1969), we suggest that the sequence important for the binding is located around segment 22-28 of the horse molecule. The inhibition studies performed in solution with tuna apo cyt c would support the idea that either residues Lys 22 or Thr 28 or both present in the horse molecule (Asn and Val in tuna cyt c) are part of the combining site since a 1000 fold decrease in binding is observed when the tuna preparation was used.

It is interesting to observe that recognition of horse peptide Tyr-11-25 occurs only when the peptide is bound to a solid phase. In solution, little or no inhibition of the binding between ^{125}I-horse apo-peptide 1-65 and the Mab is observed when the peptide was used as inhibitor.

It is, therefore, conceivable that on solid phase the two combining sites of the antibody molecule are not totally independent such that the overal binding affinity is now increased which would favor cross-reacting peptides of low affinity (Karush, 1978). The data obtained with the peptide coupled to ovalbumin lend in fact support to the idea that bivalency of the interaction is important to increase the overall binding affinity.

In the case of cyt c, partial denaturation of the molecule upon binding to the polyvinyl plate may be responsible for the recognition of the two Mab. All these cases demonstrate that data obtained from solid phase binding while very practical may not fully apply to in solution conditions.

The binding specificity of SJL2-4 Mab on antigen pulsed Mø indicate that a set of peptides similar to those recognized on solid phase is seen by the Mab. In particular it binds to peptide Tyr-11-25. Two exceptions are worth commenting. A very low degree of binding was observed when native cyt c or heme peptide 1-65 were used to pulse the Mø. One explanation is that degradation of heme peptide 1-65 and cyt c takes place and no peptides recognized by Mab SJL2-4 are then expressed on the cell surface of the Mø. Alternatively, the presence of a hydrophobic group like the heme may alter the interaction with the cell surface. For example, the heme group might penetrate the lipid bilayer rendering the adjacent segment 22-28 inaccessable for binding. On the other hand, in the case of cyt c little or no degradation or denaturation may occur upon interaction of the protein with the Mø. That this might be the case was revealed by the binding of Mab 2.61 specific for the native molecule to cyt c pulsed Mø (Demotz and Corradin, unpublished results).

Similar pattern of reactivity shown for Mab SJL2-4 were also obtained in functional studies. In fact, a T cell clone whose specificity is similar to that observed for Mab SJL2-4 (Corradin et al., 1983) is activated by apo-cyt c peptides but not by heme containing peptides or cyt c.

The capacity of the Mab to recognize peptide Tyr-11-25 on solid phase or membrane bound but not in solution has a bearing on the possibility to purify Mø processed antigenic peptides. For example, the digestion of peptide 1-65 may result in the formation of T-cell antigenic peptides which do not contain the full antigenic site recognized by SJL2-4 as is the case of Tyr-11-25 peptide and would be therefore impossible to immunoprecipitate them.

The binding constant of the interaction of apo-cyt c 1-65 and SJL2-4 is similar when the antigen is in solution or on membrane bound. But the kinetics parameters indicate that the similiratiy of the binding constant is due to different reasons; the decrease of the on-rate for the membrane bound antigen is accompanied by a decrease of the off-rate reaction. This latter is probably due to the bivalency of the interaction which occurs when the antigen is membrane bound. The on-rate association constants in solution and on Mø indicate that the antigen is most likely in different conformations. A support for this explanation is provided by circular dichroism studies. In fact, an increase of the -helical content was observed for peptide 13-25 (which is equally potent in eleciting a T cell response as peptide 11-25) upon increasing hydrophobicity of the solvent.

The capacity of the Mab SJL2-4 to block T-cell functions in numerous clones is most likely due to the high affinity interaction with the membrane bound antigen. In fact, another Mab Cyt-1-59, which recognizes the same site on apo-cyt c but with a different affinity (2×10^7 M^{-1}), is not effective of inhibiting T cell functions (Corradin et al., 1984).

Therefore, the previous failure of inhibiting antigen specific T-cell proliferation or antigen (virus) specific T cell killing by anti-antigen antibodies may be due to several different factors:

1) lack of knowledge of the exact segment recognized by the antibodies;

2) low binding affinity of the antibody for the membrane bound antigen.

If in fact a structural change occurs when antigen interacts with antigen presenting cells, it is likely that the antibody raised against the antigen in solution may recognize the membrane bound antigen poorly except in certain exceptions like ours.

The data regarding the appearance and disappearance of the antigenic site on MØ indicate that the interaction with the membrane is a fast process and while its desappearance is a slow process with a half-time of disappearance of about 24 h. Both processes are likely to be related to structural features of the peptide under investigation. But they are not mediated by the presence of class II molecules since class II negative BW5412 thymoma cells behave in a similar fashion as BM MØ. In addition, the high number of sites detected (0.5 to 4.0 x 10^6) is in much greater number than the number of class II molecule present on BM macrophages estimated to be 10-50 x 10^3 from flow cell activated cell sorter). Therefore, we would like to suggest that the first requisite of an antigenic peptide is its capacity to interact with a cell membrane independent on the presence of class II molecules. This interaction is necessary to keep the antigen attach on the presenting cells and eventually it will be able to interact with class II molecules (Babbitt et al, 1985; Babbitt et al., 1986; Buus et al., 1986). The interaction with the cell surface may be facilitated either by the capacity of the peptide to form amphiphatic structures as suggested by De Lisi and Berzofsky or by the presence in the peptide of hydrophobic segment as suggested by Corradin et al. (1987). This would explain also the long half time of disappearance of the peptide from the cell surface and could represent an advantage for the immune system to keep antigen on the cell surface for long time to facilitate the triggering of the immune system.

In agreement with this observations are the results obtained when membrane bound peptides are compared to those found in the supernatant (Demotz and Corradin, unpublished results). In general, the membrane bound peptides are eluted of higher concentration of acetonitrile than the peptides in the supernatant indicating a higher hydrophobicity of the former ones. Thus, one can envision that when a protein is pinocytosed by an antigen presenting cells, peptides of different sizes and compositions are formed and only those that can effectively interact with the membrane of the organelles where the hydrolysis occurs will be retained and reexposed on the cell surface. During this process, chemical modification of the antigenic peptide could occur as suggested by Demotz et al. (1984) and recently by Falo et al. (1986). Once on the cell surface, the peptides could then interact with class II molecules either prior, as suggested by Babbit et al. (1985 and 1986) or during recognition by antigen specific T-cell receptors.

REFERENCES

Allen, P. M., Beller, D. I., Braun, J., and Unanue, E. R., 1984, The handling of Listeria monocytogenes by macrophages: The search for an immunogenic molecule in antigen presentation, J. Immunol.,132: 323-331.

Atherton, E., Logan, C. J., and Sheppard, R. C., 1979, Peptide synthesis. Part 2. Procedure for solid phase synthesis using N - fluorenylmethoxycarbonylamino acids on polyamide supports. Synthesis of substance P and of acyl carrier 65-74 decapeptide, Biorganic Chem., 8:351-370.

Babbitt, B. P., Allen, P. M., Matsueda, G., Haber, E., and Unanue, E. R., 1985, Binding of immunogenic peptides to Ia histocompatibility molecules. Nature, 317:359-361.

Babbitt, B. P., Matsueda, G., Haber, E., Unanue, R. R., and Allen, P. M., 1985, Antigenic competition at the level of peptide-Ia binding. Proc. Natl. Acad. Sci. USA, 83:4509-4513.

Buus, S., Colon, S., Smith, C., Freed, J. H., Miles, C., and Grey, H. M., 1986, Interaction between a "processes" ovalbumin peptide and Ia molecules, Proc. Natl. Acad. Sci. USA, 83:3968-3971.

Chesnut, R. W., Colon, S. M., and Grey, H. M., 1982, Requirements for the processing of antigens by antigen-presenting B cells. I. Functional comparison of B cell tumors and macrophages, J. Immunol., 129:2382-2388.

Corradin, G., and Harbury, H. A., 1970, Cleavage of cytochrome c with cyanogen bromide. Biochim. Biophys. Acta, 221:489-496.

Corradin, G., Etlinger, E. H., and Chiller, J. M., 1977, Lymphocyte specificity to protein antigens. I. Characterization of the antigen-induced in vitro T cell-dependent proliferative response with lymph node cells from primed mice. J. Immunol., 119:1048-1053.

Corradin, G., Juillerat, M. A., Vita, C., and Engers, H. D., 1983, Fine specificity of a Balb/c T cell clone directed against beef apo-cytochrome c. Mol. Immunol., 20:763-768.

Corradin, G., and Engers, H. D., 1984. Inhibition of antigen induced T-cell clone proliferation by antigen-specific antibodies. Nature, 308:547-548.

Corradin, G., Juillerat, M. A., and Engers, H. D., 1984, Differential effects of two anti-apo-cytochrome c-specific monoclonal antibodies on the function of apo-cytochrome c-specific murine T cell clones. J. Immunol., 133:2915-2919.

Corradin, G. P., Wallace, C. J. A., Proudfoot, A. E. I., and Baumhüter, S., 1987, Murine T cell response specific for cytochrome c, "CRC", Ed. J.A. Berzofsky and E. Sercarz, (in press).

De Lisi, C., and Berzofsky, J. A., 1985, T cell antigenic site tend to be amphipathic structures, Proc. Natl. Acad. Sci. USA, 82:7048-7052.

Demotz, S., Mozzarelli, A., Baumhüter, S., and Corradin, G., 1984, Biochemical aspects of antigen degradation and presentation by macrophages, in Abstracts "6th European Immunology Meeting", Interlaken, pp. 370.

Falo, L. D., Benacerraf, Jr. B., and Rock, K. L., 1986, Phospholipase treatment of accessory cells that have been exposed to antigen selectively inhibits antigen-specific Ia-restricted, but not allo-specific, stimulation of T lymphocytes. Proc. Natl. Sci. USA, 83: 6994-6997.

Fanger, M. W., and Harbury, H. A., 1965, Trifluoroacetylated cytochrome c. Biochemistry, 4:2541-2545.

Fisher, W. R. H., Taniuchi, H., and Anfinsen, C. B., 1973, On the role of the heme in the formation of the structure of cytochrome c. J. Biol. Chem., 248:3188-3195.

Harbury, H. A., and Loach, P. A., 1960, Oxidation-linked proton functions in heme octa- and undecapeptides from mammalian cytochrome c, J. Biol. Chem., 2345:3640-3645.

Karush, F., 1978, Immunoglobulins, "Comprehensive Immunology", G. Litman and R.A. Good, eds, Plenum Publishing Corp. New York, Vol. V, pp 85-116.

Koehler, G., and Milstein, C., 1975, Continous cultures of fused cells secreting antibodies of predefined specificity. Nature, 256:495-497.

Margoliash, E., and Wasalek, O. F., 1967, Cytochrome c from vertebrate and invertebrate sources, in: "Methods in Enzymology", R. W. Estabrook and M. E. Pullman, eds, Academic Press, Inc., New York, Vol. 10, p. 339.

Meerpohl, H.-G., Lohmann-Matthes, M.-L., and Fischer, H., 1976, Studies on the activation of mouse bone marrow derived macrophages by the macrophage cytotoxicity factor, Eur. J. Immunol., 6:213-217.

Parikh, I., March, S., Cuatrecasas, P., 1974, "Methods in enzymology", W. B., Jakoby and M. Wilchek, eds, Academic Press, New York, Vol. 34, pp 77-102.

Pincus, M. R., Gerewitz, F., Schwartz, R. H., and Sheraga, H. A., 1983, Correlation between the conformation of cytochrome c peptides and their stimulatory activity in a T-lymphocyte proliferation assay, Proc. Natl. Acad. Sci. USA, 80:3297-3300.

Sela, M., 1969, Antigenicity: Some molecular aspects, Science, 166: 1365-1374.

Shimonkevitz, R., Kappler, J., Marrack, P., and Grey, H., 1983, Antigen recognition by H-2-restricted T cells. I. Cell-free antigen processing. J. Exp. Med., 158:303-316.

Shimonkevitz, R., Colon, S., Kappler, J. W., Marrack, P., Grey, H. M., 1984, Antigen recognition by H-2 restricted T cell. II. A tryptic ovalbumin peptide that substitues for processed antigen. J. Immunol., 4:2067-2074.

Wu, C. S. C., Ikeda, K., and Yang, J. T., 1981, Ordered conformation of polypeptides and proteins in acidic dodecyl sulfate solution, Biochemistry, 20:566-570.

ANTIGEN PROCESSING AND PRESENTATION AT A MOLECULAR LEVEL

Paul M. Allen and Emil R. Unanue

Department of Pathology, Washington University School of Medicine, St. Louis, Missouri 63110

The recognition of antigen by helper T-cells through their antigen specific receptor has been the center of intense investigation by many different researchers. Helper T-cells recognize antigen in association with a class II molecule on the surface of an antigen presenting cell. Unlike B-cells which generally recognize determinants found in the native form of the antigen, most T-cells recognize a non-native form of the antigen. It is this conversion of antigen from a native form to the form recognized by T-cells which has been operationally defined as antigen processing. Over the past four years, we have developed a system which utilizes the antigen hen egg-white lysozyme to determine at a molecular level 1) what antigen processing is, 2) how the determinant recognized by the T-cell is formed, and 3) what precisely is the ligand of the T-cell receptor. In this manuscript, we would like to initially review the concept of antigen processing at a molecular level and then present our results on the formation and recognition by the T-cell receptor of an antigenic determinant of HEL.

Antigen Processing

When the antigen processing requirements of two HEL specific T-cell hybridomas were examined, an interesting observation was obtained in that the definition of antigen processing was different for these two T-cell hybridomas. They both used the I-A^k molecule as their restriction element and recognized the same peptide of HEL, residues 52 to 61. However, one T-cell hybridoma, 2A11, required processing to involve a proteolytic cleavage of HEL, whereas the other T-cell hybridoma, 3A9, only required unfolding of the polypeptide chain for processing (Allen and Unanue, 1984). Thus the definition of antigen processing differed for the two T-cell hybridomas, being proteolytic cleavage for one and simply unfolding for the other.

The requirement for processing has been shown for a variety of antigens including lysozyme, myoglobin, cytochrome C, and ovalbumin. For all of these antigens, the native molecules required processing before recognition by the T-cell receptor. Myoglobin, in a similar fashion to HEL, only required unfolding of the polypeptide chain for processing (Berzofsky, 1986). All of these antigens are globular proteins and it is not surprising that they needed processing. One can define antigen processing as the biochemical changes a protein antigen must undergo to allow it to associate with an Ia molecule and to form the determinant which is recognized by the T-cell receptor. With this definition, it is conceivable that certain protein antigens can directly interact with an Ia molecule and thus not need any processing.

We wanted to examine another antigen which was not one of the small globular proteins used previously in the processing studies. The antigen we chose was human fibrinogen (hFib). As in the HEL system, we generated hFib specific T-cell hybridomas as our functional probes. When the processing requirements were determined for two of the T-cell hybridomas, the surprising finding was obtained that hFib did not require any processing (Lee, Matsueda, and Allen, Manuscript in preparation). This was demonstrated by the ability of prefixed antigen presenting cells or chloroquine treated cells to present hFib. Further evidence that strongly supported the idea that hFib did not require any processing was that 1) it was a molecule of native molecular weight (340,000 kd) which was stimulating the T-cells, 2) protease inhibitors (PMSF, DFP, Aprotinin, Leupeptin) did not prevent the presentation of hFib, and 3) the presentation of hFib to the T-cells could occur in serum free or protein free conditions. Therefore, it appears that the hFib molecule does not require any antigen processing and thus can directly interact with an Ia molecule. To further localize the determinant being recognized by the T-cell hybridomas on the hFib molecule, isolated α, β, and γ chains of hFib were tested for their ability to stimulate the T-cell hybridomas. Only the α chains could stimulate, which localized the determinant to this chain. The plasmin digestion fragment of hFib,

D_2E, did not stimulate the T-cells, which further localized the determinant to the carboxy terminal half of the α chain. Upon examining the structure of hFib, one sees the carboxy terminal portion of the α chain does not have a defined secondary structure. Since it is this portion which contains the determinant recognized by the T-cell hybridomas, one can easily envision that there is enough freedom in the conformation of this portion of the α chain that it could directly interact with the Ia molecule.

By examining the antigen processing requirements of HEL and hFib, we have seen that antigen processing can only be defined in terms of the antigen one is studying and the T-cells one is using for the functional readout. We would like to propose that antigen processing requirements can be divided into three groups from the data which is currently available (Table 1). Group I contains antigens which can directly interact with an Ia molecule and do not need any processing, with hFib being an example. Group II contains antigens for which processing is simply unfolding the polypeptide chain, an example being intact denatured HEL, CM-HEL. Finally, Group III, contains antigens which have to be proteolytic cleaved, an example being the determinant HEL(46-61). Thus, it seems very unlikely that a single molecular definition of antigen processing will emerge. The definition of antigen processing will depend upon the antigen and the T-cells studied, and will range from no changes required to proteolytic cleavage.

Table 1. Antigens and Antigenic Determinants Classified by their Processing Requirements

	Processing Requirement	Example
Group I	None	Fibrinogen
Group II	Unfolding	CM-HEL
Group III	Proteolytic Cleavage	HEL(46-61)

CM-HEL, reduced and carboxy-methylated hen egg-white lysozyme; HEL(46-61), tryptic fragment of hen egg-white lysozyme containing residues 46-61.

Dissection of an Immunogenic Peptide

Although most T cells recognized a processed form of the antigen, the precise determinant being recognized and how this determinant was actually formed was mostly unknown. Using the HEL system, we have examined in detail the determinant recognized by two HEL specific T-cell hybridomas which is composed of the peptide HEL(46-61) and an I-A^k molecule (Allen, Strydom, and Unanue, 1984, Allen et al., 1985). We have recently reported on a direct association between a purified I-A^k molecule and HEL(46-61) (Babbitt et al. 1985). Using equilibrium dialysis, we ascertained that the binding was saturable and had a K_D of 2μM. This was the first direct demonstration that an immunogenic peptide and a class II molecule could directly associate and strongly supported the theory that an antigen and an Ia molecule interacted and that this complex was then recognized by the T-cell receptor.

During the course of this investigation, we identified a series of analogue peptides of HEL(46-61) which could not stimulate the T-cells (Table 2). We then ascertained if these non-stimulatory peptides could act as antagonists by competing for the functional presentation of HEL(46-61). The two non-stimulatory peptides we examined were desTyr^{53}HEL(49-69) and Phe^{56}HEL(50-61). Both of these peptides were able to compete for the presentation of HEL(46-61), whereas an unrelated peptide did not compete. We then determined at what level this competition was occurring by using the equilibrium dialysis binding system. Both of these non-stimulatory peptides were able to compete for the binding of HEL(46-61) to I-A^k (Babbitt et al., 1986). By using these non-stimulatory analogues, we were able to demonstrate antigenic competition and show that this competition was occurring at the level of binding to I-A^k molecule.

Table 2. Dissection of HEL(52-61)

52	53	54	55	56	57	58	59	60	61
Asp	Tyr	Gly	Ile	Leu	Gln	Ile	Asn	Ser	Arg
Ia	T	-	-	T	T	Ia	-	-	Ia

The amino acid sequence of the immunogenic peptide HEL(52-61) and the assignment of each of the residues. Ia, refers to residues which contact the Ia molecule; T, refers to residues which contact the T-cell receptor; and -, refers to spacer residues.

Also, during this series of experiments, we were able to identify two amino acid residues which were being recognized by the T-cell receptor, those being Tyr^{53} and Leu^{56} (Table 2). Peptides which contained substitutions at these positions were nonstimulatory, but were still able to bind to I-A^k. Therefore, these substitutions must have affected the recognition of the peptide by the T-cell. For a peptide to be immunogenic, we reasoned that it must possess amino acid residues which contact the T-cell receptor and different amino acid residues which contact the Ia molecule. There would also be residues whose side chains are not involved in either function, and are therefore acting as spacer residues. To examine each of the residues in the shortest immunogenic peptide, HEL(52-61), we generated a series of peptides which contained single Ala substitutions at each of the 10 positions (Allen et al., Manuscript in preparation). These peptides were first tested for their ability to stimulate the T-cells. We found that at three positions, we could substitute an Ala residue and retain the ability to stimulate the T-cells, these were positions 54, 55, and 59. Using a series of peptides which contained deletions of internal residues, we found that we could remove the Ser^{60} residue and still maintain an active peptide. Thus, we had identified 4 residues which we have labelled as spacer residues in that their side chains were not involved in either contacting Ia or the T-cell receptor. Those residues were Gly^{54}, Ile^{55}, Asn^{59}, and Ser^{60}. Next we took the Ala substituted peptides which did not stimulate and tested them in the functional competition assay. The rationale was that these peptides were non-stimulatory due to either the loss of a T-cell contact residue or an Ia contact residue. If a peptide could compete for the functional presentation of HEL(46-61), then we reasoned that it could still bind to Ia, and that the residue at the position of the Ala substitution was contacting the T-cell receptor. Conversely, if the peptide could not compete, then the position of the Ala substitution must be a residue which contacted the Ia molecule. We had previously identified Tyr^{53} and Leu^{56} as T-cell contact residues and we confirmed these positions in the competition experiments. We also identified a third residue which contacts the T cell receptor, that being Gln^{57}. We also identified the three amino acids whose side chains were contacting the Ia molecule, Asp^{52}, Ile^{58}, and Arg^{61}. Thus, by this analysis, we were able to identify the contribution of each of the 10 positions in the peptide recognized by the HEL specific T-cell hybridomas. Three residues Tyr^{53}, Leu^{56}, and Gln^{57} contact the T-cell receptor, three residues Asp^{52}, Ile^{58}, and Arg^{61} contact the Ia molecule and 4 residues, Gly^{54}, Ile^{55}, Asn^{59}, and Ser^{60} were spacer residues (Table 2).

We also examined the specificity of the recognition of two of the T-cell contact residues, Tyr^{53} and Leu^{56}. Leu^{56} is the only residue which differs from the corresponding sequence in mouse lysozyme, and therefore is responsible for the "foreignness" and the specificity of this peptide. We then tested a series of peptides which examined the side chain specificity. For both the 2A11 and 3A9 T-cell hybridomas, we found tremendous specificity in the recognition. The wild type residue is a Leu and simply changing the branch point of the side chain with an Ile or a nor-Leu completely abated the ability of the resulting peptides to stimulate (Figure 1). Thus, the recognition of the Leu^{56} side chain is very specific, reminiscent of an antibody molecule. We also examined the specificity of the recognition at position 53 and found that the specificity depended upon which T-cell we used (Figure 2). The 3A9 T-cells responded to a variety of substitutions and derivatives, but it always required some type of ring structure. The 2A11 cells would only respond to the wild type residue, a Tyr. It appears then that the recognition of Tyr^{53} is not as restricted as the Leu^{56} and depends upon the T-cell used. We are currently examining the Gln^{57} residue for the specificity and we expect it to be similar to the Tyr^{53}.

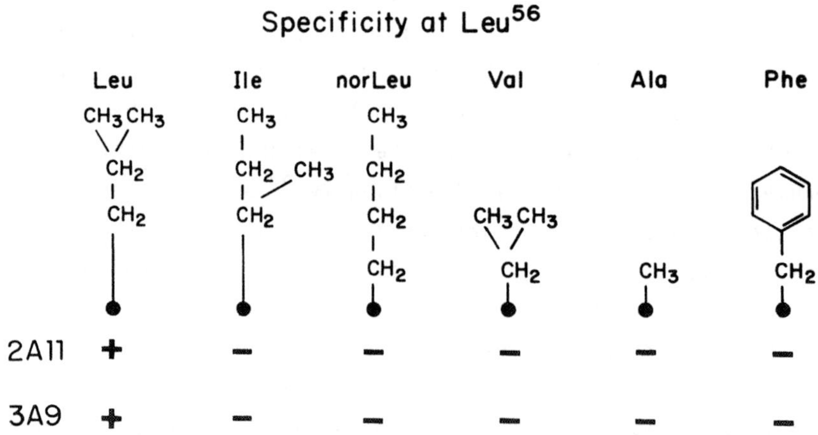

Figure 1. Specificity of the side chain recognition at position 56. The structure of the side chain of the amino acid resides at position 56 in a series of analogues of HEL (52-61) is shown. The ability of each of these single substituted peptides to stimulate either the 2A11 or 3A9 T cell hybridomas is shown. A "+" indicates a stimulatory peptide, whereas a "-" indicates a non-stimulatory peptide.

Specificity at Tyr^{53}

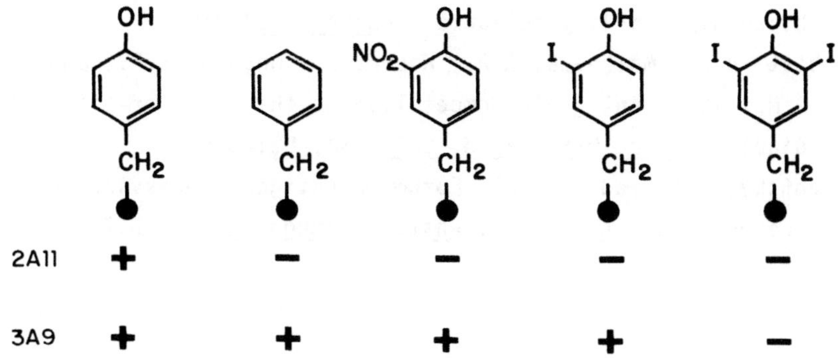

Figure 2. Specificity of the side chain recognition at position 53. The structure of the side chain of the amino acid residue at position 53 in a series of analogues of HEL (52-61) is shown. The ability of each of these single substituted peptides to stimulate either the 2A11 or 3A9 T-cell hybridomas is shown with a "+" and a "-" indicating a stimulatory and a non-stimulatory peptide respectively.

From this work we have shown a direct association between an immunogenic peptide and an Ia molecule with a K_D of 2 μM. Using several non-stimulating analogues we have also demonstrated functional competion and have shown that this competition is occurring at the level of binding to the Ia molecule. Through the use of the binding and competition assays we have now been able to completely dissect an immunogenic peptide, identifying the residues which contact the T cell receptor and those which contact the Ia molecule.

References

Allen, P.M., and Unanue, E.R., 1984, Differential requirement for antigen processing by macrophages for lysozyme-specific T cell hybridomas, J. Immunol., 132:1077.

Allen, P.M., Strydom, D.J., and Unanue, E.R., 1984, Processing of lysozyme by macrophages: Identification of the determinant recognized by two T cell hybridomas, Proc. Natl. Acad. Sci. USA, 81:2489

Allen, P.M., Matsueda, G.R., Haber, E., and Unanue, E.R., 1985, Specificity of the T cell receptor: Two different determinants are generated by the same peptide and the I-A^k molecule, J. Immunol., 135:368.

Babbitt, B.P., Allen, P.M., Matsueda, G.R., Haber, E., and Unanue, E.R., 1985, The binding of immunogenic peptides to Ia histocompatibility molecules, Nature, 317:359.

Babbitt, B.P., Matsueda, G.R., Haber, E., Unanue, E.R., and Allen, P.M., 1986, Antigenic Competition at the Level of the Peptide-I-A Binding, Proc. Natl. Acad. Sci. USA, 83:4509.

Berzofsky, J.A. (ed.), 1986, Forum on Antigen Processing and Presentation, Ann. Inst. Pasteur/Immunology, 137D:297.

THE ROLE OF SURFACE IMMUNOGLOBULIN IN THE PROCESSING AND PRESENTATION OF ANTIGEN

Lisa A. Casten and Susan K. Pierce

Department of Biochemistry, Molecular Biology and Cell Biology
Northwestern University
Evanston, IL

INTRODUCTION

Helper T-cell responses to the globular protein antigens studied to date, require the uptake and intracellular processing of the protein by an Ia expressing antigen presenting cell (APC). Processing yields a peptide fragment, containing the T-cell's antigenic determinant, which is displayed on the APC surface, where it is recognized by the helper T-cell in conjunction with Ia. Most cells which express Ia are competent APC, including macrophages, dendritic cells and B cells (Unanue, 1984). Since, with the exception of B cells, APC do not express immune receptors for antigen, processing can presumably be initiated by a nonspecific, fluid phase pinocytosis of the antigen. However, recent studies have indicated that B cells which bind antigen, or anti-Ig acting as a surrogate antigen, are far more effective APC, capable of maximally activating T-cells requiring many fold less antigen and fewer cells as compared to nonspecific B cells. The evidence suggests that the B-cell surface immunoglobulin serves to concentrate antigen for subsequent processing and/or to signal the cell to increase the level of activities required for its processing and presentation functions. However, the molecular mechanisms by which surface Ig serves to augment presentation remains largely unknown. The results of experiments described here indicate that the surface Ig is not uniquely suited to facilitate antigen processing or presentation, and that antigen artificially bound to other B-cell surface proteins, namely Class I and Class II, is also efficiently presented. In these cases, enhanced antigen presentation appears to be solely a function of the ability of the B cell surface structures to concentrate antigen for processing.

The globular protein antigen, pigeon cytochrome c(Pc) is a well characterized protein for which the major T cell antigenic determinant has been mapped to the carboxyl-terminal 10 amino acid residues. The T-cell response to Pc requires the processing and presentation of the antigen. Indeed, when APC functions are blocked by treatment with paraformaldehyde or lysosomotropic agents, the native protein antigen fails to stimulate while the peptide fragment is fully active. We report here that native Pc, covalently coupled to antibodies specific for either Ig, Class I(K^k), or Class II(I-A^k) are very effective antigens, stimulating a Pc-specific, I-E^k restricted T-cell hybrid at concentrations 50-200-fold lower than that required for P*c* alone, for P*c* coupled to antibodies which do not bind B cell surface structures, or for unmodified P*c* and antibodies. The P*c*-antibody conjugates required processing, as demonstrated by their inability to activate the P*c*-specific T cell hybrid when paraformaldehyde-fixed B-cells are used as APC. P*c* coupled to monovalent fragments of anti-Ig antibodies was nearly as effective as P*c* coupled to bivalent antibodies, indicating that phenomena mediated by bivalent binding, such as patching and capping of the surface Ig, were not required for enhanced antigen presentation.

RESULTS AND DISCUSSION

P*c* was thiolated (Jue, et al.,1978) and coupled to purified monoclonal antibodies specific for K^k(HB13), I-A^k(TIB 93), I-A^s (HB4), and to rabbit anti-mouse Ig antibodies, nonspecific rabbit Ig, or monovalent Fab fragments of rabbit anti-mouse Ig antibodies, using the heterobifunctional reagent m-maleimidobenzoyl-N-hydroxysuccinimide ester (O'Sullivan, et al., 1979). Conjugates were separated from unmodified cytochrome *c* by molecular sieve chromatography and the concentration of P*c* in the conjugates was determined by absorbance at 410nm. In each case, an average of one P*c* molecule was coupled to each antibody. The conjugates were tested for their ability to activate the I-E^k-restricted P*c*-specific T cell hybrid, TPc9.1, to IL-2 secretion when purified splenic B cells(H-2^k) were used as APC. P*c* conjugated to antibodies which bind to B cell surface I-A^k, K^k, or Ig are more effective antigens, as compared to P*c* alone or to P*c* conjugated to antibodies which do not bind the B cell surface, namely nonspecific rabbit Ig or antibodies specific for the Ia of a different MHC haplotype, I-A^s(Table 1). In addition, the monovalent fragments of rabbit anti-mouse Ig when coupled to P*c* were as effective as the divalent anti-Ig antibodies coupled to P*c* (data not shown).

Table 1. Activation of a P*c*-Specific T-Cell Hybrid by P*c*-Antibody Conjugates Presented by B Cells[1]

Conjugated Antibody: Antigen	[Pc]μM required 50% Max. Response	Unconjugated Antibody: Antigen	[Pc]μM required 50% Max. Response
P*c*	1.0	P*c*	1.4
P*c*-Anti-K^k	0.08	P*c* + Anti-K^k	1.1
P*c*-Anti-I-A^k	0.05	P*c* + Anti-I-A^k	2.0
P*c*-Anti-Ig	0.003	P*c* + Anti-Ig	2.0
P*c*-Anti-I-A^s	0.7	P*c* + Anti-I-A^s	0.9
P*c*-non-specific-Ig	>2.0	P*c* + non-specific-Ig	0.9

[1] TPc9.1 cells (5 x 10^4) were cultured in 0.2ml with purified splenic B cells (2 x 10^5) and graded concentrations of P*c* or P*c*-antibody conjugates (left panel) or graded concentrations of P*c* and unconjugated antibodies(20μg/ml) (right panel). The supernatants are assayed for the presence of IL-2 24 hours later using the CTLL indicator cell line (Casten et al., 1985). The results are expressed as the concentration required to reach the 50% maximal T-cell response achieved by the addition of P*c* alone.

The covalent attachment of Pc to the antibodies is essential to obtain the observed effect because the binding of the unconjugated antibodies to the B cell does not activate the B-cell to enhanced processing and presentation of free Pc (Table 1). We previously demonstrated that Fab fragments of anti-Ig antibodies augment the B cells' ability to present Pc independently of the internalization of the receptor-antigen complex. It was concluded that the binding of anti-Ig antibodies to surface Ig signalled for enhanced APC function. The increased efficiency of the Pc-anti-I-A^k and Pc-anti-K^k conjugates described here is apparently not a result of this phenomenon, but is more likely due to the conjugate's ability to concentrate Pc, on the B cell surface, for subsequent processing.

In all cases, the Pc-antibody conjugate required processing before TPc9.1 cells could be activated, as shown by the inability of B-cells, fixed with paraformaldehyde to block processing functions, to act as APC (Table 2). The fixation treatment did not affect the B-cell's presentation capacity, as shown by the ability of fixed B-cells to activate the TPc9.1 cells when provided with a processed form of Pc, namely the carboxyl-terminal peptide, residues 81-104(Pc81-104), which contains the T-cell antigenic determinant (Table 2). Moreover, the fixation procedure does not appear to affect the ability of the antibodies to bind the B-cells, as demonstrated using fluorescenated antibodies (data not shown). This result may be taken as evidence that the binding and attachment of native antigen to the B-cell surface is not sufficient to allow T cell activation, but that the protein antigen must be further processed to a form which can be recognized by the T-cell.

Table 2. Pc-Antibody Conjugates Require Processing to Activate TPc9.1 Cells[2]

	[Pc] (μM) Required for 50% Max. Response				
APC	Pc	Pc81-104	Pc-Anti-Ig	Pc-Anti-I-A	Pc-Anti-K
live	1.0	1.0	0.003	0.08	0.04
fixed	>100	1.0	>100	>100	>100

[2] TPc9.1 cells(5×10^4) were cultured in 0.2ml with purified splenic B-cells(2×10^5) either live or fixed with paraformaldehyde as described (Casten, et al., 1985) and graded concentrations of either Pc, Pc81-104, or Pc-antibody conjugates. The culture supernatants were tested 24 hours later for their content of IL-2. The results are expressed as the concentration of Pc or Pc81-104 required to achieve 50% maximal TPc9.1 response.

The increased effectiveness of the Pc-antibody conjugates was not attributable to an increase in the rate at which the native antigen is processed to a form recognized by T cells. Previous reports demonstrated that B-cells acquire the ability to maximally activate TPc9.1 cells after 6-8 hours incubation with native Pc (Lakey et al., 1986). The presence of Fab fragments of rabbit anti-mouse Ig antibodies, in addition to Pc, significantly increases the rate of this process in that maximal presentation is achieved by 2-4 hours (unpublished observation). In contrast, maximal presentation of the Pc-antibody conjugates is reached after 6-8 hours in culture and is indistinguishable from the unmodified Pc (see Fig. 1).

The Pc-antibody conjugates were not equivalent in their ability to activate TPc9.1 cells. Pc-Anti-Ig antibodies were consistently more effective than Pc-Anti-I-A^k antibodies, which were reproducibly more stimulatory as compared to Pc-Anti-K^k. The activity of the Pc-conjugates could not be completely accounted for by the number of antibody molecules which could be bound to the B-cell surface. The results of binding studies carried out using radiolabeled antibodies, indicated that B cells bound 6.5 x 10^5 anti-Ig antibodies, as compared to 3 x 10^5 anti-K^k antibodies versus 1 x 10^5 anti-I-A^k antibodies. Thus, the augmented presentation of the conjugates does not appear to be simply a function of their capacity to bind to B cell surfaces. Other factors which may influence the effectiveness of processing and presentation are the turnover rate of the cell surface structures to which the Pc-antibody conjugate is bound or the route of internalization of the Pc-antibody conjugate once bound to the B-cell surface.

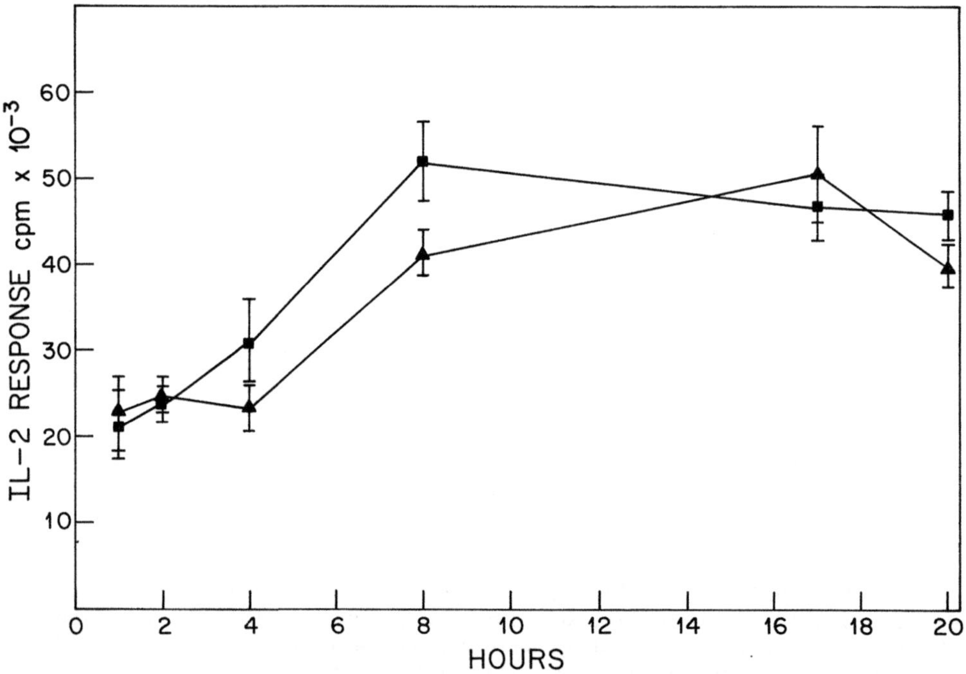

Figure 1. B-cells(2 x 10^5) were incubated for varying lengths of time with (20μM) Pc(▲) or (0.2μM) Pc-rabbit anti-mouse Ig antibody(■), washed, and co-cultured with TPc9.1 cells(5 x 10^4) Supernatants were removed 24 hours later and assayed for their IL-2 content using an IL-2 dependent cell line, CTLL. The results are expressed as the cpm of [^{3}H]-thymidine incorporated by the CTLL during a 4 hour pulse of [^{3}H]-thymidine.

In summary, the results presented here demonstrate that antigen binding to B-cell surface structures other than Ig greatly facilitates their ability to be presented to T-cells. The binding of the antigen to B cell surfaces is not sufficient to achieve T-cell activation, as the antigen-antibody conjugates, like unconjugated antigen, require antigen processing. The conjugates described here should provide the reagents to further investigate the cellular and molecular mechanism underlying B cell, surface Ig mediated, antigen processing and presentation.

This work was supported by National Institute of Health grants AI18939, AI2001 and AI23717. S.K. Pierce is a recipient of an American Cancer Society Faculty Research Award FRA 273.

REFERENCES

Casten, L. A., Lakey, E. K., Jelachich, M. L., Margoliash, E., and Pierce, S. K., 1985, Anti-immunoglobulin augments the B-cell antigen-presentation function independently of internalization of receptor-antigen complex. Proc. Natl. Acad. Sci. USA 82:5890-5894.

Jue, R., Lambert, J. M., Pierce, L. R., and Traut, R. R., 1978, Addition of sulfhydryl groups to *Escherichia coli* ribosomes by protein modification with 2-iminothioline (methyl 4-mercaptobutyrimidate), Biochemistry 25:5399-5406.

Lakey, E. K., Margoliash, E., and Pierce, S. K., 1986, Identification of a peptide binding protein which plays a role in antigen presentation, Proc. Natl. Acad. Sci. USA, (in press).

O'Sullivan, M. J., Gnemmi, E., Morris, D., Chieregatti, G., Simmons, M., Bridges, J. W. and Marks, V., 1979, Comparison of two methods of preparing enzyme antibody conjugates: application of these conjugates for enzyme immunoassay, Anal. Biochem. 100:100-108.

Unanue, E. R., 1984, Antigen-presenting function of the macrophage, Ann. Rev. Immunol. 2:395-428.

A PEPTIDE BINDING PROTEIN WHICH PLAYS A ROLE IN ANTIGEN PRESENTATION

E.K. Lakey[1], J.A. Smith[2], E. Margoliash[1] and S.K. Pierce[1]

From the [1]Department of Biochemistry, Molecular Biology and Cell Biology, Northwestern University, Evanston IL 60201 and the [2]Departments of Molecular Biology and Pathology, Massachusettes General Hospital and the Department of Pathology, Harvard Medical School, Boston Massachusetts, 02114

The helper T-cell recognition of globular protein antigens appears, in general, to require the intracellular processing of the antigen such that a peptide fragment containing the T-cell's antigenic determinant is released, is transported to and held on the surface of an Ia expressing cell. However, the molecular details underlying these phenomena are largely unknown.

In a recent report (Lakey et al., 1986a) the means by which antigenic peptides are anchored on the antigen presenting cell surface was investigated. A peptide binding protein, distinct from Ia, was described. It was isolated by its ability to bind to a C-terminal, 24-amino acid peptide fragment of pigeon cytochrome c (Pc), residues 81-104 (Pc 81-104) which includes the major antigenic determinant for B10.A mouse T cells. The peptide binding protein, PBP 72/74, affinity purified from ^{35}S-methionine labeled cells, appears as two discrete bands of approximately 72 and 74 kD M_r by SDS/PAGE. PBP 72/74 is eluted from the affinity column with equivalent and relatively high concentrations of either the antigenic pigeon cytochrome c peptide or the corresponding non-antigenic peptide of mouse cytochrome c, Mc 81-104. However, it does not bind to the native pigeon protein nor the native mouse protein even though the antigenic peptide is exposed as an alpha helix on the "back" surface of the protein, and is available for binding by antibodies (Hannum, 1986). In this regard, PBP 72/74 appears to recognize some structure or sequence available only in the free peptides. That this protein plays a role in antigen presentation is evidenced by the ability of rabbit antibodies raised against it to block the antigen dependent activation of a Pc-specific, I-E^k-restricted T-cell hybrid by antigen presenting cells (APC) and Pc, but not stimulation by the mitogen, concanavalin A. The expression of PBP 72/74 is not MHC restricted in that the blocking activity of the rabbit antisera can be absorbed on spleen cells from both CBA/J (H-2^k) and C57Bl/10 (H-2^b) mice. Moreover, the protein is expressed by a variety of cells, not just APC, as it has been isolated from B-cells, T-cells and fibroblasts. It is suggested that this peptide binding protein belongs to a class of molecules which facilitate the anchoring of processed peptides on the cell surface and may play a role in antigen presentation by facilitating the interaction of antigenic peptides with Ia and/or the T-cell receptor.

The ability of PBP 72/74 to bind to the antigenic peptide of Pc as well as to the corresponding non-antigenic peptide of the mouse protein, but not to the native cytochromes c, is reminiscent of the properties of the cellular system. Thus, when APC processing functions are blocked by gentle paraformaldehyde fixation, Pc 81-104 is capable of stimulating T-cells, and related non-stimulatory peptides can block this activation. However, the native cytochromes c, whether antigenic or not, have no influence whatsoever. Studies published elsewhere (Lakey et al., 1986b) have described this cellular phenomenon in detail. Briefly, cytochromes c and their corresponding C-terminal fragments which are not capable of stimulating Pc-specific T cells, including the autologous Mc 81-104, were demonstrated to block the T-cells' response to Pc. In contrast, non-stimulatory N-terminal peptides of Pc, which share no homology with the antigenic peptide, and C-terminal peptides of fewer than 9 residues, do not block. Blocking is observed when the nonstimulatory cytochromes c or peptides are present in culture with the live APC and nonsaturating concentrations of Pc and it can be overcome with supraoptimal concentrations of Pc. With tobacco hormworm moth cytochrome c (THMc) as antigen, a protein for which the T-cell has a higher functional affinity, the response of T cells cannot be blocked by the non-stimulatory cytochromes c or by peptides even when limiting concentrations of THMc are used.

A different cellular phenomenon is observed when paraformaldehyde-fixed APC are employed. No native cytochrome c can stimulate the T-cells, including THMc, which with live APC is effective at 50 to 100-fold lower concentrations than Pc. However, with fixed APC, the T-cells are stimulated by the C-terminal fragments of these proteins, Pc 81-104 and THMc 81-103, as readily and with the same relative efficiencies as the native proteins presented by live APC. The non-stimulatory peptides, but not the native cytochromes c block T-cell activation by Pc pulsed-fixed APC, indicating that the non-stimulatory peptides compete with the stimulatory pigeon cytochrome c peptides produced by processing within the APC. This competition appears to be due to non-stimulatory peptides which associate at the APC surface and not to those acting from solution, because APC which have been incubated with Pc and non-stimulatory peptides and washed free of excess antigen and peptides, remain blocked in their ability to stimulate the T-cell.

It was concluded that the activation of Pc-specific T-cells, which recognize a peptide fragment on the surface of an APC, can be blocked by an excess of a non-stimulatory homologous peptide which is also associated with the surface of the APC. The ability to block T-cell activation does not appear to be competition for processing of the native molecule but may represent competition for specific peptide binding sites on the APC, such as PBP 72/74, or on the T-cell receptor.

If all protein antigens must ultimately be fragmented or denatured to allow their recognition by T-cells on APC surfaces, then the peptide anchoring machinery of APC must be capable of binding a diverse set of peptides. To determine the range of peptides which can bind to PBP 72/74, advantage was taken of the antigen, staphylococcal nuclease (Nase). A series of overlapping 20-amino acid peptides corresponding to and spanning nearly the length of the entire 149 residue chain have been synthesized and used by Finnegan et al. (1986) to examine the fine specificity of mouse T-cell response to Nase. Although each peptide fragment of the bacterially derived Nase has the potential to be antigenic, by virtue of it having no obvious homolog in mice, an

Table I. Amino-acid sequence of selected peptides and their effect on Pc-specific T-cell activation.

		stim.[a)]	block[b)]	MHC[c)]
Pc 81-104	I F A G I K K K A E R A D L I A Y L K Q A T A K	+	-	I-E[k]
THMc 81-103	V F A G L K K A N E R A D L I A Y L K Q A T K	++	-	I-E[k]
Mc 81-104	I F A G I K K K G E R A D L I A Y L K K A T N E	-	+	-
Mc 66-80	E Y L E N P K K Y I P G T K M	-	-	-
Nase 1-20	A T S T K K L H K E P A T L I K A I D G	-	-	-
Nase 11-30	P A T L I K A I D G D T V K L M Y K G Q	-	-	-
Nase 41-60[d)]	T P G T K H P K K G V E K Y G P E A S A	-	-	-
Nase 51-70	V E K Y G P E A S A F T K K M V E N A K	-	-	I-E[k]
Nase 61-80	F T K K M V E N A K K I E V E F D K G Q	-	+	I-E[d]
Nase 71-90	K I E V E F D K G Q R T D K Y G R G K A	-	-	-
Nase 81-100	R T D K Y G R G K A Y I R A D F K M V N	-	-	I-E[k]
Nase 91-110	Y I R A D F K M V N E A L V R Q G L A K	-	+	I-A[b]
Nase 101-120	E A L V R Q G L A K V A Y V Y K P N N T	-	-	-
Nase 111-130	V A Y V Y K P N N T H E Q H L R K S E A	-	-	-
Nase 121-140	H E Q H L R K S E A Q A K K E K L N I W	-	-	-
Nase 131-149	Q A K K E K L N I W S E D N A D S G Q	-	-	-

a) A plus indicates that the Pc-specific T-cell hybrid, TPc9.1, is activated to produce IL-2 when incubated with either the native protein or the peptide fragment shown. A minus indicates that the peptide is not stimulatory at concentrations as high as 250µM.

b) A plus indicates that the peptide blocks the TPc9.1 response to Pc-pulsed APC. A minus indicates that it does not block at concentrations in excess of 100µM. If the peptide has been demonstrated to serve as a T cell antigen, its MHC restriction is indicated. A minus indicates that the peptide has not yet been demonstrated to act as a T-cell antigen.

c) It is not possible to measure a blocking effect of peptides which are stimulatory.

d) Nase 21-40 is not soluble and Nase 31-50 is lytic to mouse lymphocytes, thus these peptides could not be examined in this system.

exhaustive survey identified only three peptides as T-cell antigens. This finding suggested that the mere presence of a potential antigenic determinant is not sufficient to create a T-cell antigen from a native protein. Furthermore, the MHC haplotype of the mouse strain employed predicted which of the three peptides would be antigenic. This panel of Nase peptides were tested for their ability to block the activation of P*c*-specific T-cells. Among the twelve Nase peptides tested, three were found to block the response of a P*c*-specific T-cell hybrid to P*c*-pulsed APC (Table I). Two of the three blocking peptides were among those previously identified as T-cell antigens, both in the context of I-A^b, while only one of the nine peptides which were not T-cell antigens, resulted in blocking. Thus there may be a correlation between the peptides' ability to be a T-cell antigen and to block the response of P*c*-specific T-cells. This suggests a common mechanism for antigen presentation, presumably involving some unknown primary or secondary structural features of the peptides.

Neither of the Nase peptides which are recognized in the context of I-E^k, Nase 81-100 and Nase 51-70, block the P*c*-specific, I-E^k restricted T cell from responding to P*c*. The lack of correlation between the ability of a peptide to block and its MHC restriction suggests that the blocking phenomenon is not due to competition for binding to Ia. The present data also indicate that the ability of the Nase peptides to block does not reflect their potential to generate a response in the context of the I-E molecule as compared to the I-A molecule. Experiments are in progress to examine the binding of these peptides to PBP 72/74. If blocking the P*c* response is found to correlate with binding to PBP 72/74, this would further indicate that PBP 72/74 is involved in a mechanism which allows certain peptides of globular protein antigens, produced by antigen processing, to be expressed on the APC surface for effective T-cell activation.

This work was supported by NIH grants AI 18939, AI 12001, AI 23717 and GM 19121. E. K. Lakey was supported by USPHS training grant GM 80861. J. A. Smith was supported by a grant from Hoechst Aktiengesellschaft. S. K. Pierce was a recipient of an American Cancer Society Faculty Research Award FRA 273.

REFERENCES

Finnegan, A., Smith, M. A., Smith, J. A., Berzofsky, J., Sachs, D. H., and Hodes, R. J., 1986, The T cell repertoire for recognition of a phylogenetically distant protein antigen, J. Exp. Med., 164:897-910.

Hannum, C., Matis, L. A., Schwartz, R. H., and Margoliash, E., 1985, The B10.A mouse B cell response to pigeon cytochrome *c* is directed against the same area of the protein that is recognized by B10.A T cells in association with the E^k_β:E^k_α Ia molecule, J. Immunol. 135:3314-3322.

Lakey, E. K., Margoliash, E., and Pierce, S. K., 1986a, Identification of a peptide binding protein which plays a role in antigen presentation. Proc. Natl. Acad. Sci. USA, in press.

Lakey, E. K., Margoliash, E., Fluoret, G., and Pierce, S. K., 1986b, Peptides related to the antigenic determinant block T cell recognition of the native protein as processed by antigen-presenting cells, Eur. J. Immunol. 16:721-727.

T-CELL CLONES SPECIFIC FOR SYNTHETIC POLYPEPTIDES IN CELLULAR COLLABORATIONS

Edna Mozes, Heidy Zinger and Ofra Axelrod

Department of Chemical Immunology
The Weizmann Institute of Science
Rehovot 76100, Israel

INTRODUCTION

The establishment of antigen specific T-cell clones of murine and human origins and the means for propagating them for prolonged periods in vitro facilitated several kinds of investigations such as T-cell heterogeneity and functional repertoires with regard to immunoregulatory and effector activities, the characterization of the molecular nature of the T cell receptor and the nature of T-cell collaborations with other cell types for the generation of immune reactions (Mozes and Apte, 1986).

Most of the information on the functional requirements for T-cell cellular interactions were performed with proliferating T-cell clones (Fathman and Kimoto, 1981; Sredni and Schwartz, 1981), however little information has been available on the mechanism of T-B cell collaborations leading to antibody responses, and the nature of the regulatory role of T helper cells and the physiological significance of their antigen specific secreted factors are still awaiting their elucidation

Synthetic polypeptide antigens as well as their ordered defined analogues have contributed significantly to our knowledge and understanding of the cellular events associated with immune phenomena (McDevitt and Sela, 1965; Mozes, 1975; Mozes and Apte, 1986). It thus appeared that T cell lines and clones specific to synthetic polypeptide antigens with distinct biological activities should provide the appropriate tool for the understanding of the mechanism of T cell functions and for the comparison of the requirements for the generation of the different immunological reactions.

The role of anti-idiotypic antibodies in the regulation of immune responses has been shown in different antigenic systems (Eichman and Rajewsky, 1975; Sy et al., 1980; Strassmann et al., 1980; Lifshitz et al., 1981; Weissberger et al., 1983; Rajewsky and Takemori, 1983). The effect of anti-idiotypic antibodies on helper T cell induction or suppression (Rajewsky and Takemori, 1983) has been demonstrated as well. However, the information on the characteristics of anti-idiotype stimulated T cells, their mechanism of action and capacity to recognize the original antigen, is very limited. The development of T-cell clones specific to monoclonal anti-idiotypic antibodies against idiotypes to a well characterized antigenic system, is the direct approach to this problem.

The antigenic system of the well characterized multichain synthetic polypeptide antigen poly(Tyr,Glu)-poly(DLALA)--poly(Lys) abbreviated as (T,G)-A--L (Sela et al., 1962), its closely related analogues (Fuchs and Sela, 1964; Mozes et al., 1974), monoclonal antibodies (idiotypes) against it (Parhami-Seren et al., 1983, 1984) and the anti-idiotypic antibodies (polyclonal, Axelrod et al., 1985b) or monoclonal) produced against it appeared to be ideal for studies aimed at the elucidation of the above raised problems.

T-CELL LINES AND CLONES SPECIFIC TO (T,G)-A--L

In the past we established and characterized T-cell helper lines specific to (T,G)-A--L. These antigen specific helper T-cell lines were constitutive secretors of T-cell helper factors which were partially purified and analysed as the representatives of the T-cell recognition units (Apte et al., 1981, Lifshitz et al., 1983). To understand better the mechanism by which T-cells interact with other cell populations for the elucidation of immune reactions we have further established T-cell lines which possess (T,G)-A--L specific proliferative and helper activities and secrete IL-2 following stimulation with antigen (Axelrod and Mozes, 1986).

Two (T,G)-A--L specific T-cell lines were developed from (T,G)-A--L immunized C3H.SW ($H\text{-}2^b$, high responser) lymph modes. The two lines proliferated efficiently upon stimulation with (T,G)-A--L. The proliferative responses were H-2 restricted as only $H\text{-}2^b$ spleen cells or homogeneous thymic derived macrophages could present (T,G)-A--L to the proliferating cells (Axelrod et al., 1985a). One of the lines designated TPB1 was very restricted in the specificity of its response and proliferated only in the presence of (T,G)-A--L. The second line, TPB2, on the other hand, showed a broader specificity and proliferated following stimulation with the random polypeptide poly (Phe,Glu)-poly(DLAla)--poly(Lys), (Phe,G)-A--L, with the ordered synthetic antigen (Tyr-Glu-Tyr-Glu)-poly(DLAla)--poly(Lys) (T-G-T-G)-A--L and to a lesser degree with (Tyr-Tyr-Glu-Glu)-poly(DLAla)--poly(Lys), (T-T-G-G)-A--L. It should be noted that antibodies elicited with (T,G)-A--L cross-reacted to a very limited extent with (T-G-T-G)-A--L in contrast to their high cross reactivity with (T-T-G-G)-A--L (Mozes et al., 1974). It appears that the fine specificity of (T,G)-A--L specific antibodies is not identical to that of (T,G)-A--L specific T cells.

The T-cell lines provided efficient help to (T,G)-A--L stimulated B cells of C3H.SW origin in an in vitro antibody production system. Antibody responses were determined in culture supernatants by a solid phase radioimmunoassay. Figure 1 represents the (T,G)-A--L specific responses obtained with the TPB1 T cells. As can be seen at the optimal antigen dose 3.68 μg/ml (T,G)-A--L specific antibodies were produced (Fig. 1),

Enriched (T,G)-A--L immunized B-cells (0.5 x 10^6) were cultured with 10^4 TPB1 T cells and antigen presenting cells in the presence of different doses of (T,G)-A--L (●—●, o—o), or RSA (▲—▲, Δ—Δ) for 8 days. Supernatants diluted 1:40 were assayed for anti-(T,G)-A--L antibodies in a solid phase radioimmunoassay. Results are expressed as cpm (mean ± SD, ●—●, ▲—▲) or μg antibodies/ml (o—o, Δ—Δ).

in comparison to 0.3 μg/ml determined in supernatants of cultured mixtures of immunized spleen and lymph node cells (data not shown). No significant antibody responses were triggered with the non-relevant antigen-rabbit serum albumin (RSA).

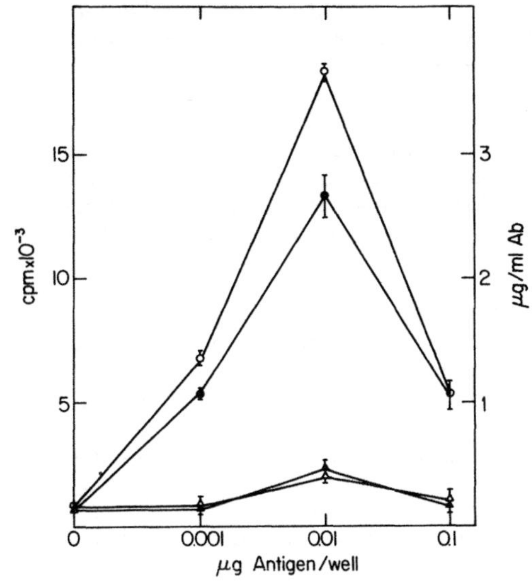

Fig. 1. In vitro anti-(T,G)-A--L response induced with the help of TPB1 T-cells.

The same fine specificity observed for the proliferative responses of the two T cell lines could be observed for their helper activity. Thus, TPB1 T-cells could provide help only in the presence of (T,G)-A--L, the original stimulating antigen, whereas TPB2, T-cells reacted with synthetic polypeptide antigens closely related to (T,G)-A--L. Although restricted for stimulation, TPB1 cells could collaborate with (Phe,G)-A--L primed B cells for antibody production. However, the latter response could be obtained only when (T,G)-A--L was present in the culture as shown in Table 1.

Table 1. Collaboration of TPB1 cells with (Phe,G)-A--L immunized B-cells.

Cells \ Antigen	-	(T,G)-A--L	(Phe,G)-A--L	RSA
Primed B cells + APC	5768 ± 86	4713 ± 209	5031 ± 113	4385 ± 273
Primed B cells + APC + TPB1	4298 ± 10	16431 ± 21	5287 ± 323	5827 ± 33

Enriched (Phe,G)-A--L immunized B cells (0.5×10^6) were cultured with 10^4 TPB1 cells and antigen presenting cells in the presence of 0.01 μg/well antigen for 8 days. Culture supernatants were assayed for anti-(T,G)-A--L antibodies in a solid phase radioimmunoassay. Results are expressed as mean ± SD.

It should be noted that although TPB1 provided help to (T,G)-A--L or (Phe,G)-A--L primed B cells only in the presence of (T,G)-A--L, the antibodies produced cross-reacted with the closely related synthetic polypeptides as demonstrated for in vivo elicited antibodies (McDevitt and Chinitz, 1969).

Since the TPB2 T-cell line exhibited several biological activities and cross-reacted with polypeptides closely related to (T,G)-A--L, it has been a suitable source for clones which enabled the determination of the specificity and functional potential of monoclonal T-cells. Mainly two types of T-cell clones were obtained from the TPB2, T-cell line; high proliferative cells with weak helper activity, and efficient helper T-cells with low proliferative capacity. Among the proliferative T cells we could distinguish between those that proliferated in the presence of (T,G)-A--L only and between clones that required the addition of 10% of Concanavalin A (Con A) supernatant to the antigen for their proliferative responses. Table 2 demonstrates the proliferative responses of representative clones belonging to the different groups. It should be noted that clones like C.28 (efficient helpers) did not proliferate well even in presence of the Con A supernatant.

Table 3 shows the helper activity of 2 clones C.4 and C.28. As can be seen C.4 which proliferated efficiently in the presence of (T,G)-A--L was not capable of collaborating with (T,G)-A--L immunized B-cells for the production of specific antibodies. In contrast, C.28 which proliferated poorly when triggered with (T,G)-A--L helped efficiently B cells in the process of the induction of (T,G)-A--L specific antibodies. It is not clear whether the clones with the distinct functions originated from cells already committed to one of the above functions, or that they were cloned at a specific stage of differentiation that enabled them to efficiently perform just one function.

Table 2. Proliferative capacity of TPB2 T cell line derived clones.

Clones \ Antigen	-	(T,G)-A--L
C.1	100 ± 50	800 ± 100
C.1 with 10% Con A Supernatant	2000 ± 100	32000 ± 3000
C.4	280 ± 44	25200 ± 1800
C.28	353 ± 10	839 ± 59

Cells of the individual clones (10^4) were cultured with 0.5 x 10^6 syngeneic irradiated spleen cells in the presence of 100 μg antigen. At the end of 48 hr incubation period 0.5 μCi of [^{3}H] thymidine was added. Sixteen hr later cells were harvested and radioactivity was counted. Results are expressed as mean cpm of triplicates ± SD.

It is noteworthy that the requirements for T-cell proliferation and for induction of helper activity are different. Thus, T-cell proliferation requires 1000-10000 times more (T,G)-A--L than helper induction, indicating differences in the mechanisms leading to these reactions.

Since the TPB2 line proliferated in the presence of (T,G)-A--L, (Phe,G)-A--L, (T-G-T-G)-A--L and to a lesser extent (T-G-T-G)-A--L, it was of interest to find out whether a single clone will respond to more than one antigen. Table 4 summarizes the fine specificity of the proliferative response of 6 clones. A variety of patterns of proliferative responses could be observed. Whereas clones 4, 13 and 32 proliferated to (T,G)-A--L only, clones 2 and 19 proliferated to (Phe,G)-A--L and (T-G-T-G)-A--L as well and clone 8 proliferated to (T-G-T-G)-A--L and weakly to (T-T-G-G)-A--L in addition to its proliferative response to

Table 3. Helper activity of TPB2 derived T-cell clones

Clone	-	(T,G)-A--L μg/well 0.001	0.01	0.1
C.28	6000 ± 550	12780 ± 320	28800 ± 1660	22775 ± 830
C.4	555 ± 25	1110 ± 87	890 ± 35	975 ± 120

Enriched (T,G)-A--L immunized B-cells (0.5x10^6) were cultured together with antigen presenting cells, 10^4 T cells of the clones, and different concentrations of antigen. Supernatants of the cultures were assayed for anti-(T,G)-A--L antibodies in a solid phase radioimmunoassay. Results are expressed as mean cpm ± SD.

Table 4. Fine Specificity of the proliferation responses of (T,G)-A--L specific T-cell clones

Antigen / Clone	-	(T,G)-A--L	(Phe,G)-A--L	(T-T-G-G)-A--L	(T-G-T-G)-A--L
C.2	367 ± 81	4617 ± 285	2447 ± 122	525 ± 32	3602 ± 134
C.4	185 ± 33	10648 ± 700	266 ± 2	270 ± 22	205 ± 1
C.8	223 ± 30	8282 ± 162	721 ± 97	1874 ± 729	4000 ± 685
C.13	264 ± 12	9706 ± 375	530 ± 47	318 ± 9	326 ± 17
C.19	179 ± 5	11218 ± 1024	9388 ± 1676	555 ± 17	3729 ± 15
C.32	275 ± 67	61571 ± 593	353 ± 23	336 ± 41	820 ± 91

Cells of the individual clones (10^4) were cultured with 0.5×10^6 syngeneic irradiated spleen cells in the presence of 100 μg antigen. At the end of 48 hr incubation period 0.5 μCi of (^{3}H) thymidine was added. Sixteen hr later cells were harvested and radioactivity was counted. Results are expressed as mean cpm of triplicates ± S D.

(T,G)-A--L. It thus appears that one clone is capable of reacting with cross reactive antigenic determinants. The recognition of more than one specificity by monoclonal T cells has been reported previously (Ben-Nun et al., 1983; Leeman and Cantor, 1983).

IL-2 secretion by a variety of T cell lines and clones as a result of antigenic stimulation has been reported in many systems that were studied (Kappler et al., 1981; Kelso and Glasebrook, 1984). Furthermore, the ability to produce IL-2 upon a specific antigenic stimulation has been frequently used as a measurement for helper activity. Since the TPB1 and TPB2 T cell lines were found to secrete IL-2, it was of interest to find out whether all the clones have the capacity to secrete IL-2 and whether IL-2 secretion correlates with the other functions of the clones. All the clones tested secreted different levels of IL-2 following stimulation with (T,G)-A--L. However, no direct correlation was found between the efficiency of IL-2 secretion and either the helper or proliferative capacity of the T-cell clones. We thus concluded that IL-2 secretion cannot be used as a measure for T-cell functions.

H-2 RESTRICTION REQUIREMENTS FOR PROLIFERATIVE AND HELPER RESPONSES

Most of the information on H-2 restriction in cellular collaborations of T cells have been provided on the interactions between T cells and antigen presenting cells (APC) leading to T-cell proliferation (Fathman and Kimoto, 1981, Sredni and Schwartz, 1981). Studies with T-cell clones of F1 origin led to the most interesting results since their use enabled the demonstration that different T-cells could recognize a soluble antigen with different Ia determinants. The information on the H-2 restriction of the T-B collaboration in the process of antibody production is very limited because of the complexity of this process and the lack of appropriate assay systems. Since, as described above, we established an in vitro system by which we could evaluate the helper capacity of single T-cell clones specific for (T,G)-A--L, we have developed cloned T-cells of (C57BL/6 x C3H/HeJ)F1, ($H\text{-}2^b$ x $H\text{-}2^k$)F1 origin specific to the closely related polypeptide (Phe,G)-A--L to which both the $H\text{-}2^b$ and $H\text{-}2^k$ mice are high responders. These clones were used for the comparison of the genetic restriction of the collaboration between T and B cells to the H-2 restriction of the interaction between T-cells and APC which leads to proliferation.

The genetic restriction of the proliferative responses of the F1 derived clones was similar to that reported previously (Kimoto and Fathman, 1981). Thus 3 kinds of clones differing from each other in their H-2 restriction were observed. One group of clones was found to be restricted to the $H\text{-}2^b$ haplotype and they proliferated when antigen was presented on $H\text{-}2^b$ or ($H\text{-}2^b$ x $H\text{-}2^k$)F1 APC. The clones of the second class were restricted to the $H\text{-}2^k$ haplotype in their proliferative response and the clones in the third group were restricted to determinants of the F1 hybrid ($H\text{-}2^b$ x $H\text{-}2^k$), and thus proliferated in the presence of antigen presented on APC of the F1 hybrid exclusively. The (Phe,G)-A--L specific T cell clones were also tested for their ability to secrete IL-2 upon antigenic stimulation. The same H-2 restriction demonstrated for the proliferative responses was observed for IL-2 secretion.

Two of the T-cell clones that manifested weak proliferative responses were found to provide efficient help for antibody production. This finding is in agreement with our above described observation that (T,G)-A--L specific helper T cell clones had a low potential to proliferate in response to antigen. One of these clones was restricted in its proliferative response to F1 APC exclusively. However, it could help in the presence of (Phe,G)-A--L immunized B-cells and APC of C3H/HeJ (H-2^k) in addition to the help provided to B-cells of F1 origin. The second clone was restricted to H-2^b APC in its (Phe,G)-A--L specific proliferative response. However it could provide help to (Phe,G)-A--L primed B-cells of H-2^b, H-2^k and F1 origin (Axelrod and Mozes, 1986). It thus appears that the H-2 restriction requirements for the successful collaboration between T-cells and B-cells are less stringent than those for the T-APC interaction. The stringent H-2 restriction and the high dose of antigen required for the proliferative responses indicate that for the triggering of proliferation a stronger interaction between the cells is necessary.

(T,G)-A--L SPECIFIC HELPER T-CELL FACTORS

Antigen specific regulatory T-cell factors that are the product of effector T-cells (Tada and Okumura, 1979; Mozes and Apte, 1986) provide an ideal tool for studies aimed at the understanding of the events occurring when T-cells are activated on one hand, and in the collaboration between T-cells and B-cells on the other hand. Both the TPB1 and TPB2, (T,G)-A--L specific T-cell lines were found to secrete, upon stimulation with antigen, T cell helper factors which could provide help to immunized B cells in the process of antibody production. The lines could be stimulated to produce the factors by a low dose of antigen - 2 µg/ml as well as by a high antigen dose of 150 µg/ml. However, as demonstrated with factors produced by the TPB1 T cell line, the factors induced by the low dose of antigen, shown in Figure 2, were very restricted and provided help just in the presence of (T,G)-A--L, like the secreting T-cell line.

In contrast, the factors induced by the high dose of antigen had a broader specificity and helped also in the presence of closely related polypeptides such as (Phe.G)-A--L. The secretion of the factors by the T cells did not require their proliferation since no proliferation of the TPB1 T-cells was observed at a concentration of 2 µg/ml (T,G)-A--L. This dose of antigen could not stimulate the secretion of IL-2 by the TPB1 cells as well.

The (T,G)-A--L specific T-cell clones derived from the (T,G)-A--L specific T cell line, TPB2, were found to secrete antigen specific helper factors. Representative results of 2 clones are demonstrated in Table 5. All the tested clones were found to secrete helper factors including clones which their helper activity was very weak and could be detected only when 10^5 rather 10^4 helper cells were used (C.2 Table 5). The latter findings suggest a physiological role for the antigen specific T cell helper factors.

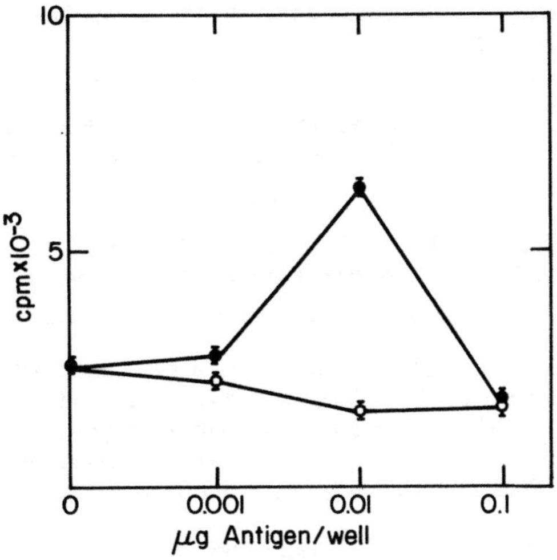

Fig. 2. The fine antigenic specificity of the low dose antigen induced helper factor of TPB1.

Cells ($3x10^6$) of the TPB1 T-cell line were incubated for 24 hr in enriched medium supplemented with 2 μg/ml (T,G)-A--L in the presence of irradiated syngeneic spleen cells. The cells were then washed and incubated in enriched medium for an additional period of 48 hr. Thereafter cells were spun down and the supernatants were collected and tested for helper activity. Enriched (T,G)-A--L immunized B-cells were cultured with the TPB1 derived helper factors (diluted 1:4). Culture were set up in the presence of APC and different concentrations of (T,G)-A--L (●——●) or (Phe,G)-A--L (o---o). Supernatants of the cultures were assayed for anti-(T,G)-A--L antibodies in a solid phase radioimmunoassay. Results are expressed as mean cpm ± SD.

The helper T-cell factors were H-2 restricted in their collaboration with the B-cells and interacted successfully with syngeneic B cells only. However, in contrast to the T cells which required APC for their helper activity, the secreted factors could collaborate successfully with syngeneic immunized B-cells for antibody production in the absence of detectable APC. This difference between the helper cells and the helper factors might be due to the fact that the factors are the final product of the activated T-cells, while the APC are required for the T-cell activation. Alternatively, it is possible that the function of the APC in T-B collaboration is a supply of factors which are necessary for B cell differentiation and maturation. As the helper factors are the product of interactions between T-cells and APC the supernatants containing the antigen specific factors might include also the other non-specific factors required. It was indeed reported recently that APC can be replaced by Con A supernatants in the secondary low dose T-dependent antibody responses in vitro (Ishihara et al., 1986).

Table 5. The ability of T-cell clones to secrete antigen specific T-cell helper factors.

Clone No.	Helper cells -	Helper cells (T,G)-A--L	Helper factor -	Helper factor (T,G)-A--L
C.2	644 ± 24	3944 ± 196	209 ± 1	3000 ± 98
C.34	2258 ± 70	20702 ± 118	3844 ± 54	7838 ± 372

Enriched (T,G)-A--L immunized B-cells were cultured with APC, (T,G)-A--L (0.01 μg/well) and either T-cells of the clones (10^5 cells of C.2 and 10^4 cells of C.34) or their derived helper factors. Supernatants of the cultures were assayed for anti-(T,G)-A--L antibodies in a solid phase radioimmunoassay. Results are expressed as mean cpm ± SD.

Some of the T cell factors secreted by the TPB1 T-cell line or by the T cell clones were inefficient in the triggering of B-cells for antibody production. It was found that Con A supernatants could restore the activity of the inefficient helper factors. In an attempt to find out whether IL-2 was the active factor in the Con A supernatant, we have used recombinant IL-2 (r-IL-2) for restoring the activity of an inefficient helper factor. We have demonstrated that an inactive factor preparation together with r-IL-2 which by itself had no helper activity induced (T,G)-A--L specific antibody responses. It thus appears that for successful triggering of B cells for antibody production a non-specific signal, provided by IL-2, is required in addition to the specific signal provided by the antibody specific T cell factors.

T-CELL LINES AND CLONES SPECIFIC TO MONOCLONAL ANTI-IDIOTYPIC ANTIBODIES

Despite the availability of monoclonal anti-idiotypic reagents and the know-how of establishing cloned T-cell lines, little information has been accumulated on the specificity and mode of interaction with other cells of anti-idiotype stimulated T-cells. To this end we have attempted the production of monoclonal anti-idiotypic antibodies against monoclonal antibodies to the synthetic polypeptide (T,G)-A--L. The monoclonal idiotypes used for the production of the anti-idiotypic antibodies - McAb103, were demonstrated to express the major idiotypes of conventional (T,G)-A--L specific antibodies (Parhami-Seren et al., 1983, 1984). As a result of two fusion experiments performed with C57BL/6 derived spleen cells immunized with McAb103, 9 monoclonal anti-idiotypic antibodies were obtained that bound specifically McAb103. The monoclonal anti-idiotypes were all of the IgM isotype and varied in their capacity to bind conventional (T,G)-A--L specific antibodies of C3H.SW origin. One of the monoclonal anti-idiotypic antibodies, McAbA-6, that bound efficiently McAb103 and cross-reacted the best with polyclonal (T,G)-A--L specific antibodies produced in C3H.SW mice was chosen for attempts to establish a T cell line and clones. The T cell line, TA-6, established from McAbA-6 immunized lymph nodes of C3H.SW mice is maintained in culture in medium containing 10% Con A supernatant and is periodically stimulated (every 14-18 days) with McAbA-6. The T-cell line proliferated efficiently and specifically when triggered with

McAbA-6. A low but significant proliferation could be obtained in presence of (T,G)-A--L. These results suggest a cross reaction on the level of recognition between the anti-idiotypes and (T,G)-A--L.

It was of interest to find out whether the TA-6 T cells could collaborate with (T,G)-A--L primed B-cells for the production of (T,G)-A--L specific antibodies. It was reproducibly shown that the TA-6 T cell line could help (T,G)-A--L immunized B cells for the production of (T,G)-A--L specific antibodies in the presence of either (T,G)-A--L or McAbA-6 in the culture.

Since the TA-6 T-cell line receptors were shown to recognize (T,G)-A--L, the cloning of the TA-6 line was performed in presence of either the anti-idiotypic antibodies McAbA-6 used for the stimulation of the line or in the presence of (T,G)-A--L. When the T-cell clones were tested for their ability to proliferate following triggering with either McAbA-6 or (T,G)-A--L it has been demonstrated that both type of clones, those growing in presence of McAbA-6 and those stimulated with (T,G)-A--L, proliferated efficiently only in the presence of McAbA-6, as represented by the 2 clones shown in Table 6.

Since the T-cell clones could not proliferate following a stimulus with (T,G)-A--L, it was of interest to find out whether (T,G)-A--L could inhibit the proliferative response observed with McAbA-6. Table 7 demonstrates the results of a representative inhibition experiment performed with a (T,G)-A--L stimulated clone (C.115) which proliferated efficiently following triggering with McAbA-6 (see Table 6). As can be seen in Table 7, (T,G)-A--L could inhibit specifically the proliferative response to McAbA-6. Thus 125 μg of (T,G)-A--L could inhibit 73% of the proliferative response whereas the same dose of either the related polypeptide (H,G)-A--L or the non-related antigen ribonuclease did not affect the proliferative response.

Table 6. Proliferative responses of the TA-6 line derived T-cell clones.

Clone \ Antigen	-	McAbA-6	(T,G)-A--L
C.34	260 $\pm$ 22	25550 $\pm$ 2190	280 $\pm$ 35
C.115	262 $\pm$ 20	22950 $\pm$ 2250	290 $\pm$ 3

Cells (10^4) of the McAbA-6 (C.34) and of the (T,G)-A--L (C.115) propagated clones were cultured with 0.5 x 10^6 syngeneic irradiated spleen cells in the presence of 50 μg McAbA-6 or 100 μg (T,G)-A--L. At the end of 48 hr incubation period 0.5 μCi of [^{3}H] thymidine was added. Sixteen hr later cells were harvested and radioactivity was counted. Results are expressed as mean cpm of triplicates $\pm$ SD.

Table 7. (T,G)-A--L inhibits specifically the proliferative response of clone 115 to McAbA-6

μg/well \ Inhibitor	(T,G)-A--L	(H,G)-A--L	Ribonuclease
	% Inhibition		
250	88%	35%	34%
125	73%	0%	0%
62.5	20%	0%	0%

Cells (10^4/well) of C.115 were cultured together with 0.5 x 10^6 syngeneic irradiated spleen cells, McAbA-6 (12.5 μg/well) and the various antigens used as inhibitors at different concentrations. At the end of 48 hr incubation period 0.5 μCi of [^{3}H] thymidine was added. Sixteen hr later cells were harvested and radioactivity was counted. The results are expressed as percentage of inhibition of the proliferative response stimulated by McAbA-6.

Both types of clones were tested also for their capacity to collaborate with (T,G)-A--L immunized B-cells for the production of (T,G)-A--L specific antibodies. A large number of the clones helped in the induction of (T,G)-A--L specific antibodies as demonstrated for the two representative clones, C.34 and C.115, in Table 8. It thus appears that (T,G)-A--L is recognized by the McAbA-6 specific T-cell receptors on the T cell clones. It is not clear yet why (T,G)-A--L cannot trigger the T-cell clones to efficient proliferation in vitro although it can serve as a stimulating antigen for antibody production in vitro.

Table 8. Helper activity of the TA-6 line derived T-cell clones

Clone	-	(T,G)-A--L μg/well 0.001	0.01	0.1
C.34	4790 ± 70	7320 ± 60	12230 ± 950	3580 ± 205
C.115	1550 ± 20	11640 ± 1760	4195 ± 1360	4390 ± 1070

Enriched (T,G)-A--L immunized B cells (0.5 x 10^6) were cultured together with antigen presenting cells, different concentrations of (T,G)-A--L and 10^4 T-cells of either the clone stimulated in culture with McAbA-6 (C.34) or the (T,G)-A--L propagated clone (C.115). Supernatants of the cultures were assayed for anti-(T,G)-A--L antibodies in a solid phase radioimmunoassay. Results are expressed as mean cpm ± SD.

It is possible that (T,G)-A--L is recognized with a lower affinity than McAbA-6 by the T cell clones due to the fact that the anti-idiotypes were used for the initial in vivo/in vitro stimulation of the T-cells utilized for the establishment of the line.

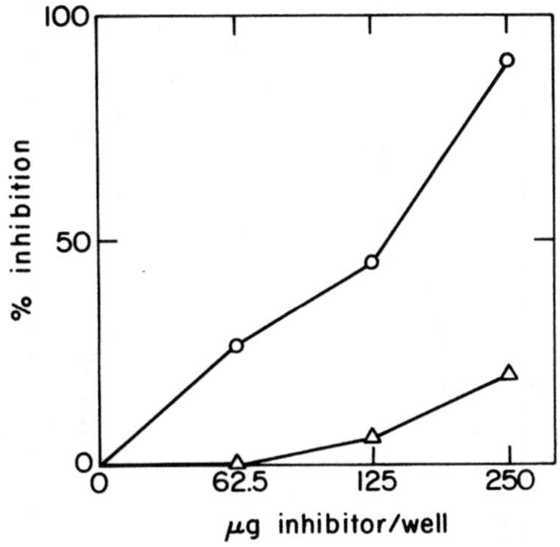

Fig. 3. Inhibition of (T,G)-A--L stimulated proliferative response of TPB1 cells by McAbA-6.
TPB1 cells (10^4/well) were cultured with irradiated syngeneic spleen cells ($0.5x10^6$/well) and 50 μg/well (T,G)-A--L. Either McAbA-6 (o—o) or NMIg (Δ-Δ) which were used as inhibitors were added to the cultures at different doses. At the end of a 48 hr incubation period 0.5 μCi of [^{3}H] thymidine was added. Sixteen hr later cells were harvested and radioactivity was counted. Results are expressed as percentage of inhibition of the proliferative response stimulated by (T,G)-A--L.

It should be noted that similar results were observed when the (T,G)-A--L specific TPB1 T-cell line was tested for its reaction with the McAbA-6. Since McAbA-6 are against an idiotype (McAb103) specific to (T,G)-A--L, it was of interest to find out whether the anti-idiotypes will recognize and react with the TPB1 T-cell line. No proliferation could be observed with the TPB1 line in the presence of McAbA-6. However, the proliferative response induced by (T,G)-A--L could be efficiently and specifically inhibited as demonstrated in Figure 3.

McAbA-6 could also induce the production of (T,G)-A--L specific antibodies when added to a mixture of (T,G)-A--L primed B cells and TPB1 T cells as demonstrated in Figure 4. Thus, (T,G)-A--L stimulated T-cells

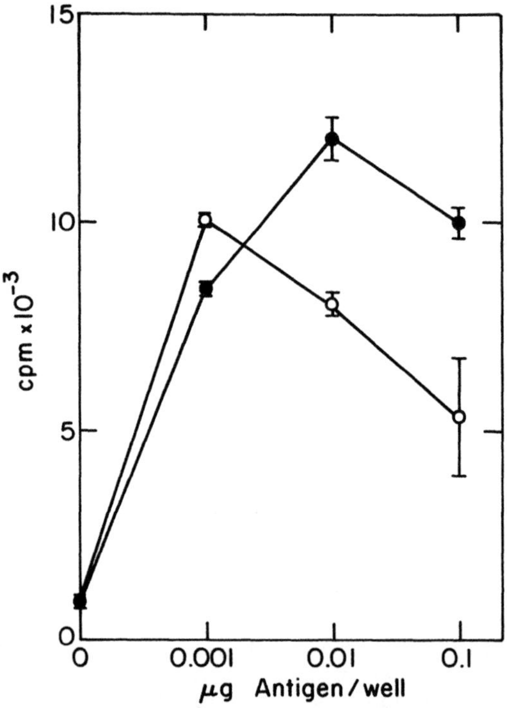

Fig. 4. In vitro anti-(T,G)-A--L response induced by the help of TPB1 cells.
Enriched (T,G)-A--L immunized B cells were cultured together with antigen-presenting cells and TPB1 cells in the presence of (T,G)-A--L (●—●) or McAbA-6 (o—o). After 7 days, supernatants were assayed for anti-(T,G)-A--L antibodies in a solid phase radioimmunoassay. Results are expressed as mean cpm ± S.D.

recognize monoclonal anti-idiotypic antibodies and are triggered by the latter to provide help. Nevertheless, McAbA-6 could not stimulate the proliferation of the (T,G)-A--L specific T cell line.

One of the interesting questions is the relation of the monoclonal anti-idiotypic antibodies McAbA-6 to the receptor of the TA-6 line as well as to the receptor of the (T,G)-A--L specific T-cell line-TPB1. Immunoblotting experiments performed with lysates of cells of the TA-6, TPB1 lines and of a line specific to RSA indicated that McAbA-6 reacted with ~ 40,000 molecular weight bands of the reduced lysates of the TA-6 and TPB1 cells but not of the RSA specific T-cell line.

CONCLUDING REMARKS

The analysis of T-cell clones specific to the synthetic polypeptide antibodies (T,G)-A--L and (Phe,G)-A--L and to monoclonal anti-idiotypes contributed to our knowledge on the fine specificity of monoclonal T-cells, the requirement for T cell interactions for proliferation and helper activity and the number of functions that are manifested by a single T cell clone.

It has been demonstrated that a single clone could not manifest both efficient (T,G)-A--L specific proliferation and help. Monoclonal T-cells were shown to be capable of reacting with antigenic determinants that are cross reactive with the major determinant of (T,G)-A--L. Different clones vary in their fine antigenic specificities.

Secretion of antigen specific helper T cell factors was found to be a general feature of helper T cells since all of the helper T-cell clones tested, with no exception, secreted helper factors suggesting a physiological role for these soluble molecules. The use of the T-cell replacing factors enabled a better insight into the mechanism of T-B cell interactions leading to antibody production.

Many differences were observed between the requirements for cellular interactions resulting in T-cell proliferation and those leading to T-cell help for antibody production. T-cell proliferation requires 1000-10000 times more antigen than helper induction. A more stringent H-2 restriction was shown to be necessary for proliferation and as shown with the McAbA-6 anti-idiotype stimulated T-cell clones, (T,G)-A--L could induce helper activity but not proliferation. The inability of a T-cell clone to efficiently proliferate following a stimulation with an antigen might be due to lack or excess of non-specific signals provided by factors like IL-1, IL-2, etc. It is also possible that a high frequency of antigen specific or non-specific receptors is crucial for a proliferative reaction.

Based on the newly described phenomenon of IL-1 production by certain T-cell clones (Tartakovsky et al., 1986) we attempted the comparison of (T,G)-A--L specific proliferative T-cell clones to helper clones. Preliminary results suggest that IL-1 production is associated with the helper T-cell activity. Furthermore, preliminary in situ hybridization and Northern blot techniques were used to compare (T,G)-A--L specific proliferating clones with helper clones for mRNA T cell receptor expression. The proliferating clones appeared to express consistently higher levels of mRNA coding for T-cell receptor than helper clones (Tartakovsky, Ben-Nun, Axelrod and Mozes, unpublished data). Further studies using the above approaches will hopefully lead to elucidation of the mechanisms underlying both antigen specific help and proliferation.

Finally, the monoclonal anti-idiotypic antibodies, serving as an antigen for the stimulation of T-cell clones could also been used as an antibody in immunoblotting experiments and reacted with both the T-cell receptor on the TA-6 - McAbA-6 specific line and the TPB1- (T,G)-A--L specific line. Experiments aimed at the comparison of the T-cell receptor which is bound t clonotypic antibodies with that reactive with the anti-idiotypic antibodies - McAbA-6 are under progress.

REFERENCES

Apte, R.N., Löwy, I., De Baetselier, P., and Mozes, E., 1981, Establishment and characterization of continuous helper T cell line specific to poly(LTyr,LGlu)-poly(DLAla)--poly(Lys), J. Immunol., 127:25.

Axelrod, O., and Mozes, E., 1986a, Analysis of the biological functions and fine specificity of (T,G)-A--L specific T cell clones, Immunobiol., 172:99.

Axelrod, O., and Mozes, E., 1986b, Functional requirements of (Phe,G)-A--L specific T cell clones of (H-2^b x H-2^k)F1 origin, Immunogenetics, in press.

Axelrod, O., Mozes, E., and Gallily, R., 1985a, Antigen presentation by proliferating thymic macrophages to (T,G)-A--L specific T cell line in an H-2 restricted manner, Immunol. Lett., 10:21.

Axelrod, O., Stanislawski, M., and Mozes, E., 1985b, Establishment and biological activity of a proliferative anti-idiotype activated T cell line, Immunol. Lett., 10:347.

Ben-Nun, A., Lando, Z., Dorf, M.E., and Burakoff, S.J., 1983, Analysis of cross-reactive antigen specific T cell clones. Specific recognition of two major histocompatibility complex (MHC) and two non-MHC antigens by a single clone, J. Exp. Med., 157:2147.

Eichmann, K., and Rajewsky, K., 1975, Induction of T and B cell immunity by anti-idiotypic antibodies, Eur. J. Immunol., 5:661.

Fathman, C.G., and Kimoto, M., 1981, Studies utilizing murine T cell clones: Ir genes, Ia antibodies and MLR stimulating determinants, Immunol. Rev., 54:57.

Fuchs, S., and Sela, M., 1964, Antigenicity of some new synthetic polypeptides and polypeptidyl gelatins, Biochem. J., 98:566.

Ishihara, T., Takahara, S., and Fathman, G., 1986, IL-2 restores memory B cell activation by antigen-specific T cell clone variants, J. Immunol., 136:39.

Kappler, J.W., Skidmore, B., White, J., and Marrack, P., 1981, Antigen inducible, H-2 restricted, interleukin-2 producing T cell hybridomas, J. Exp. Med., 153:1198.

Kelso, A., and Glasebrook, A.L., 1984, Secretion of interleukin 2, macrophage activating factor, interferon, and colony-stimulating factor by alloreactive T lymphocyte clones, J. Immunol., 132:2924.

Kimoto, M., and Fathman, C.G., 1981, Antigen reactive T cell clones. II. Unique homozygous and (high responder x low responder)F1 hybrid antigen presenting determinants detected using poly(Tyr,Glu)-poly(DLAla)--poly(Lys) reactive T cell clones, J. Exp. Med., 153:375.

Leeman, S.R.A., and Cantor, H., 1983, Specificity of T cell clones for antigen and autologous major histocompatibility complex products, J. Exp. Med., 158:428.

Lifshitz, R., Apte, R.N., and Mozes, E., 1983, Partial purification and characterization of an antigen specific helper factor synthesized by a T cell continuous line, Proc. Natl. Acad. Sci. USA., 80:5689.

Lifshitz, R., Parhami, B., and Mozes, E., 1981, Enhancing effect of murine anti-idiotypic serum on the proliferative response specific for poly(LTyr,LGlu)-poly(DLAla)--poly(LLys) [(T,G)-A--L], Eur. J. Immunol., 11:27.

McDevitt, H.O., and Chinitz, A., 1969, Genetic control of the antibody response and histocompatibility (H-2) type, Science., 163:1207.
McDevitt, H.O., and Sela, M., 1965, Genetic control of the antibody response. I. Demonstration of determinant specific differences in response to synthetic polypeptide antibodies in two strains of inbred mice, J. Exp. Med., 122:517.
Mozes, E., 1975, Expression of immune response (Ir) genes in T and B cells, Immunogenetics, 2:397.
Mozes, E., and Apte, R.N., 1986, Nature and function of antigen specific T cell lines and their products, Physiol. Rev., 66:653.
Mozes, E., Schwartz, M., and Sela, M., 1974, Antibody response of inbred mouse strains to ordered tetrapeptides of tyrosine and glutamic acid attached to multichain polyalanine and polyproline. Tyr-Tyr-Glu-Glu is the major antigenic determinant of the random poly(Tyr,Glu)-poly(DLAla)-poly(Lys), J. Exp. Med., 140:349.
Parhami-Seren, B., Eshhar, Z., and Mozes, E., 1983, Fine specificity and idiotypic expression of monoclonal antibodies directed against poly(Tyr,Glu)-poly(DLAla)--poly(Lys) and its ordered analogue (Tyr-Tyr-Glu-Glu)-poly(DLAla)--poly(Lys), Immunology, 49:9.
Parhami-Seren, B., Eshhar, Z., and Mozes, E., 1984, Serological analysis of idiotypic determinants on monoclonal antibodies specific to poly(Tyr,Glu)-poly(DLAla)--poly(Lys) and its ordered analogue (Tyr-Tyr-Glu-Glu)-poly(DLAla)--poly(Lys), Immunology, 51:367.
Rajewsky, K., and Takemori, T., 1983, Genetics, expression and function of idiotypes, Ann. Rev. Immunol., 1:569.
Sela, M., Fuchs, S., and Arnon, R., 1962, Studies on the chemical basis of the antigenicity of proteins. V. Synthesis, characterization and immunogenicity of some multichain and linear polypeptides containing tyrosine, Biochem. J., 85:223.
Sredni, B., and Schwartz, R.H., 1981, Antigen specific proliferating T lymphocyte clones. Methodology, specificity, MHC restriction and alloreactivity, Immunol. Rev., 54:187.
Strassmann, G., Lifshitz, R., and Mozes, E., 1980, Elicitation of delayed-type hypersensitivity responses to poly(LTyr,LGlu)-poly(DLAla)--poly(LLys) by anti-idiotypic antibodies, J. Exp. Med., 152:1448.
Sy, M.S., Brown, A.R., Benacerraf, B., and Greene, M.I., 1980, Antigen and receptor driven regulatory mechanisms. III. Induction of delayed-type hypersensitivity to azobenzearsonate with anti-cross reactive idiotypic antibodies, J. Exp. Med., 151:896.
Tada, T., and Okumura, R., 1979, The role of antibody-specific factors in the immune response, Adv. Immunol., 28:1.
Tarkakovsky, B., Kovacs, E.J., Takacs, L., and Durum, S.K., 1986, T cell clone producing an IL-1 like activity after stimulation by antigen-presenting B cells, J. Immunol., 137:160.
Weissberger, H.Z., Shenk, R.R., and Dickler, H.B., 1983, Anti-idiotype stimulation of antigen specific antigen independent antibody response in vitro. I. Evidence for stimulation of helper T lymphocyte function, J. Exp. Med.., 158:465.

MODULATION OF T-CELL FUNCTIONS BY PEPTIDE HORMONES

Christopher J. Krco, Tu T. Nguyen* and Vay Liang W. Go*

Department of Immunology and *Gastroenterology Unit
Mayo Clinic Clinic and Medical School
Rochester, MN 55905

INTRODUCTION

An immune response is a net result of a myriad set of cellular interactions, each interaction having multiple regulatory points. Although the nature of the regulatory factors is not fully known, the role of genetics, age, nutrition and circadium rhythm in affecting immunocompetence has been described (Rogers et al, 1979). More recently, it has been suggested that psychoneurological components may also be a potential source of immunomodulatory influences (Solomon, 1981; Riley, 1981; Fauman, 1982). Circumstantial evidence collected as a result of measuring the effects of central nervous system lesions, sympathectomy and emotional status on immunity have led to the concept of nerve mediated regulation of immune responses (Solomon, 1981; Riley, 1981; Jankovic and Isakovic, 1973). Whether denoted as "psychoimmunology", "psychoneuroimmunology" or "neuroimmunomodulation", the common denominator is the prediction that lymphoid cell function may be modulated as a consequence of the release of neuropeptides within the lymphoid tissue microenvironment. Innervation of lymph nodes, spleen, and thymus have been described in several species. In vitro experimentation have indicated that some neuropeptides can augment or inhibit immune responses (Payan and Goetzl, 1985). While these data suggest that neuroendocrine substances may serve as immunomodulators there are discrepancies in the literature concerning the effects mediated by some neuropeptides. Although this line of investigation is promising, systematic analyses of the effects of a variety of neuropeptides on a battery of immunologic assays within a given species has not been reported. In particular, the effects of neuropeptides on mouse lymphoid cell function is not well known. We summarize here results of testing in vitro ten neuropeptides present in intrinsic nerves on immunologic reactions in the mouse.

MATERIALS AND METHODS

Details of in vitro cultures have been previously published (Krco et al, 1986a, 1986b).

RESULTS

Initial investigations were directed towards determining the effects of exogenously adding β-endorphin and vasoactive intestinal peptide (VIP) on the response of lymph node cells stimulated with Con A (Table 1). It was observed that VIP would modulate the Con A induced blastogenesis (as measured as ^{3}H-thymidine incorporation) in a dose dependent manner from 10^{-6} (46% of control) to 10^{-11} M (89% of control) while under identical conditions β-endorphin modulation the response is less than 10%. Failure to detect a more pronounced effect of β-endorphin was not attributable to kinetic shifts, inappropriate cell density, or Con A concentration (data not shown).

Table 1. Comparison of the Ability of β-Endorphin and VIP to Modulate Con A Induced Proliferation of Lymph Node Cells

	% Control	
[Neuropeptide] M	β-Endorphin	VIP
10^{-6}	91	46
10^{-7}	91	59
10^{-8}	91	78
10^{-9}	92	95
10^{-10}	98	90
10^{-11}	93	89

Delaying the addition of VIP from 0 hr (40% of control) to 36 hr rendered the cultures refractory to the immunomodulatory effects of VIP (Table 2). In contrast there was no alteration of the Con A induced response if the addition of β-endorphin was delayed.

Table 2. Effect of Delaying the Addition of Neuropeptides to Con A Stimulated Lymph Node Cells

Time of Neuropeptide (10^{-6} M) Addition	% Control	
	β-Endorphin	VIP
0 hr	84	40
12 hr	86	56
24 hr	100	80
36 hr	100	100

Having demonstrated that VIP was a stronger immunomodulator than β-endorphin of mitogen activation of T-cells, the effects of exogenously adding four other neuropeptides (substance P, met-enkephalin, bombesin and somatostatin) on Con A mediated activation of lymph node cells was determined (Table 3). All of these additional peptides failed to affect (less than 10% modulation) the Con A response in the range of 10^{-6} to 10^{-11} M. As observed earlier, VIP (70% of control) but not β-endorphin (90% of control) inhibited T-cell activation.

Table 3. Ability of Neuropeptides to Modulate Con A Cultures (n=6)

[Neuropeptide] M	% Control: VIP	β-Endorphin	Substance P	Met-Enkephalin	Bombesin	Somatostatin
10^{-6}	48±2	89±3	91±4	95±4	82±6	84± 8
10^{-7}	57±4	87±3	88±5	94±2	80±9	77± 6
10^{-8}	74±2	86±4	90±3	86±2	82±7	87± 5
10^{-9}	82±2	84±4	91±3	88±5	79±7	77± 7
10^{-10}	80±4	87±5	87±4	89±5	82±9	78± 8
10^{-11}	80±3	87±6	89±5	93±4	74±9	74±10

The specificity of VIP for T-cells was suggested by the observation (data not shown) that LPS stimulated spleen cells were refractory to modulation by VIP or any other of the five neuropeptides (less than 10% modulation). Furthermore, if PHA was used to stimulate lymphoid cells then essentially the same titration curves for VIP and β-endorphin were obtained (data not shown) indicating that the modulation measured is indeed T-cell dependent and was not a pecularity of the Con A culture system.

VIP is considered to be a member of the secretin-glucagon family of gastrointestinal peptides which include secretin, glucagon, gastric inhibitory peptide (GIP) and peptide having NH_2-terminal histidine and COOH-terminal isoleucine (PHI) (Table 4). It has been reported that glucagon receptors exist on human mononuclear cells (Bhathena et al. 1982, 1982). While the effects of GIP, PHI and glucagon on mouse lymphoid cell function have not been reported, the effects of secretin on immune reactions, although largely unexplored, are thought to be weak (Ottaway and Greenberg, 1984). Therefore, the effects of adding these structurally related peptides to Con A stimulated cells was determined (Table 5). Both GIP and glucagon were ineffective as immunomodulators in that neither peptide had a major effect on the Con A induced blastogenesis (mean value of 80±2% of control) throughout the titration range of 10^{-6} to 10^{-16} M. In contrast, VIP exhibited a dose response inhibition beginning at 10^{-6} M (60% of control) which was lost at 10^{-16} M (78% of control) as did the closely related peptide PHI (48% of control at 10^{-6} M). Secretin was immunomodulatory only at 10^{-6} M (62% of control).

Table 4. Amino Acid Sequences of the Secretin-Glucagon Family of Peptides

```
              N-Terminus                                  C-Terminus
                 1   5    10   15   20   25   30   35   40

SECRETIN         HSDGTFTSELSRLRDSARLQRLLQFLV
GLUCAGON         HSQGTFTSDYSKYLDSRRAQDFVQWLMDT
VIP              HSDAVFTDNYTRLRKWQMAVKKYLNSILN
PHI              HADGVFTSDFSFLLGQLSAKKYLESLI
GIP              YAEGTFISDYSIMDKIRQQDFVNWLLAQKGKKSDWKHNITQ
```

Table 5. Ability of Secretin-Glucagon Family of Peptides to Inhibit Con A Cultures (n=3)

[Neuropeptide] M	% Control VIP	PHI	Secretin
10^{-6}	59± 2	48±1	62±6
10^{-8}	55± 3	57±1	86±9
10^{-10}	64±11	74±3	78±2
10^{-12}	67± 4	70±5	78±2
10^{-14}	72±10	79±2	79±2
10^{-16}	73± 1	78±1	80±2

The experiments described above did not demonstrate that the inhibition was a result of a VIP directly interacting with T-cells. Rather, it suggested that the inhibition was T-cell dependent. It was possible that other cells (e.g. macrophages) might be affected in such a way as to inhibit T-cell but not B-cell function. In an attempt to answer this question, a VIP receptor binding assay was developed (Nguyen et al, submitted for publication). The results of binding analyses are summarized in Table 6. It was possible to demonstrate that lymph node cells (6% specific binding) but not thymocytes or B-cells (3% specific binding) have appreciable numbers of VIP binding sites. Nylon wool purified T-cells (98% Thy-1^+) exhibited significant binding (14%). These receptor results coupled with the functional observation that VIP inhibits Con A but not LPS activation of lymphoid cells is consistent with the direct inhibition of T-cell activation as a consequence interaction with binding sites on the T-cell surface.

Table 6. Characteristics of ^{125}I-VIP Binding to Different Lymphocyte Populations

Cells	% Specific Binding	Kd (nM)
Lymph node	6	3.5
Thymocytes	2	4.8
T-cells	14	4.0
B-cells	3	-

DISCUSSION

We have demonstrated that VIP is an immunomodulator of Con A and PHA, but not LPS mediated, activation of T-cells. Furthermore, the demonstration of VIP binding sites on T-cells but not B-cells is consistent with the notion that VIP may directly inhibit T-cells. Consistent with this interpretation are the reports that VIP increases adenyl cyclase activity in human tumor cells, an event associated with inhibition of lymphocyte activation. Furthermore, the report that VIP also inhibits the activation of BALB/c spleen cells by Con A (Ottaway and Greenberg, 1984) would also be consistent with the concept that VIP is a neuromodulatory with immunosuppressive properties.

In contrast to the results obtained using VIP, β-endorphin was ineffective as a an immunomodulator of either Con A or LPS activation of lymphoid cells. Thus, our results using β-endorphin are in conflict with other reports demonstrating immunoenhancing (Gilman et al. 1982) or immunosuppressive (McCain et al. 1982) properties of β-endorphin on mitogen activation of cells from rat or human, respectively. Whether the reported differences in susceptibility to neuropeptide-mediated immunomodulation are in vitro cultural artifacts or indeed reflect species differences is not known. The possibility nevertheless does exist for genetic differences affecting the expression of VIP receptors.

The functional data suggesting that some neuropeptides affect lymphocyte function is supported by anatomical evidence for the localization of sympathetic nerve fibers in the corticomedullary thymic boundary, perivascular areas as well as the medullary, capsular and high endothelial venules of the splenic white pulp. That such innervation has functional significance to immune function has been supported by cholingeric and adrengeric stimulation experiments (Schiavi et al. 1975; Besendovsky et al. 1979), as well as chemically and surgically induced sympathectomy (Besedovsky et al. 1979).

An understanding of the effects of neuropeptides on lymphoid elements may contribute new perspectives into the pathophysiology of diseases having an immunologic component. For example, does the increase in VIP levels observed in pulmonary disease, duodenal ulcers, coeliac disease and some lung cancers impair pulmonary or gut-associated lymphoid tissue function? The more recent reports that structural and functional homologies may exist between neurohormones and lymphokines (Smith and Blalock, 1981) offer new avenues of thought and may provide a context in which to integrate immune and neuroendocrine functions.

REFERENCES

1. Besedovsky, H.O., Del Rey, A., De Prada, M. and Keller, H.H., 1979, Immunoregulation mediated by the sympathetic nervous system, Cellul. Immunol., 48:346.
2. Bhatena, S.J., Louie, J., Schechter, G.P., Redman, R., Wahl, L. and Recant, L., 1981, Identification of human mononuclear leukocytes bearing receptors for somatostatin and glucagon, Diabetes, 30:127.
3. Bhatena, S.J., Gazdar, A.F., Schechter, G.P., Russell, E.K., Soehnlen, F.E., Gritsman, A. and Recant, L., 1982, Expression of glucagon receptors on T- and B-lymphoblasts: comparison with insulin receptors, Endocrinol., 111:684.
4. Fauman, M.A., 1982, The central nervous system and the immune system, Biol. Psychol., 17:1459
5. Gilman, S.C., Schwartz, R.J., Milner, R.J., Bloom, F.E. and Geldman, J.D., 1983, β-endorphin enhances lymphocyte proliferative responses, Proc. Natl. Acad. Sci. (USA), 79:4226.
6. Jankovic, B.D. and Isakovic, K., 1973, Neuro-endocrine correlates of immune response, Int. Arch. Allergy Appl. Immunol., 45:360.
7. Krco, C.J., Gores, A. and Go, V.L.W., 1986, Gastrointestinal regulatory peptides modulate in vitro immune reactions of mouse lymphoid cells, Clin. Immuno. Immunopath., 39:308.

8. Krco, C.J., Gores, A. and Go, V.L.W., 1986, Gastrointestinal regulatory peptides modulate mouse lymphocyte functions under serum-free conditions in vitro, Immunol. Invest., 15:103.
9. McCain, H.W., Lamster, I.B., Bozone, J.M. and Grbic, J.T., 1982, β-endorphin modulates human immune reactivity via non-opiate receptor mechanisms, Life Sci., 31:1619.
10. Ottaway, C.A. and Greenberg, G.R., 1984, Interaction of vasoactive intestinal peptide with mouse lymphocytes: Specific binding and the modulation of mitogen responses, J. Immunol., 132:417.
11. Payan, D.G. and Goetzl, E.J., 1985, Modulation of lymphocyte function by sensory neuropeptides, J. Immunol., 135:783s.
12. Riley, V., 1981, Psychoneuroendocrine influences on immunocompetence and neoplasia, Science (Washington, D.C.), 212:1100.
13. Rogers, M.P., Devendra, D. and Reich, P.,1979, The influence of the psyche and brain on immunity and disease susceptibility: A critical review, Psychosom. Med., 41:147.
14. Schiavi, R.C., Macris, N.T., Camerino, M.S. and Stein, M., 1975, Effect of hypothalamic lesions on immediate hypersensitivity, Amer. J. Physiol., 228:596.
15. Smith, E.M. and Blalock, J.E., 1981, Human lymphocyte production of corticotropin and endorphin-like substances: Associaiton with leukocyte interferon, Proc. Natl. Acad. Sci. (USA), 78:7530.
16. Solomon, G.F., 1981, Psychoneurological effects on the immune response, Ann. Rev. Microbiol., 35:155.

ENDOSOME ACIDIFICATION AND THE PATHWAYS OF RECEPTOR-MEDIATED ENDOCYTOSIS

Frederick R. Maxfield and Darrell J. Yamashiro

Department of Pharmacology
New York University School of Medicine
550 First Avenue
New York, NY 10016

INTRODUCTION

Receptor-mediated endocytosis serves a variety of physiologically significant purposes (Goldstein et al., 1985). These include regulation of surface receptors, clearance of various macromolecules from the circulation, uptake of nutrients, transport of macromolecules across cells, cholesterol homeostasis, infection by some viruses, and penetration into the cytoplasm by certain toxins. Many basic steps in the endocytic pathways have been elucidated, but some of the essential features of this process remain poorly understood. Several organelles have been identified as being involved in endocytic events. However, in many cases the characteristics and function of these organelles are uncertain. Few proteins have been identified which are highly enriched in the individual endocytic compartments, and virtually nothing is known of the molecular recognition signals which govern targeting of proteins to specific endocytic or membrane recycling compartments.

One of the characteristic features of endocytic compartments is the regulation of the vesicle contents to an acidic pH (Tycko and Maxfield, 1982; Yamashiro et al., 1984). Internal acidity is maintained by an ATP-dependent proton pump which is in the membrane of endosomes (Mellman et al., 1986; Yamashiro et al., 1983). Studies of various endocytic processes have revealed that acidification plays a key role in many endocytic processes (Yamashiro and Maxfield, 1984). In this paper the kinetics of endosome acidification are described along with a discussion of the mechanisms by which acidification is responsible for carrying out key steps in the endocytic pathway. Recent studies have shown that different compartments on the endocytic pathway are regulated to different pH values. This regulation may determine when and where various sorting events take place within the cell.

ORGANELLES INVOLVED IN ENDOCYTOSIS AND RECYCLING

The pathways of receptor-mediated endocytosis have been described in several cell types. A schematic description of the pathway in the Chinese hamster ovary (CHO) cell line is shown in Figure 1. The endocytic processes in these cells are very similar to those observed in many other cell types. In our laboratory and others, these cells have been studied extensively because of their convenience for obtaining stable mutant cell lines.

Organelles along the endocytic pathway are easily identified by following the uptake of exogenously added tracers. For light microscopy, fluorescent probes (usually fluorescein or rhodamine) are generally used. For electron microscopy, ligands can be conjugated with horseradish peroxidase, ferritin, or colloidal gold. Alternatively, the

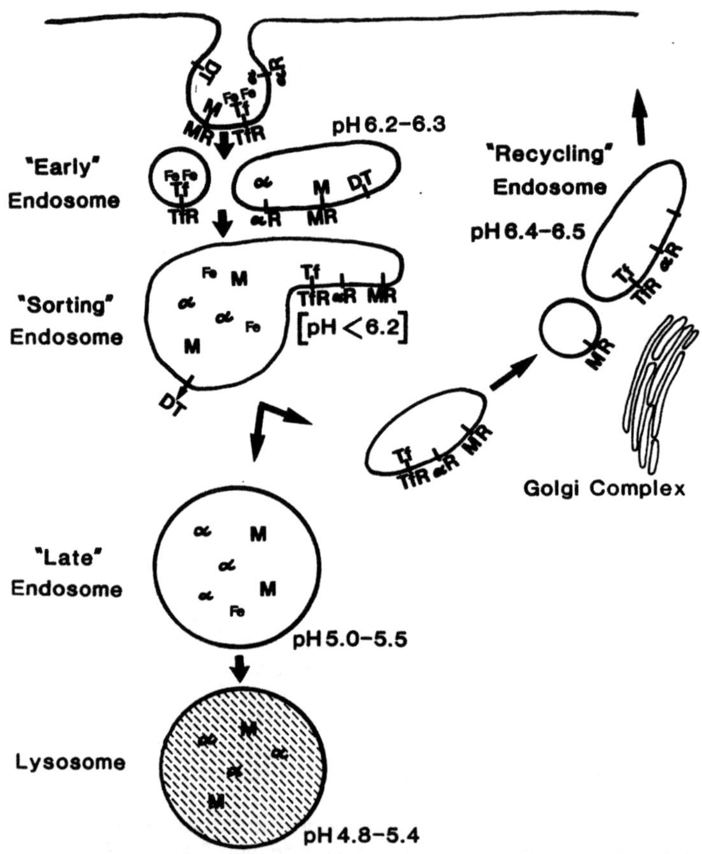

Figure 1. Schematic model for endocytosis and recycling in CHO cells. Various ligands bind to receptors which collect in clathrin coated pits. These include diphtheria toxin (DT), lysosomal enzymes with mannose–6–phosphate (M), transferrin (Tf), and α_2–macroglobulin (α). Within two minutes, these ligands are found in the early endosome compartment of small vesicles and tubules. In the sorting endosome, acidification releases iron (Fe) from Tf. Lysosomal enzymes and α_2–macroglobulin dissociate from their receptors and are delivered to lysosomes. Apo–Tf remains bound to its receptor and returns to the surface via a recycling endosome.

native molecules can be internalized by cells and then localized within intracellular compartments by immunofluorescence or immunoelectron microscopy. For biochemical studies, radiolabeled ligands can be used to follow endocytosis, recycling, and degradation in lysosomes. The kinetics of passage through organelles can also be followed using density gradient centrifugation of cell homogenates to identify specific compartments. The use of all of these methods has produced a basic description of many of the organelles involved in endocytosis.

The schematic diagram shown in Figure 1 is a current working model for the endocytic and recycling pathways in CHO cells. We have concentrated our work on two ligands: α_2–macroglobulin, which is internalized and degraded in lysosomes (Tycko et al., 1982), and transferrin, which returns to the cell surface intact (Klausner et al., 1983; Dautry–Varsat et al., 1983). The α_2–macroglobulin serves as a marker of the pathway leading to lysosomes. Transferrin remains associated with its receptor within the cell (Enns et al., 1983; Yamashiro et al., 1984). Thus, transferrin is a convenient tracer of receptor recycling pathways.

At very early incubation times, occupied receptors can be observed concentrated over clathrin–coated pits. Within 5 minutes after binding, essentially all of the occupied receptors have been cleared from the surface. Using electron microscopic tracers, two compartments become labeled during a 5 minute chase period (Yamashiro et al., 1984). One of these is a large electron lucent vesicle which is often irregularly shaped and is approximately 200–300 nm in diameter. The other compartment is made up of small vesicles or tubules which are approximately 80 nm in diameter. At early times, both α_2–macroglobulin and transferrin are seen in the small vesicles and tubules (Table I). These early small vesicles and tubules are predominantly near the cell surface. With further incubation, nearly all of the α_2–macroglobulin moves into the larger endocytic vesicles (Table I). The final destination of α_2–macroglobulin is lysosomes where it is degraded (Yamashiro et al., 1984). In contrast, most of the transferrin remains in small vesicles and tubules. Over a 5–15 minute chase period, the distribution of the labeled small vesicles becomes more localized, with a heavy concentration near the Golgi complex. Subsequently, transferrin and its receptor exit this compartment, and they are returned to the cell surface. The vesicles used for transport to the cell surface are not well characterized at present.

Table I. Characterization of Structures Containing Transferrin and α_2–Macroglobulin

	Distribution of Tf–Fer		Distribution of α_2M–Gold	
Conditions*	SV/T§	LV¶	SV/T	LV
5 min incubation no chase	79%	21%	47%	53%
5 min incubation 5 min chase	80%	20%	16%	84%
5 min incubation 10 min chase	75%	25%	10%	90%

* Cells were incubated with transferrin–ferritin conjugates (Tf–Fer) and α_2–macroglobulin–colloidal gold (α_2M–Gold) at 37°C for the indicated times and processed for electron microscopy. The data for each point were obtained from 200 electron micrographs containing between 350 and 1300 particles. A complete description of the method is in Yamashiro et al. (1984).

§ Small vesicles and tubules (SV/T) were structures with diameters less than 120 nm. Most of these were approximately 80 nm in diameter.

¶ Large endocytic vesicles (LV) were defined as having diameters greater than 120 nm. These included multivesicular bodies. At these times, less than 20% of the vesicles were lysosomes, as identified by acid phosphatase cytochemistry.

KINETICS OF ENDOSOME ACIDIFICATION

At this time, relatively little is known of the molecular recognition signals which govern intracellular routing during endocytosis. For example, it is not known how receptors (and in many cases only the occupied receptors) are concentrated over clathrin coated pits. Nor is it understood why many receptors recycle, whereas some receptors are degraded inside the cell after internalization.

One of the events which is now clearly associated with sorting processes is the acidification of endocytic compartments (Tycko et al, 1983; Yamashiro and Maxfield, 1984). Exposure to pH values between 5.0 and 7.0 has dramatic effects on many of the molecules brought into the cell by endocytosis. Many ligands dissociate from their receptors at pH values below 7. In the case of the epidermal growth factor receptor and the asialoglycoprotein receptor, we have shown that a large scale conformational change in the receptor accompanies the loss of affinity (DiPaola and Maxfield, 1984; Figure 2). At pH values below 6.0, diferric transferrin releases iron (Princiotto and Zapolski, 1975; Aisen and Listowsky, 1980). The apo-transferrin remains receptor-associated at low pH values, but it dissociates at the neutral pH encountered when the complex returns to the cell surface (Dautry-Varsat et al., 1983; Klausner et al., 1983).

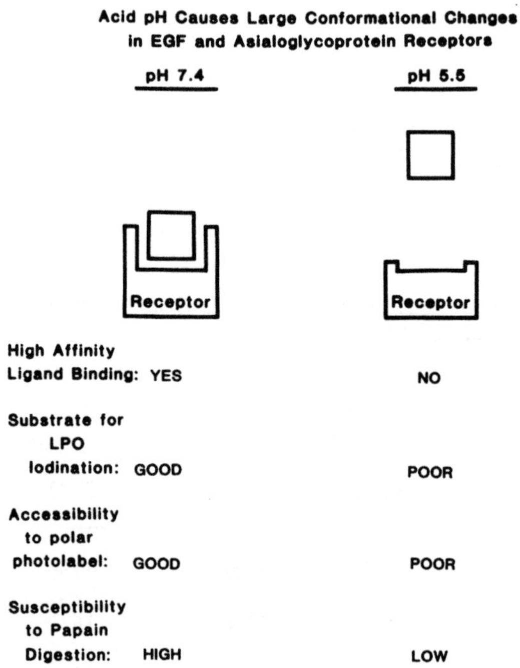

Figure 2. Effects of pH on biochemical properties of the epidermal growth factor (EGF) and asialoglycoprotein receptors. EGF receptors were examined in living A-431 cells. Purified asialoglycoprotein receptors were incorporated into phosphatidylcholine liposomes. As shown schematically, three methods were used to detect possible conformational changes between pH 7.4 and pH 5.5. Both receptors were less efficiently iodinated by lactoperoxidase (LPO) at pH 5.5, even though the enzyme is more active at the mildly acidic pH. At acidic pH, the receptors were less heavily labeled by a nonspecific, highly polar photo label (NAP-taurine) which only labels the outer surface of proteins. They were also less susceptible to proteolysis by papain at low pH. These results suggest that both receptors undergo a conformational change which reduces overall exposure to the medium at pH 5.5 (DiPaola and Maxfield, 1984).

Some viruses and toxins undergo significant changes in conformation when exposed to acidic pH. Diphtheria toxin acquires the ability to insert into lipid membranes (Olsnes and Sandvig, 1983). This insertion is an important step in the translocation of the enzymatic portion of the toxin into the cytosol. Coat proteins of enveloped viruses such as influenza or Semliki Forest virus also undergo conformational changes (Kielian and Helenius, 1985). These changes facilitate fusion of the virus membrane with various target membranes (White et al., 1980). In an endosome, this fusion allows the virus nucleocapsid to escape into the cytosol (Marsh et al., 1983).

Many of these pH-dependent processes occur over relatively narrow pH ranges. For example, pH-dependent membrane fusions mediated by viruses are apparently regulated over a range of approximately 0.3 pH units (White et al., 1980). Different ligands dissociate from their receptors at different pH values. For example, α_2-macroglobulin is nearly completely dissociated by pH 6.5 (Maxfield, 1982), but lysosomal enzymes bound to the mannose-6-phosphate receptor require pH values below 6.0 for efficient dissociation (Gonzalez-Noriega et al., 1980). These results suggest the possibility that sorting events could be differentially regulated by progressive exposure of internalized receptors to increasingly acidic pH values. In order to determine whether this occurs, it is necessary to measure the pH of endocytic compartments as a function of time. It is also necessary to determine the pH of specific types of organelles. Changes in the pH surrounding an internalized molecule could occur as a result of pH changes within an organelle, or the changes could result from transfer to a new type of organelle.

The pH in endocytic compartments can be measured using fluorescein-labeled ligands (Ohkuma and Poole, 1978; Tycko and Maxfield, 1982). Fluorescein fluorescence

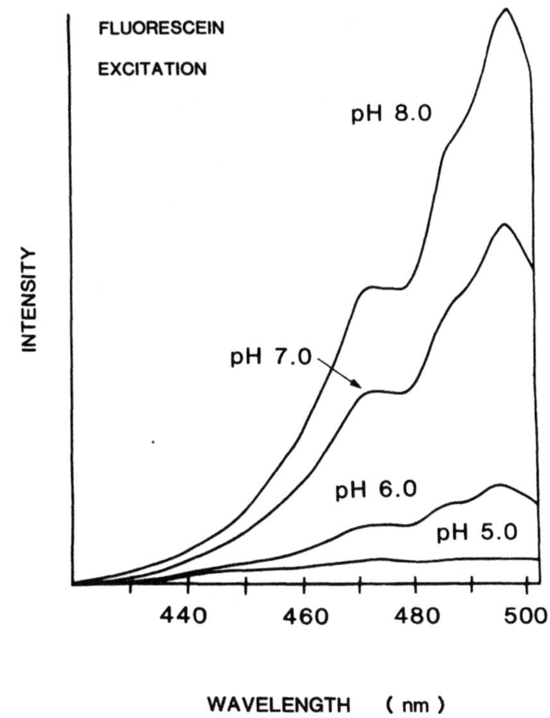

Figure 3. pH dependence of fluorescein fluorescence. α_2-macroglobulin was labeled with fluorescein-isothiocyanate. Fluorescence excitation spectra (emission at 520 nm) were obtained in buffers between pH 5.0 and pH 8.0. The excitation profile is strongly pH dependent in this range.

intensity increases dramatically between pH 5.0 and pH 7.0 (Figure 3). Thus, changes in fluorescence intensity can be used as an assay for changes in pH. Using the ratio of fluorescence intensities at two wavelengths (450- and 490-nm) the actual pH values can be obtained. These properties have been used in several studies to measure the pH of lysosomes and the pH of the large, prelysosomal endocytic vesicles. In various cell types, lysosomes have pH values between 4.6 and 5.2, and the large, endocytic vesicles have pH values between 5.0 and 5.5 (Ohkuma and Poole, 1978; Tycko and Maxfield, 1982; Tycko et al., 1983; Yamashiro et al., 1984).

For technical reasons it has been difficult to make accurate pH measurements in the earliest endocytic compartments. Two problems are encountered. First, at very early times there is relatively little fluorescent probe internalized. Thus, the signal is weak compared to cellular autofluorescence. A second problem results from nonsynchronous internalization. Any fluorescein left on the surface (pH 7.4) will fluoresce with greater relative intensity than fluorescein inside an acidic endocytic compartment. This can lead to serious underestimates of the acidification of endocytic vesicles. In order to circumvent these problems, we have developed a new null point method which provides accurate pH measurements as early as 2-3 minutes after the start of endocytosis. The steps in this procedure are shown in Table II. Measurements are made using a microscope spectrophotometer (Maxfield, 1985).

Using three different fluorescein-labeled probes, we have measured the kinetics of endosome acidification in CHO cells (Table III). In the wild type cells, compartments labeled with the fluid phase marker fluorescein-dextran reach an average pH of 6.3 within three minutes. Within 10 minutes, the average pH drops below 6.0. Rapid acidification of vesicles containing α_2-macroglobulin is also observed. In the case of transferrin, rapid acidification is observed, but on further incubation the average pH increases. This increase in pH corresponds to the movement of transferrin to the para-Golgi small vesicles and tubules which have been shown to have a pH of 6.4 in CHO cells.

Table II. Measurement of Average pH in Endocytic Compartments by Null Point Method

Step	Measurements and Interpretation
1. Incubate with fluorescein-labeled ligand, rinse exhaustively.	Total cell-associated fluorescence is measured. Includes intracellular and surface fluorescein plus cellular autofluorescence.
2. Change buffer to a non-permeant buffer at test pH (e.g., pH 6.4).	Total fluorescence decreases due to reduced fluorescence from extracellular dye at the lower pH. Intracellular fluorescein and autofluorescence are unaffected.
3. Change to a membrane permeant buffer at the same test pH.	Extracellular fluorescence and autofluorescence are unaffected. Only the intracellular fluorescein fluorescence is changed. If the intensity rises at this step, the average pH of the intracellular compartments is below the test pH. If the intensity falls, the average pH is above the test pH.

Table III. Time Dependence of Acidification of Endocytic Compartments

Fluorescent* Probe	Conditions Pulse / Chase	pH Wildtype WTB	pH Mutants DTG 1–5–4	pH Mutants DTF 1–5–1
F–Dextran	2 min / 1 min	6.3 ± 0.2	n.d.	n.d.
	5 min / 1 min	6.2 ± 0.1	6.7 ± 0.1	6.7 ± 0.1
	5 min / 5 min	<6.0	6.5 ± 0.2	6.4 ± 0.1
	5 min / 10 min	<6.0	6.1 ± 0.3	<6.0
F–α_2M	9 min / 1 min	6.0 ± 0.1	6.8 ± 0.3	6.4 ± 0.2
	9 min / 6 min	<6.0	6.4 ± 0.2	6.0 ± 0.3
F–Transferrin	5 min / 1 min	6.2 ± 0.1	6.7 ± 0.1	6.3 ± 0.2
	18 min / 2 min	6.5 ± 0.1	6.6 ± 0.1	6.5 ± 0.1

* The pH of F–Dextran, F–α_2M, and F–Transferrin containing compartments were measured using a null point method as described in the text. A full description of this method will be presented (Yamashiro and Maxfield, in preparation).

In addition to the wild type cells we have also made measurements with two mutant CHO cell lines. These lines are resistant to diphtheria toxin, and they are defective in the release of iron from transferrin and the internalization of lysosomal enzymes (Robbins et al., 1983, 1984; Klausner et al., 1984). Thus, they appear to be excellent candidates for defects in acidification. As shown in Table III, both cell lines do exhibit defects in acidification of early endocytic compartments. However, in both mutants acidification to pH 6.0 or below is observed within a few minutes.

pH IN MORPHOLOGICALLY DEFINED COMPARTMENTS

As described above, ligands pass through a series of distinct compartments during endocytosis and recycling. In order to measure the pH in these separate compartments, we have developed image analysis methods in conjunction with image intensification fluorescence microscopy to measure the pH within individual endocytic compartments. Using these methods, it is possible to measure the pH in single large endocytic vesicles (Tycko et al., 1983) or in the para–Golgi small vesicle and tubule compartment which becomes filled with fluorescein transferrin (Yamashiro et al., 1984). Measurements made on these compartments are summarized in Table IV.

In the wild type cells, the average pH of the large endocytic vesicles is always at or below pH 5.8. Even at very early times, when the average pH of all compartments is above pH 6.0, these large vesicles maintain a more acidic pH. The difference in pH between the early and late endosomes is more striking in the mutant cells. In both mutants, we find that acidification of large endocytic vesicles and lysosomes is essentially the same as in wild type cells at all incubation times. Thus, it appears that the defect in the mutant cells is limited to the early endocytic compartments.

The finding that only the acidification of early compartments is affected in the mutants provides important information about mechanisms of pH regulation and about the intracellular organelles where pH–dependent sorting processes occur. First, it is clear that pH regulation can be maintained by different mechanisms in the two prelysosomal endocytic compartments. This is also shown for wild type cells by the observation that the pH in large endocytic vesicles at early times is lower than the average pH of all endocytic compartments. Furthermore, the pH of the para–Golgi

Table IV. pH Measurement in Morphologically Identifiable Compartments

Fluorescent* Probe	Compartment	pH Wildtype WTB	Mutants DTG 1–5–4	DTF 1–5–1
F–Dextran	Large, Prelysosomal Vesicle	5.8 ± 0.1	5.9 ± 0.2	6.0 ± 0.1
	Lysosome	5.3 ± 0.1	5.2 ± 0.3	5.3 ± 0.1
F–α_2M	Large, Prelysosomal Vesicle	5.4 ± 0.1	5.7 ± 0.1	5.6 ± 0.3
F–Transferrin	Para–Golgi Vesicles and Tubules	6.4 ± 0.1	6.3 ± 0.1	6.4 ± 0.1

* The pH of various endocytic endocytic compartments were measured using image intensified fluorescence microscopy and digital image processing (Tycko et al., 1983; Yamashiro et al., 1984). A full description of the measurements will be presented (Yamashiro and Maxfield, in preparation).

compartment is higher than the pH of large endocytic vesicles. The pH of this compartment is the same in the two mutants and wild type. The mechanisms responsible for the differences in pH are not clear at this time. One possibility is that the ATP–dependent proton pumps or a regulatory subunit are different in the various compartments. Alternatively, the differences may be due to other ion transport proteins. These could affect the pH directly (i.e., by transporting protons) or indirectly (by changing the membrane potential against which the electrogenic proton pump must work).

The step–wise exposure to an acidic pH can be important for physiological processes. When cells are exposed to Semliki Forest virus, there is a lag of a few minutes before cytoplasmic penetration occurs (Kielian et al., 1986). The early kinetics of penetration by this virus are the same in wild type cells as in the DTF or DTG mutants (A. Helenius, I. Mellman, and M. Marsh, personal communication). Thus, it appears that the pH achieved in the early endosomes of wild type cells is not sufficiently acidic to cause the conformational change in the virus coat protein. The pH found in the large endocytic vesicles of mutant or wild type cells is sufficiently low to allow penetration. Viruses with a higher pH threshold would be expected to penetrate from the earlier endocytic compartment.

Relatively little transferrin enters the large endocytic compartment (Table I). In the wild type cells, the acidification of the early small vesicles and tubules may be sufficient to release iron from transferrin. In the mutant cells, iron is released from only about 25% of the internalized transferrin molecules (Yamashiro and Maxfield, unpublished). This confirms that in the mutants most of the transferrin does not pass through the highly acidic large endocytic vesicle. It also suggests that the early small vesicle and tubule compartment (or the brief fusion of these with the large endocytic vesicle) may be the site of iron release in the wild type cells.

The resistance of the mutant cells to diphtheria toxin indicates that exposure to low pH in a large endocytic vesicle is not sufficient to cause penetration into the cytoplasm. Recent studies have suggested that factors in addition to low pH are required for diphtheria toxin penetration (Olsnes and Sandvig, 1983).

Delivery of α_2–macroglobulin to lysosomes is the same in the mutant cells and in the wild type cells (Yamashiro and Maxfield, unpublished). However, delivery of lysosomal enzymes is defective in DTG and DTF (Robbins et al., 1983, 1984). Our pH measurements show that the pH of the early endocytic compartment will dissociate α_2-macroglobulin, but not lysosomal enzymes, from the receptor. In the mutant cells, the lysosomal enzymes appear to remain receptor-associated, so they recycle rather than being delivered to lysosomes.

SUMMARY AND CONCLUSIONS

Acidification of endocytic compartments occurs within 2–3 minutes following internalization. In CHO cells, three kinetically and morphologically distinct endocytic or recycling compartments can be identified. Measurements of the pH in these compartments show that the acidity of the compartments is regulated independently, although some parts of the acidification mechanism may be shared. The pH values found in these compartments provide a satisfactory explanation for various required steps in the endocytosis and recycling pathways. Further work is required to understand the biochemical basis for the pH regulation in various intracellular organelles.

ACKNOWLEDGEMENTS: We are grateful to Dr. Tim McGraw for helpful discussions. This work was supported by grant DK-27083 from the National Institutes of Health.

REFERENCES

Aisen, P. and Listowsky, I., 1980, Iron transport and storage proteins, Ann. Rev. Biochem., 49:367.

Dautry-Varsat, A., Ciechanover, A. and Lodish, H.F., 1983, pH and the recycling of transferrin during receptor-mediated endocytosis, Proc. Natl. Acad. Sci. USA, 80:2258.

DiPaola, M. and Maxfield, F.R., 1984, Conformational changes in the receptor for epidermal growth factor and asialoglycoproteins induced by the mildly acidic pH found in endocytic vesicles, J. Biol. Chem., 259:9163.

Enns, C.A., Larrick, J.W., Suomalainen, H. Schroder, J. and Sussman, H.H., 1983, Co-migration and internalization of transferrin and its receptor on K562 cells. J. Cell Biol., 97:579.

Goldstein, J.L., Brown, M.S., Anderson, R.G.W., Russell, D.W. and Schneider, W.J., 1985, Receptor-mediated endocytosis: Concepts emerging from the LDL receptor system, Ann. Rev. Cell Biol., 1:11.

Gonzalez-Noriega, A., Grubb, J.H., Talkad, V. and Sly, W.S., 1980, Chloroquine inhibits lysosomal enzyme pinocytosis and enhances lysosomal enzyme secretion by impairing receptor recycling, J. Cell Biol.,85:839.

Kielian, M.C. and Helenius, A., 1985, pH-induced alterations in the fusogenic spike protein of Semliki Forest virus, J. Cell Biol., 101:2284.

Kielian, M.C., Marsh, M. and Helenius, A., 1986, Kinetics of endosome acidification detected by mutant and wild-type Semliki Forest virus, EMBO J., 5:3103.

Klausner, R.D., van Renswoude, J., Ashwell, G., Kempf, C., Schechter, A.N., Dean, A. and Bridges, K.R., 1983, Receptor-mediated endocytosis of transferrin in K562 cells, J. Biol. Chem., 258:4715.

Klausner, R.D., van Renswoude, J., Kempf, C., Rao, K., Bateman, J.L. and Robbins, A.R., 1984, Failure to release iron from transferrin in a Chinese hamster ovary cell mutant pleiotropically defective in endocytosis, J. Cell Biol., 98:1098.

Marsh, M., Bolzau, E. and Helenius, A., 1983, Penetration of Semliki Forest virus from acidic prelysosomal vacuoles, Cell, 32:931.

Maxfield, F.R., 1982, Weak bases and ionophores rapidly and reversibly raise the pH of endocytic vesicles in cultured mouse fibroblasts, J. Cell Biol., 95:676.

Maxfield, F.R., 1985, Acidification of endocytic vesicles and lysosomes, in: "Endocytosis," I. Pastan and M.C. Willingham, eds., Plenum Press, New York, pp. 235–257.
Mellman, I., Fuchs, R. and Helenius, A., 1986, Acidification of the endocytic and exocytic pathways, Ann. Rev. Biochem., 55:663.
Ohkuma, S. and Poole, B., 1978, Fluorescence probe measurement of the intralysosomal pH in living cells and the perturbation of pH by various agents, Proc. Natl. Acad. Sci. USA, 75:3327.
Olsnes, S. and Sandvig, K., 1983, Entry of toxic proteins into cells, in: "Receptor–mediated endocytosis: Receptors and Recognition," P. Cuatrecasas and T.F. Roth, eds., Chapman and Hall, London, pp. 187–236.
Princiotto, J.V. and Zapolski, E.J., 1975, Difference between the two iron–binding sites of transferrin, Nature, 255:87.
Robbins, A.R., Peng, S.S. and Marshall, J.L., 1983, Mutant Chinese hamster ovary cells pleiotropically defective in receptor–mediated endocytosis, J. Cell Biol., 96:1064.
Robbins, A.R., Oliver, C., Bateman, J.L., Krag, S.S., Galloway, C.J. and Mellman, I., 1984, A single mutation in Chinese hamster ovary cells impairs both Golgi and endosomal function, J. Cell Biol., 99:1296.
Tycko, B. and Maxfield, F.R., 1982, Rapid acidification of endocytic vesicles containing α_2–macroglobulin, Cell, 28:643.
Tycko, B., Keith, C.H. and Maxfield, F.R., 1983, Rapid acidification of endocytic vesicles containing asialoglycoprotein in cells of a human hepatoma line, J. Cell Biol., 97:1762.
White, J., Kartenbeck, J. and Helenius, A., 1980, Fusion of Semliki Forest Virus with the plasma membrane can be induced by low pH, J. Cell Biol., 87:264.
Yamashiro, D.J., Fluss, S.R. and Maxfield, F.R., 1983, Acidification of endocytic vesicles by an ATP–dependent proton pump, J. Cell Biol., 97:929.
Yamashiro, D.J. and Maxfield, F.R., 1984, Acidification of endocytic compartments and the intracellular pathways of ligands and receptors, J. Cell. Biochem., 26:231.
Yamashiro, D.J., Tycko, B., Fluss, S.R. and Maxfield, F.R., 1984, Segregation of transferrin to a mildly acidic (pH 6.5) para–Golgi compartment in the recycling pathway, Cell, 37:789.

INTRACELLULAR TRAFFIC OF THE MANNOSE 6-PHOSPHATE RECEPTOR AND ITS LIGANDS

Catherine M. Nolan and William S. Sly

Biochemistry Department, St. Louis University School of Medicine, 1402 S. Grand Blvd., St. Louis, MO 63104

Eukaryotic cells are compartmentalized, increasing the efficiency of the cell by allowing the existence of microenvironments of unique properties and by segregating potentially incompatible biochemical reactions. The targeting of newly synthesized macromolecules to their correct location within the cell and the maintenance of the distinctive macromolecular composition of these compartments is an important feature of cellular organization. The mechanisms by which cells direct the intracellular traffic of macromolecules are the subject of much investigation in cell biology. One well-studied example of intracellular sorting and trafficking is the mannose 6-phosphate-mediated transport of lysosomal enzymes.

LYSOSOMES

The lysosome is a membrane-enclosed intracellular organelle which contains numerous hydrolytic enzymes. These are the products of unlinked genes and include proteases, nucleases, glycosidases, lipases, phospholipases, phosphatases and sulfatases. All of these enzymes have acidic pH optima. A pH of approximately 5.0 is maintained within the lysosome by means of a membrane-bound, ATP-dependent proton pump. Lysosomes are a heterogeneous group of organelles and are often classified for convenience into two groups: primary lysosomes, which contain only newly synthesized acid hydrolases, and secondary lysosomes, in which newly synthesized enzymes have been brought into contact with substrate material, for example through endocytosis. This classification is, of course, an oversimplification.

The lysosome plays an important role in degradative cellular metabolism. Its significance in the physiology of the whole organism is reflected in the numerous inherited disorders of lysosomal metabolism which have been described. Most of them have severe consequences for affected patients. These disorders usually result from the deficiency of a single acid hydrolase, with the consequent accumulation of the undegraded substrate within the lysosome. The study of these diseases has been helpful in elucidating the physiological role of these enzymes and the routes of intracellular transport of acid hydrolases.

ACID HYDROLASES SHARE A COMMON "RECOGNITION MARKER"

The transport of acid hydrolases to lysosomes is part of the more general phenomenon whereby the cell regulates the protein composition of its intracellular compartments. The study of I-cell disease fibroblasts, cells which secrete to excess a large number of acid hydrolases and in which the lysosomes are deficient in these enzymes, led to the hypothesis that the transport of acid hydrolases was dependent on a common "recognition marker" present on a large number of lysosomal enzymes (Hickman and Neufeld, 1972). This marker was subsequently shown to be carbohydrate in nature and sensitive to acid phosphatase treatment, and was identified as mannose 6-phosphate (M6P) (Kaplan et al., 1977). The identification of M6P as the recognition marker for the targeting of acid hydrolases to lysosomes provoked the search for a protein capable of recognizing this sugar determinant on acid hydrolases. An integral membrane protein fulfilling these requirements was identified and termed the phosphomannosyl receptor (PMR) (Rome et al., 1979; Fischer et al., 1980a).

BIOSYNTHESIS OF ACID HYDROLASES

Precursor lysosomal enzymes, together with many other secretory and membrane proteins, are synthesized on endoplasmic reticulum-bound ribosomes. These proteins have been shown to have a signal sequence which mediates their interaction with the signal recognition particle (SRP). This interaction is followed by binding of the complex to the SRP-receptor (docking protein) and translocation of the nascent protein into the lumen of the ER, with subsequent cleavage of the signal peptide. These reactions are common to many proteins and have been the subject of a recent review (Walter and Lingappa, 1986).

As seen with non-lysosomal glycoproteins, acid hydrolases are modified in the ER by the addition of a high mannose oligosaccharide from a dolichol pyrophosphate intermediate (Kornfeld and Kornfeld, 1985). This oligosaccharide is then subjected to the typical "trimming" reactions which have been shown to occur in the ER. Following this, they are transferred to the Golgi apparatus, where further trimming and modification of the oligosaccharide side chains take place. A unique modification, which occurs only in the case of lysosomal enzymes and not with other non-lysosomal proteins, is the addition of the mannose 6-phosphate recognition marker.

GENERATION OF THE MANNOSE 6-PHOSPHATE MARKER

The M6P marker is added to newly synthesized acid hydrolases in a two-step reaction (see Figure 1) (Reitman and Kornfeld, 1981; Varki and Kornfeld, 1981; Waheed et al., 1981, 1982a). The first step in this process is the addition of an N-acetylglucosamine 1-phosphate residue to the six position of a selected mannosyl moiety of an oligosaccharide side chain on the precursor acid hydrolase. This gives rise to a phosphodiester intermediate. The reaction is catalyzed by the enzyme, UDP-N-acetylglucosamine:lysosomal enzyme N-acetylglucosaminyl-1-phosphotransferase (termed the phosphotransferase), and it is this enzyme that is defective in I-cell disease (Mucolipidosis II [ML II]) and in pseudo-Hurler polydystrophy (ML III) (Reitman et al., 1981). In the second step of the reaction, the N-acetylglucosamine residue is removed. This secondary reaction, catalyzed by N-acetylglucosamine-1-phosphodiester α-N-acetyl-glucosaminidase (the Man 6P GlcNAc glucosaminidase), exposes the M6P marker, which can then be recognized by the PMR.

Only lysosomal enzymes receive this M6P recognition marker. The question of how lysosomal enzymes are selectively recognized by the phosphorylating enzymes is of major importance. Analysis of the oligosaccharide units of several lysosomal enzymes revealed that they are no different from those found on many glycoproteins which are poor substrates for the phosphorylating enzymes (Hasilik et al., 1980; Goldberg and Kornfeld, 1981; Takahashi et al., 1983). It is the protein portion of the lysosomal enzyme which contains the major determinant responsible for their recognition by the phosphotransferase. Deglycosylated lysosomal enzymes are potent inhibitors of the phosphotransferase (Lang et al., 1984). This determinant does not apparently reside in the primary sequence alone. It is sensitive to treatments that destroy the tertiary structure of the enzymes, such as

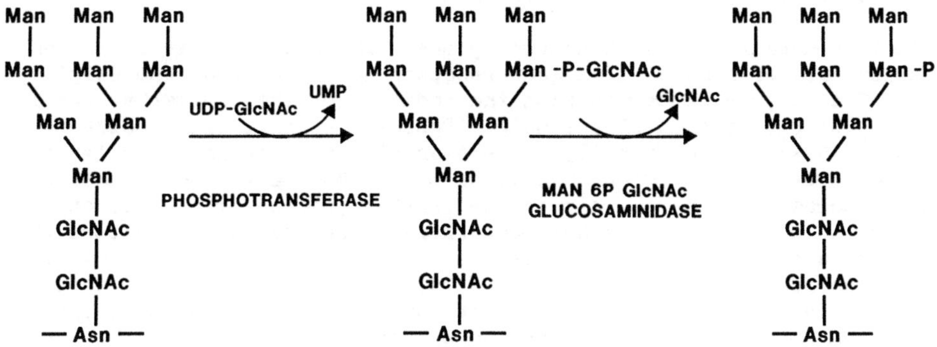

Fig. 1. Generation of the mannose 6-phosphate recognition marker by a two-step reaction.

proteolysis and heat denaturation (Lang et al., 1984). The phosphotransferase appears to possess not only a catalytic site which recognizes the acceptor oligosaccharide, but also a site capable of recognizing some common feature of the conformation of many lysosomal enzymes. Recently, several lysosomal enzymes have been cloned and sequenced and it is likely that many more will be cloned in the near future (Faust et al., 1985; Fukushima et al., 1985; Myerowitz et al., 1985; Bishop et al., 1986; Korneluk et al., 1986; Nishimura et al., 1986; Tsuji et al., 1986; Oshima et al., 1987). To date, however, a common signal for processing of acid hydrolases by the phosphotransferase has not become clear from the sequence information. The application of the techniques of molecular biology to this question will undoubtedly help in our understanding of this important feature of the transport of lysosomal enzymes.

ACID HYDROLASES ARE SEGREGATED FROM OTHER GLYCOPROTEINS IN A RECEPTOR-DEPENDENT MANNER

Following exposure of the M6P marker, lysosomal enzymes may be recognized by and bind to the PMR. This is then followed by their segregation from glycoproteins bound for other destinations in the cell or for secretion. Prior to delivery of the acid hydrolases to the lysosome, dissociation of ligand from the receptor occurs, under the influence of an acidic environment (receptor-ligand complexes dissociate rapidly below pH 5.7) (Fischer et al., 1980a). The compartment in which ligands dissociate from their receptors has been called the compartment of uncoupling of receptors and ligand (CURL) (Geuze et al., 1983). It has been suggested that, prior to enzyme delivery to the lysosome, the ligand-receptor complexes become transiently associated with the plasma membrane and subsequently reinternalized, since acid hydrolases have been found to be associated with the cell surface (von Figura and Voss, 1979; Geuze et al., 1985). However, the growth of cells in culture over several generations in the presence of mannose 6-phosphate (which should promote dissociation of ligand-receptor complexes at the cell surface) does not result in lower levels of lysosomally-associated acid hydrolases (von Figura and Weber, 1978; Sly et al., 1981). Thus, the majority of acid hydrolases probably reach the lysosome without trafficking through the plasma membrane.

Another detail in this transport process which is unclear at present is the exact site of removal of ligand-receptor complexes from the Golgi apparatus. The enzymes concerned with the addition of the M6P marker are located in the cis portion of the Golgi (Pohlmann et al., 1982; Goldberg and Kornfeld, 1983). Theoretically, diversion of acid hydrolases to lysosomes could occur from this region. Addition of the M6P marker to an antenna of an oligosaccharide side chain prevents further processing of that antenna (Goldberg et al., 1984). It has been shown by several investigators that acid hydrolases isolated from lysosomes contain complex- or hybrid-type oligosaccharides (van Elsen and Leroy, 1979; Vladutiu, 1983) and this was taken as evidence that the enzymes must have passed through the trans portion of the Golgi apparatus, where the enzymes responsible for the assembly of these types of oligosaccharides are located (Dunphy et al., 1981; Roth and Berger, 1982; Goldberg and Kornfeld, 1983). However, a problem with these experiments was the possibility that the presence of the complex- or hybrid-type oligosaccharides in lysosomally-associated enzymes was due to the presence in lysosomes of acid hydrolases which had been endocytosed from the extracellular environment. To address this possibility, we have recently grown cells defective in β-galactosidase activity (and therefore defective in one of the initial steps in the lysosomal degradation of glycoproteins) in the presence of M6P, to prevent endocytosis of secreted enzymes (Fedde and Sly, 1985). The lysosomes of such cells possess acid hydrolases in which the carbohydrate composition is very similar to that found in secreted acid hydrolases which are thought to have passed through the trans portion of the Golgi apparatus.

It seems, then, that acid hydrolases may in fact traverse the entire structure of the Golgi apparatus. As will be discussed later, this suggestion is supported by immunocytochemical observations on the subcellular localization of acid hydrolases and the phosphomannosyl receptor. It is not clear, however, if transport through the trans region of the Golgi is necessary for their correct sorting to lysosomes.

In lysosomes, the proforms of most acid hydrolases are proteolytically processed to yield the lower molecular weight mature forms. These processing reactions have been recently reviewed (Hasilik and von Figura, 1984). The significance of this processing is not clear. It may be that it serves to activate or stabilize some enzymes in the lysosome.

Acid hydrolases which fail to receive the M6P marker are not segregated to the lysosome and are generally secreted through the constitutive secretion pathway, as is a small proportion of enzymes which are phosphorylated but escape segregation by the PMR.

A SECOND M6P-DEPENDENT PATHWAY EXISTS FOR TRANSPORT OF ACID HYDROLASES

A second pathway by which acid hydrolases may be transported within the cell also exists. In some cells, including fibroblasts, phosphomannosyl receptors are expressed on the plasma membrane. These cell surface receptors are capable of binding M6P-containing acid hydrolases present in the extracellular medium. These enzymes are then internalized through a process of receptor-mediated endocytosis. Receptor and ligand dissociate in a pre-lysosomal acid compartment. The ligand is transferred to the lysosome and the receptor recycles to the cell surface. It appears that the plasma membrane receptor and the PMR in the intracellular pool are in equilibrium with each other.

It is not clear if this second transport pathway is vital to the cell. One case in which it appears to be of significance in maintaining normal levels of acid hydrolase is in female carriers of Hunter disease. This is an X-linked lysosomal disorder which is the result of a deficiency of iduronate sulfatase. Carriers of the disorder carry two populations of cells, one of which is defective in iduronate sulfatase, due to the inactivation of the X-chromosome carrying the normal allele. The phenotype of the carrier, and the morphology of her tissues, are normal, however. This has been explained by the transfer of iduronate sulfatase from normal cells to the defective cells by receptor-mediated endocytosis (McKusick and Neufeld, 1983). Similar _in vitro_ cross-correction of fibroblasts deficient in lysosomal enzymes, by normal fibroblasts, was of importance in elucidating the receptor-mediated transport of acid hydrolases (reviewed in Creek and Sly, 1984).

The transport of acid hydrolases, both from the plasma membrane and from the ER to the lysosome, is represented in cartoon fashion in Figure 2.

TWO PHOSPHOMANNOSYL RECEPTORS

The identification of mannose 6-phosphate as the common recognition marker on many lysosomal hydrolases prompted the search for a protein capable of binding lysosomal enzymes in an M6P-specific manner. Two such proteins, termed phosphomannosyl receptors (PMR), have now been identified and purified (Rome et al., 1979; Fischer et al., 1980a; Sahagian et al., 1981; Hoflack and Kornfeld, 1985a,b). These differ from each other in terms of binding characteristics and molecular weight and are also immunologically unrelated. The cation-independent PMR has a molecular weight of 215kD, does not require the presence of cations for binding activity and recognizes, in addition to the mannose 6-phosphate monoester, the so-called "covered" phosphates (methylphosphomannosyl diesters) found on acid hydrolases from the slime mold _D. discoideum_ (Fischer et al., 1980a; Freeze et al., 1980; Sahagian et al., 1981; Gabel et al., 1984). The cation-dependent receptor shows a molecular weight of 46 kD, has an absolute requirement for divalent cations for binding activity, and does not recognize the methylphosphomannosyl moiety, but only binds the phosphomonoesters (Hoflack and Kornfeld, 1985a,b). The cation-independent PMR was the first to be discovered and most of what is known of the M6P-mediated transport of acid hydrolases is derived from studies of this receptor. The role of the cation-dependent receptor in the transport of acid hydrolases is not yet clear and will not be further discussed in this article.

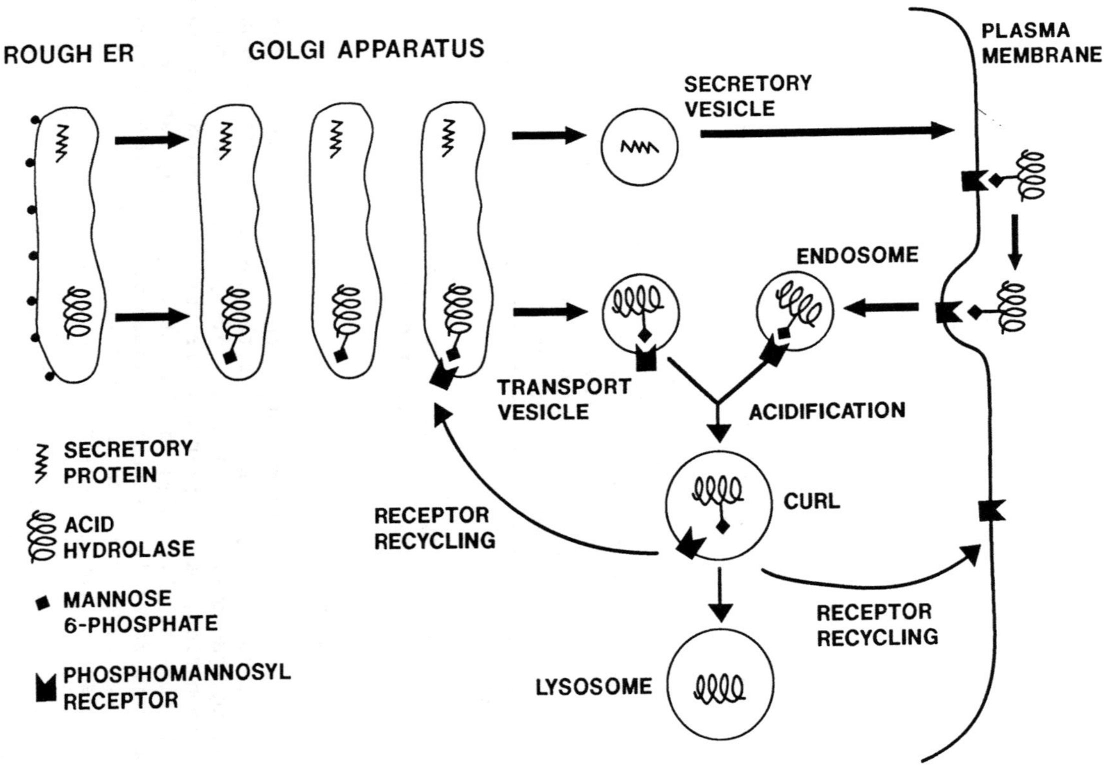

Figure 2. The mannose 6-phosphate-dependent transport of acid hydrolases within the cell.

THE CATION-INDEPENDENT PMR

The cation-independent PMR is an integral membrane glycoprotein with a molecular weight of 215 kD (Sahagian et al., 1981). It appears to be composed of a single polypeptide chain, though there is one report of it being composed of subunits of lower molecular weight (Mitchell et al., 1984). The C-terminal portion of the molecule is located toward the cytosolic side of the membrane, while the lysosomal enzyme binding site of the receptor faces the luminal or extracellular side (Sahagian and Steer, 1985; von Figura et al., 1985). Binding of acid hydrolases to the receptor is competitively inhibited by M6P and by the phosphomonoester phosphomannan fragment from H. holstii (Kaplan et al., 1977). Binding is specific for "high uptake" forms of lysosomal enzymes, i.e. prior treatment of the enzymes with alkaline phosphatase, or with endoglycosidase H, greatly reduces their binding to the receptor (Fischer et al., 1980a,c). Dissociation of bound enzymes from membrane receptors is very slow at neutral pH but is accelerated by addition of M6P or by lowering the pH to levels comparable to intralysosomal pH (Fischer et al., 1980a).

The receptor has been isolated from several sources, including bovine liver (Sahagian et al., 1981), Swarm rat chondrosarcoma membranes (Steiner and Rome, 1982), rat liver (Geuze et al., 1984) and human liver (von Figura et al., 1984). Antibodies have been raised to the receptor by several investigators (Sahagian et al., 1982; Creek and Sly, 1983; Geuze et al., 1984; von Figura et al., 1984) and have been used to study its biosynthesis, turnover, subcellular location and role in the transport of acid hydrolases. In monolayer cultures of fibroblasts and of CHO cells, the receptor is turned over slowly, with a half-life of 20-29 hours (Creek and Sly, 1983) and 16 hours (Sahagian and Neufeld, 1983) respectively. The site of degradation is not known. It does not appear to occur in the lysosome as it is not significantly affected by incubation of cells with ammonium chloride (NH_4Cl), leupeptin or saturating concentrations of ligand (Creek and Sly, 1983). It does seem to be enhanced on treatment of fibroblasts with certain anti-receptor antibodies (von Figura et al., 1984; Gartung et al., 1985; our unpublished results).

The PMR was first identified as a cell surface receptor which facilitated the uptake of acid hydrolases from the extracellular medium. Early studies of the receptor emphasized its role in pinocytosis, but more recently the central importance of the receptor in targeting newly synthesized acid hydrolases to lysosomes has been shown.

SUBCELLULAR LOCATION OF THE PMR

The subcellular location of the receptor has been studied using subcellular fractionation of cells or tissues, followed by examination of membranes for M6P-dependent binding of ligands. In both human fibroblasts and rat liver, only 10-20% of receptors are found on the plasma membrane with the remainder being intracellular. In rat liver, the intracellular location was reported to be mainly in the ER, Golgi apparatus, and lysosomes (80, 7 and 5% respectively) with negligible amounts in nuclei and mitochondria (Fischer et al., 1980b).

Several groups have looked at the subcellular distribution of the receptor by immunocytochemical methods. While confirming the presence of the majority of the PMR in intracellular locations, these latter investigations have yielded contradictory evidence to some extent.

Using an immunoperoxidase technique, Brown and Farquhar (1984) localized the PMR to the Golgi cisternae, coated vesicles, endosomes and lysosomes. However, with the Golgi apparatus, the PMR was restricted in distribution to one or two cisternae on the cis side of the stacks and was not found in the trans region or in GERL. Based on the high concentration of the receptor at the cis face of the Golgi apparatus, they proposed that it is in this region that the segregation of lysosomal enzymes from secretory proteins occur. Using a colloidal gold-protein A labeling technique, Geuze et al. (1984) found the receptor in the plasma membrane, in coated pits and coated vesicles, in CURL and throughout the Golgi complex. An essentially similar distribution of PMR in CHO cells had been reported by Willingham et al. (1983). In addition, Geuze et al. (1984) showed that the lysosomal enzyme, cathepsin D, co-localized with the PMR throughout the Golgi cisternae. They con-cluded from these results that lysosomal enzymes traversed the entire Golgi complex en route to lysosomes.

The reasons for the discrepancy in the ultrastructural location of the PMR are not clear at present. It may be a reflection of the different labeling techniques or antibody preparations used by the different investigators. In any case, it is important to resolve the discrepancy in order to further define the site of PMR binding to lysosomal enzymes and the site of segregation of the latter from the secretory pathway.

RECYCLING OF PHOSPHOMANNOSYL RECEPTORS

During pinocytosis of lysosomal enzymes by fibroblasts, the number of molecules of ligand internalized far exceeds the number of cell surface receptors. Calculations based on the maximum rate of uptake of ligand and on the amount of enzyme maximally bound to the cell surface suggested that under these conditions, receptors must be replaced or reutilized every five minutes (Gonzalez-Noriega et al., 1980; Rome et al., 1979). A constant rate of enzyme uptake was maintained even when cells were incubated with cycloheximide for up to three hours, suggesting that synthesis of new receptors was not necessary, and that either a very large pool of intracellular receptors existed (containing at least 36 times the number present on the cell surface) or that receptors were re-utilized (Gonzalez-Noriega et al., 1980). Examination of the binding of ligand to cell surfaces and to total cellular membrane preparations has shown that there is in fact an intracellular pool of receptor (Fischer et al., 1980a). The size of this pool, however, is inadequate to explain the observed level of enzyme internalization without invoking re-utilization of receptors.

The long half-life of the receptor suggested that receptor re-utilization also occurred following delivery of newly synthesized acid hydrolases to lysosomes. Brown et al. (1986) have provided direct evidence for such re-utilization, by immunocytochemical means.

AMINES INHIBIT RECYCLING OF PMR

The treatment of normal fibroblasts with lysosomotropic amines, such as chloroquine or ammonium chloride, has provided much information on the mechanism of receptor re-utilization. Treatment of fibroblasts with NH_4Cl has three effects on the cells: (1) greatly enhanced secretion of newly synthesized acid hydrolases; (2) depletion of enzyme binding sites at the cell surface; and (3) inhibition of pinocytosis of exogenous enzyme (Gonzalez-Noriega et al., 1980). Only the third effect was seen in I-cell fibroblasts. These amines cause an elevation of the pH of acidic compartments such as endosomes and lysosomes (De Duve et al., 1974; Ohkuma and Poole, 1978). The observed pH dependence of acid hydrolase-PMR binding (Fischer et al., 1980a) suggested a mechanism whereby amines act. According to this model, in amine-treated cells, receptors become "trapped" because they are unable to dissociate from their ligands and therefore are not able to recycle. Both pathways of enzyme transport, from the plasma membrane to lysosomes and from the ER and Golgi apparatus to lysosomes, were disrupted by these amines, suggesting the involvement of acid compartments in both of these processes.

Further evidence of the importance of acidic compartments in the recycling of PMR came from studies of mutant cells which are defective in the ability to acidify their endosomes (Robbins et al., 1983; Sly et al., 1983). These cells are deficient in the uptake of lysosomal enzymes via cell surface PMR. They also show decreased PMR activity reflected in enhanced secretion of acid hydrolases into the medium, with decreased intracellular levels of these enzymes. Brown et al. (1984, 1986) have provided visual evidence, using immunocytochemistry, of the "trapping" of receptors by showing a redistribution of PMR along the sorting pathway in amine-treated cells and their accumulation at the presumptive delivery site. Both these studies and those of Gonzalez-Noriega et al. (1980) suggested that ligand-binding by receptors triggers movement of receptor-ligand complexes to endosomes or lysosomes and that ligand dissociation triggered the return of receptors to the sorting areas of the cell (Golgi apparatus and plasma membrane). The defective sorting of acid hydrolases in cells deficient in endosome acidification suggested that the endosome might be the site of dissociation of ligand from receptor. Recently, Brown et al. (1986) have identified the delivery site for newly synthesized acid hydrolases as an endosome rather than a lysosome, and have shown that M6P-induced ligand dissociation can trigger PMR recycling, even in amine-treated cells.

ANTIBODIES INHIBIT THE FUNCTION OF THE PMR

Antibodies to the PMR have been shown to inhibit both functions of the PMR (Creek et al., 1983; Creek and Sly, 1983; von Figura et al., 1984; Gartung et al., 1985). In antibody-treated cells, pinocytosis of acid hydrolases is decreased and the sorting of newly synthesized acid hydrolases is disrupted, as reflected in the enhanced secretion of precursor acid hydrolases into the medium. The mechanism of inhibition, however, seems to depend on the particular antibody used. Von Figura and co-workers have shown that their antibody inhibits ligand binding by the receptor and that this can account for the observed inhibition of function (Gartung et al., 1985). We have found that our antibody does not significantly affect binding of ligand by the PMR (unpublished results). Rather it seems that cross-linking of receptors by antibody prevents normal recycling of the receptor to the sorting sites, such that the cell surface is depleted of receptors and the intracellular receptor is redistributed from its normal ER/Golgi location to a more distal site along the sorting pathway, presumably similar to the endosome delivery site observed in NH_4Cl-treated cells (Brown et al., 1986). This interpretation was supported by the fact that monovalent anti-PMR Fab fragments were less inhibitory than intact anti-PMR IgG, but that their effectiveness in inhibition could be increased by incubation of Fab fragment-treated cells with a second cross-linking antibody, which, by itself, had no effect on the function of the PMR.

Antibodies to the PMR may be useful as reagents with which to study the transport of acid hydrolases. For example, anti-receptor antibodies might affect the sorting of individual lysosomal enzymes to different extents. It would also be of interest to compare the effects of antibodies to the cation-independent PMR with those of antibodies raised to the cation-dependent receptor on acid hydrolase sorting, in an attempt to study the contribution of both of these receptors to targeting.

Table I. Questions which need to be addressed regarding the transport of acid hydrolases to lysosomes.

1. What is the basis for the recognition of numerous acid hydrolases by the phosphotransferase?

2. Where are newly synthesized acid hydrolases segregated from proteins destined for secretion?

3. What are the signals involved in the direction of receptor-ligand complexes from one compartment to the next in the transport pathways?

4. Following receptor-ligand dissociation, how are receptors and ligands differentially targeted, with ligands being delivered to lysosomes and receptors continuing to recycle?

5. What are the relative contributions of the cation-independent and cation-dependent phosphomannosyl receptors in the transport of acid hydrolases?

6. What is the nature of the mannose 6-phosphate independent pathway of transporting acid hydrolases?

AN M6P-INDEPENDENT PATHWAY OF TRANSPORT OF ACID HYDROLASES MUST ALSO EXIST

It is evident that a pathway of transport of acid hydrolases which is independent of M6P must also exist. This has come from the study of I-cell fibroblasts. As mentioned above, these cells are defective in the synthesis of the M6P marker. The lysosomes in these cells are deficient in the majority of acid hydrolases. Some lysosomal enzymes, however, are present at relatively high levels in these cells, and it seems that these must be targeted by an alternate pathway (Hasilik and Neufeld, 1980; Lemansky et al., 1985). Other tissues in patients with I-cell disease have normal levels of lysosomal enzymes in spite of the deficiency of the phosphotransferase (Owada and Neufeld, 1982; Waheed et al., 1982b). There is also evidence that membrane-associated lysosomal enzymes are transported in an M6P-independent manner (Tager, 1985). At present, there is no information available on the nature of this alternative pathway.

SUMMARY

The role of the mannose 6-phosphate recognition marker and the phosphomannosyl receptor in the intracellular transport of acid hydrolases is well established. Several details of the process, however, are presently unclear and warrant further investigation (Table 1). The development of *in vitro* systems for the reconstitution of receptor-mediated endocytosis and intracellular transport, together with the application of the techniques of molecular biology to this field, should lead to major advances in our understanding of the targeting of enzymes to lysosomes.

REFERENCES

Bishop, D.F., Calhoun, D.H., Bernstein, H.S., Hantzopoulos, P., Quinn, M., and Desnick, R. J., 1986, Human α-galactosidase A: Nucleotide sequence of a cDNA clone encoding the mature enzyme, Proc. Natl. Acad. Sci. USA, 83:4859-4863.

Brown, W.J., Constantinescu, E., and Farquhar, M.G., 1984, Redistribution of mannose 6-phosphate receptors induced by tunicamycin and chloroquine, J. Cell Biol., 99:320-326.

Brown, W.J., and Farquhar, M.G., 1984, The mannose 6-phosphate receptor for lysosomal enzymes is concentrated in *cis* Golgi cisternae, Cell, 36:295-307.

Brown, W.J., Goodhouse, J., and Farquhar, M.G., 1986, Mannose 6-phosphate receptors for lysosomal enzymes cycle between the Golgi complex and endosomes, J. Cell Biol., 103:1235-1247.

Creek, K.E., Grubb, J.H., and Sly, W.S., 1983, Immunological inactivation of receptor-mediated uptake and intracellular sorting of lysosomal enzymes, J. Cell Biol., 97:253a (abstract).

Creek, K.E., and Sly, W.S., 1983, Biosynthesis and turnover of the phosphomannosyl receptor in human fibroblasts, Biochem. J., 214:353-360.

Creek, K.E., and Sly, W.S., 1984, The role of the phosphomannosyl receptor in the transport of acid hydrolases to lysosomes, *in*: "Lysosomes in Biology and Pathology," J.T. Dingle, R.T. Dean, and W.S. Sly, eds., Elsevier, Amsterdam.

De Duve, C., De Barsy, T., Poole, B., Trouet, A., Tulkens, P., and van Hoof, F., 1974, Lysosomotropic agents, Biochem. Pharmacol., 23:2495-2531.

Dunphy, W.G., Fries, E., Urbani, L.J., and Rothman, J.E., 1981, Early and late functions associated with the Golgi apparatus reside in distinct compartments, Proc. Natl. Acad. Sci. USA, 78:7453-7457.

Faust, P.L., Kornfeld, S., and Chirgwin, J.M., 1985, Cloning and sequence analysis of cDNA for human cathepsin D, Proc. Natl. Acad. Sci. USA, 82:4910-4914.

Fedde, K.N., and Sly, W.S., 1985, Ricin-binding properties of acid hydrolases from isolated lysosomes implies prior processing by terminal transferases of the *trans*-Golgi apparatus, Biochem. Biophys. Res. Commun., 133:614-620.

Fischer, H.D., Gonzalez-Noriega, A., and Sly, W.S., 1980a, β-glucuronidase binding to human fibroblast membrane receptors, J. Biol. Chem., 255:5069-5074.

Fischer, H.D., Gonzalez-Noriega, A., Sly, W.S., and Morre, D.J., 1980b, Phosphomannosyl-enzyme receptors in rat liver, J. Biol. Chem., 255:9608-9615.

Fischer, H.D., Natowicz, M., Sly, W.S., and Bretthauer, R.K., 1980c, Fibroblast receptor for lysosomal enzymes mediates pinocytosis of multivalent phosphomannan fragment, J. Cell Biol., 84:77-86.

Freeze, H.H., Miller, A.L., and Kaplan, A., 1980, Acid hydrolases from *Dictyostelium discoideum* contain phosphomannosyl recognition markers, J. Biol. Chem., 255:11081-11084.

Fukushima, H., de Wet, J.R., and O'Brien, J.S., 1985, Molecular cloning of a cDNA for human α-L-fucosidase, Proc. Natl. Acad. Sci. USA, 82:1262-1265.

Gabel, C.A., Costello, C.E., Reinhold, V.N., Kurtz, L., and Kornfeld, S., 1984, Identification of methylphosphomannosyl residues as components of the high mannose oligosaccharides of *Dictyostelium discoideum* glycoproteins, J. Biol. Chem., 259:13762-13769.

Gartung, C., Braulke, T., Hasilik, A., and von Figura, K., 1985, Internalization of blocking antibodies against mannose 6-phosphate specific receptors, EMBO J., 4:1725-1730.

Geuze, H.J., Slot, J.W., Strous, G.J.A.M., Hasilik, A., and von Figura, K., 1984, Ultrastructural localization of the mannose 6-phosphate receptor in rat liver, J. Cell Biol., 98:2045-2054.
Geuze, H.J., Slot, J.W., Strous, G.J.A.M., Hasilik, A., and von Figura, K., 1985, Possible pathways for lysosomal enzyme delivery, J. Cell Biol., 101:2253-2262.
Geuze, H.J., Slot, J.W., Strous, G.J.A.M., Lodish, H.F., and Schwartz, A.L., 1983, Intracellular site of asialoglycoprotein receptor-ligand uncoupling: double-labeling immunoelectron microscopy during receptor-mediated endocytosis, Cell, 32:277-287.
Goldberg, D., Gabel, C., and Kornfeld, S., 1984, Processing of lysosomal enzyme oligosaccharide units, in: "Lysosomes in Biology and Pathology," J.T. Dingle, R.T. Dean, and W.S. Sly, eds., Elsevier Press, New York.
Goldberg, D.E., and Kornfeld, S., 1981, The phosphorylation of β-glucuronidase oligosaccharides in mouse P388D$_1$ cells, J. Biol. Chem., 256: 13060-13067.
Goldberg, D.E., and Kornfeld, S., 1983, Evidence for extensive subcellular organization of asparagine-linked oligosaccharide processing and lysosomal enzyme phosphorylation, J. Biol. Chem., 258:3159-3165.
Gonzalez-Noriega, A., Grubb, J.H., Talkad, V., and Sly, W.S., 1980, Chloroquine inhibits lysosomal enzyme pinocytosis and enhances lysosomal enzyme secretion by impairing receptor recycling, J. Cell Biol., 85: 839-852.
Hasilik, A., Klein, U., Waheed, A., Strecker, G., and von Figura, K., 1980, Phosphorylated oligosaccharides in lysosomal enzymes: Identification of α-N-acetylglucosamine(1)phospho(6)mannose diester groups, Proc. Natl. Acad. Sci. USA, 77:7074-7078.
Hasilik, A., and Neufeld, E.F., 1980, Biosynthesis of lysosomal enzymes in fibroblasts, J. Biol. Chem., 255:4937-4945.
Hasilik, A., and von Figura, K., 1984, Processing of lysosomal enzymes in fibroblasts, in: "Lysosomes in Biology and Pathology," J.T. Dingle, R.T. Dean, and W.S. Sly, eds., Elsevier, Amsterdam.
Hickman, S., and Neufeld, E.F., 1972, A hypothesis for I-cell disease: Defective hydrolases that do not enter lysosomes, Biochem. Biophys. Res. Commun., 49:992-999.
Hoflack, B., and Kornfeld, S., 1985a, Lysosomal enzyme binding the mouse P388D$_1$ macrophage membranes lacking the 215-kDa mannose 6-phosphate receptor: Evidence for the existence of a second mannose 6-phosphate receptor, Proc. Natl. Acad. Sci. USA, 82:4428-4432.
Hoflack, B., and Kornfeld, S., 1985b, Purification and characterization of a cation-dependent mannose 6-phosphate receptor from murine P388D$_1$ macrophages and bovine liver, J. Biol. Chem., 260:12008-12014.
Kaplan, A., Achord, D.T., and Sly, W.S., 1977, Phosphohexosyl components of a lysosomal enzyme are recognized by pinocytosis receptors on human fibroblasts, Proc. Natl. Acad. Sci. USA, 74:2026-2030.
Korneluk, R.G., Mahuran, D.J., Neote, K., Klavins, M.H., O'Dowd, B.F., Tropak, M., Willard, H.F., Anderson, M.J., Lowden, J.A., and Gravel, R.A., 1986, Isolation of cDNA clones coding for the α-subunit of human β-hexo-saminidase, J. Biol. Chem., 261:8407-8413.
Kornfeld, R., and Kornfeld, S., 1985, Assembly of asparagine-linked oligosaccharides, Ann. Rev. Biochem., 54:631-664.
Lang, L., Reitman, M.L., Tang, J., Roberts, R.M., and Kornfeld, S., 1984, Lysosomal enzyme phosphorylation, J. Biol. Chem., 259:14663-14667.
Lemansky, P., Gieselmann, V., Hasilik, A., and von Figura, K., 1985, Synthesis and transport of lysosomal acid phosphatase in normal and I-cell fibroblasts, J. Biol. Chem., 260:9023-9030.
McKusick, V.A., and Neufeld, E.F., 1983, The mucopolysaccharide storage diseases, in: "The Metabolic Basis of Inherited Disease," fifth edition, J.B. Stanbury, J.B. Wyngaarden, D.S. Frederickson, J.L. Goldstein, and M.S. Brown, eds., McGraw-Hill, New York.

Mitchell, D.C., Maler, T., and Jourdian, G.W., 1984, Detergent dissociation of bovine liver phosphomannosyl binding protein, J. Cell. Biochem., 24:319-330.
Myerowitz, R., Piekarz, R., Neufeld, E.F., Shows, T.B., and Suzuki, K., 1985, Human β-hexosaminidase α chain: Coding sequence and homology with the β chain, Proc. Natl. Acad. Sci. USA, 82:7830-7834.
Nishimura, Y., Rosenfeld, M.G., Kreibich, G., Gubler, U., Sabatini, D.D., Adesnik, M., and Andy, R., 1986, Nucleotide sequence of rat preputial gland β-glucuronidase cDNA and in vitro insertion of its encoded polypeptide into microsomal membranes, Proc. Natl. Acad. Sci. USA, 83:7292-7296.
Ohkuma, S., and Poole, B., 1978, Fluorescence probe measurement of the intralysosomal pH in living cells and the perturbation of pH by various agents, Proc. Natl. Acad. Sci. USA, 75:3327-3331.
Oshima, A., Kyle, J.W., Miller, R.D., Hoffmann, J.W., Powell, P.P., Grubb, J.H., Sly, W.S., Tropak, M., Guise, K.S., and Gravel, R.A., 1987, Cloning, sequencing, and expression of cDNA for human β-glucuronidase, Proc. Natl. Acad. Sci. USA, 84:685-689.
Owada, M., and Neufeld, E.F., 1982, Is there a mechanism for introducing acid hydrolases into liver lysosomes that is independent of mannose 6-phosphate recognition? Biochem. Biophys. Res. Commun., 105:814-820.
Pohlmann, R., Waheed, A., Hasilik, A., and von Figura, K., 1982, Synthesis of phosphorylated recognition marker in lysosomal enzymes is located in the cis part of Golgi apparatus, J. Biol. Chem., 257:5323-5325.
Reitman, M.L., and Kornfeld, S., 1981, UDP-N-Acetylglucosamine: Glycoprotein N-acetylglucosamine-1-phosphotransferase, J. Biol. Chem., 256:4275-4281.
Reitman, A.L., Varki, A., and Kornfeld, S., 1981, Fibroblasts from patients with I-cell disease and pseudo-Hurler polydystrophy are deficient in uridine 5'-diphosphate-N-acetylglucosamine: Glycoprotein N-acetylglucosaminylphosphotransferase activity, J. Clin. Invest., 67:1574-1579.
Robbins, A.R., Peng, S.S., and Marshall, J.L., 1983, Mutant Chinese hamster ovary cells pleiotropically defective in receptor-mediated endocytosis, J. Cell. Biol., 96:1064-1071.
Rome, L.H., Weissman, B., and Neufeld, E.F., 1979, Direct demonstration of binding of a lysosomal enzyme, α-L-iduronidase, to receptors in cultured fibroblasts, Proc. Natl. Acad. Sci. USA, 76:2331-2334.
Roth, J., and Berger, E.G., 1982, Immunocytochemical localization of galactosyltransferase in HeLa cells: Codistribution with thiamine pyrophosphatase in trans-Golgi cisternae, J. Cell Biol., 93:223-229.
Sahagian, G.G., Distler, J., and Jourdian, G.W., 1981, Characterization of a membrane-associated receptor from bovine liver that binds phosphomannosyl residues of bovine testicular β-galactosidase, Proc. Natl. Acad. Sci. USA, 78:4289-4293.
Sahagian, G.G., Distler, J., and Jourdian, G.W., 1982, Membrane receptor for phosphomannosyl residues, Methods Enzymol., 83:392-396.
Sahagian, G.G., and Neufeld, E.F., 1983, Biosynthesis and turnover of the mannose 6-phosphate receptor in cultured Chinese hamster ovary cells, J. Biol. Chem., 257:7121-7128.
Sahagian, G.G., and Steer, C.J., 1985, Transmembrane orientation of the mannose 6-phosphate receptor in isolated clathrin-coated vesicles, J. Biol. Chem., 260:9838-9842.
Sly, W.S., Fischer, H.D., Gonzalez-Noriega, A., Grubb, J.H., and Natowicz, M., 1981, Role of the 6-phosphomannosyl-enzyme receptor in intracellular transport and adsorptive pinocytosis of lysosomal enzymes, in: "Basic Mechanisms of Cellular Secretion," A.R. Hand and C. Oliver, eds., Academic Press, New York.

Sly, W.S., Merion, M., Schlesinger, P., Moehring, J.M., and Moehring, T.J., 1983, Defective endosome acidification in mammalian cell mutants "cross-resistant" to certain toxins and viruses, in: "Protein Synthesis," A.K. Abraham, T.S. Eikhom, and I.F. Pryme, eds., The Humana Press, Clifton, NJ.
Steiner, A.W., and Rome, L.H., 1982, Assay and purification of a solubilized membrane receptor that binds the lysosomal enzyme α-L-iduronidase, Arch. Biochem. Biophys., 214:681-687.
Tager, J.M., 1984, Biosynthesis and deficiency of lysosomal enzymes, Trends Biochem. Sci., 10:324-326.
Takahashi, T., Schmidt, P.G., and Tang, J., 1983, Oligosaccharide units of lysosomal cathepsin D from porcine spleen, J. Biol. Chem., 258:2819-2830.
Tsuji, S., Choudary, P.V., Martin, B.M., Winfield, S., Barranger, J.A., and Ginns, E.J., 1986, Nucleotide sequence of cDNA containing the complete coding sequence for human lysosomal glucocerebrosiolase, J. Biol. Chem., 261:50-53.
van Elsen, A.F., and Leroy, J.G., 1979, Lysosomal enzymes in fibroblasts: Lectin affinities, in: "Models for the Study of Inborn Errors of Metabolism," F.A. Hommes, ed., Elsevier/North-Holland Biomedical Press, Amsterdam.
Varki, A., and Kornfeld, S., 1981, Purification and characterization of rat liver α-N-acetylglucosaminyl phosphodiesterase, J. Biol. Chem., 256: 9937-9943.
von Figura, K., Gieselmann, V., and Hasilik, A., 1984, Antibody to mannose 6-phosphate specific receptor induces receptor deficiency in human fibroblasts, EMBO J., 3:1281-1286.
von Figura, K., Gieselmann, V., and Hasilik, A., 1985, Mannose 6-phosphate specific receptor is a transmembrane protein with a C-terminal extension oriented towards the cytosol, Biochem. J., 225:543-547.
von Figura, K., and Weber, E., 1978, An alternative hypothesis of cellular transport of lysosomal enzymes in fibroblasts, Biochem. J., 176:943-950.
Vladutiu, G.D., 1983, Effect of the co-existence of galactosyl and phosphomannosyl residues of β-hexosaminidase on the processing and transport of the enzyme in MLI fibroblasts, Biochim. Biophysica Acta, 760:363-370.
Waheed, A., Hasilik, A., and von Figura, K., 1981, Processing of the phosphorylated recognition marker in lysosomal enzymes, J. Biol. Chem., 256: 5717-5721.
Waheed, A., Hasilik, A., and von Figura, K., 1982a, UDP-N-acetylglucosamine: Lysosomal enzyme precursor N-acetylglucosamine-1-phosphotransferase, J. Biol. Chem., 257:12322-12331.
Waheed, A., Pohlmann, R., Hasilik, A., von Figura, K., van Elsen, A., and Leroy, J.G., 1982b, Deficiency of UDP-N-acetylglucosamine: Lysosomal enzyme N-acetylglucosamine-1-phosphotransferase in organs of I-cell patients, Biochem. Biophys. Res. Commun., 105:1052-1058.
Walter, P. and Lingappa, V.R., 1986, Mechanism of protein translocation across the endoplasmic reticulum membrane, Ann. Rev. Cell Biol., 2:499-516.
Willingham, M.C., Pastan, I.H., and Sahagian, G.G., 1983, Ultrastructural immunocytochemical localization of the phosphomannosyl receptor in Chinese hamster ovary (CHO) cells, J. Histochem. Cytochem., 31:1-11.

USE OF SYNTHETIC PEPTIDES IN THE DELINEATION OF THE ROLE OF NON-ANTIGEN RECEPTORS IN MAST CELL SIGNALLING PROCESSES

D.R. Stanworth

Rheumatology and Allergy Research Unit
University of Birmingham
Birmingham B15 2TJ
United Kingdom

INTRODUCTION

On first sight a paper on mast cell signalling processes would seem to be out of place amongst contributions which are mainly concerned with T cell receptor-ligand interactions. As I hope will become apparent, however, our observations on the manner in which IgE antibodies initiate the release of mediators of immediate-type allergy from mast cells could be more than a little relevant to a better understanding of T cell recognition and trigger processes.

Our long term objective has been to define the precise role of anaphylactic antibodies of the IgE class in the sensitisation and subsequent triggering of mast cells in response to allergen challenge with the ultimate aim of, hopefully, devising more effective anti-allergy compounds.

Initially, we adopted a fragmentation approach, using both proteolytic and chemical cleavage products of the first to be discovered myeloma form of IgE in inhibition PK (Stanworth et al, 1968) and PCA (Stanworth, 1973) tests aimed at establishing the location of the site(s) through which the sensitising antibody binds to the mast cell plasma membrane. These studies provided the first evidence for the presence of Fc receptors on mast cells. Interestingly, we have shown recently (Coleman et al, 1985) that a human immunoglobulin ε-chain fragment synthesised in Escherichia coli as a result of gene cloning is likewise capable of blocking the binding of IgE to receptors on human mast cells (lung) in vitro.

But, there are obvious limitations to the use of cleavage procedures in attempts to retrieve active fragments of immunoglobulins in which particular Fc functional activities have survived. For this reason, some years ago we turned to an alternative strategy, namely, the synthesis of peptides representative of continuous amino acid sequences constituting putative Fc effector sites. Moreover, we have recently been extending this approach to the production of specific antisera (both polyclonal and monoclonal) against the synthetic Fc region peptides, thereby providing an additional means of probing the structure of this part of the IgE molecule, and the manner in which it interacts with receptors on mast cells and initiates the release of mediators of inflammation.

DELINEATION OF THE ROLE OF THE ANTIBODY IN THE ELICITATION OF MEDIATOR RELEASE FROM MAST CELLS

IgE antibody molecules are involved at two consecutive stages in the elicitation of release of mediators of immediate-type allergic reactions from mast cells. Firstly, in bringing about sensitisation of the effector cells by binding with high affinity to Fc receptors (FcεR) on their plasma membranes. Secondly, in facilitating the initiation of endocytosis of the mast cell granules, with the non-cytolytic secretion of various formed and non-formed mediators, following the cross-linking of adjacent cell bound antibody molecules by antigen (allergen).

Short chain peptides representative of continuous ε-chain amino acid sequences have been employed in attempts to identify and structually characterise those Fc effector sites which are implicated in the expression of these complementary functions of anaphylactic antibodies of the IgE class.

1. Characterisation of an Fc effector site capable of providing a triggering signal to IgE sensitised mast cells

A popular concept of the immunological triggering of mast cells, particularly prominent in the USA, is that the IgE antibody molecule plays a passive role; merely acting as a link through which the allergen brings about cross-linking of the Fc(ε)R. This conclusion is based on the observation (Ishizaka and Ishizaka, 1978) that anti-FcεR antibody is likewise capable of effecting mediator secretion. In contrast, I have hypothesised (Stanworth, 1971, 1973) that the antibody is actively involved in the elicitation of mediator release, by providing a triggering signal to a second (ie other than FcεR) "receptor" on the mast cell plasma membrane.

In order to obtain experimental evidence in support of this idea, structure-activity studies were initially performed on model histamine releasing polypeptides, synthetic ACTH analogues and melittin cleavage fragments; the capacity of these ligands to elicit histamine release from purified normal rat peritoneal mast cells in vitro being determined by automated spectrofluorometric assay (Jasani et al, 1973, 1979). The finding indicated that the cluster of basic amino acids in these two polypeptides (Lys-Lys-Arg-Arg in ACTH, and Lys-Arg-Lys-Arg in melittin) was an essential requirement for direct mast cell triggering activity, which was enhanced by the presence of neighbouring hydrophobic residues and the blocking of the C-terminal carboxyl group (eg by amidation); whereas, on the other hand, the presence of a free C-terminal carboxyl group or nearby dicarboxylic acid residues led to a considerable diminution in histamine releasing activity. Moreover, further studies on analogues of a synthetic peptide intermediate with potent histamine releasing activity indicated that there was a stereo selectivity of this form of ligand (Roy et al, 1980). This was interpreted as evidence that the so-called second "receptor" on mast cells resembled a polypeptide hormone receptor. But, as will become apparent, subsequent experimental evidence has suggested that this is not a conventional type of receptor.

Armed with this information on the likely structural characteristics of an IgE antibody mast cell triggering effector site, it was of considerable interest to inspect the complete amino acid sequence of the Fc region of human IgE (reported by Bennich and Bahr-Lindstrom, 1978) and ascertain whether any continuous part of the ε-chains fulfilled such requirements. The sequence spanning residues 496-506 within the $C_{\varepsilon}4$ domains (viz, Arg-Lys-Thr-Lys-Gly-Ser-Gly-Phe-Phe-Val-Phe) was the only one which showed such structural features, and the additional one of

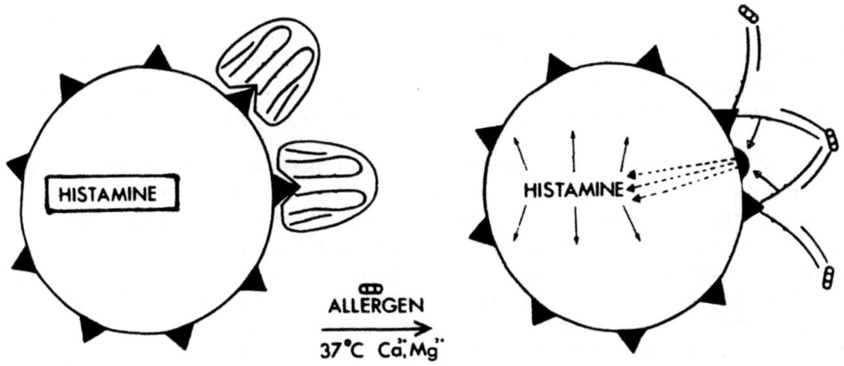

Figure 1. Postulated manner in which a conformational change, brought about within mast cell IgE antibody molecules as a result of bridging by specific allergen, could lead to the triggering of a "second receptor" on the plasma membrane (reproduced from Stanworth, 1971).

accessibility, inasmuch as it was not close to a cysteine residue (involved in disulphide bridging). Consequently, short chain peptides composed of sequences representative of this region of the human ε-chain were synthesised (at that time by classical procedures), and tested over suitable dose ranges for their ability to elicit non-cytolytic release of histamine from purified rat mast cells in vitro. An octapeptide (496-504), a nonapeptide and a decapeptide (497-506) all showed dose-dependent histamine release over a peptide concentration range of 1-100μλM in a manner which manifested many of the features of the IgE antibody-allergen induced mediator release process (Stanworth et al, 1979).

Detailed structure-activity studies (Stanworth et al, 1984) have been subsequently undertaken on a whole range of peptides incorporating this region of the human ε-chain, and various analogues, synthesised by the solid phase procedure of Merrifield et al (1963); on this occasion 5-hydroxy tryptamine release (which parallels histamine release) was measured, by means of a radio-isotopic technique. These observations confirmed and extended our earlier findings from the model peptide studies, providing valuable information on the precise structural requirements for the direct elicitation of mediator release. As will be seen from Figure 2, the essential structural features of this ligand are a positively charged (i.e. cationic) amino acid "head" separated by three residues from a hydrophobic "tail". Significantly, such structural characteristics are not found in the corresponding Fc regions of the other four human immunoglobulin classes. They are, however, very similar to

ε-Chain peptide	Lys-Thr-Lys-	Gly-Ser-Gly-	Phe-Phe-Val-Phe-NH_2
Substance P	Arg-Pro-Lys-	Pro-Gln-Gln-	Phe-Phe-Gly-Leu-Met-NH_2

Figure 2. Comparison of the primary structures of substance P and the histamine-releasing synthetic ε-chain decapeptide, showing them both to possess cationic N-terminal regions and hydrophobic C-terminal regions.

those of substance P, a neuropeptide which is released from primary afferent neurones in response to antidromic impulses and is capable of eliciting histamine release from neighbouring mast cells (manifested as a flare response in skin reactions), as will also be seen from Figure 2.

It is of interest to speculate on the possible mode of action of such peptide ligands on the mast cell plasma membrane. One might expect, perhaps, that the hydrophobic C-terminal "tail" would readily insert into the lipid bilayer, leaving the cationic N-terminal region within the polar environment on the exterior of the cell membrane where it could interact electrostatically with polar membrane components, thereby affording a triggering signal. It was fascinating to find, therefore, that there was a close correlation between the capacity of different ε-chain peptides to initiate 5-HT release from isolated rat mast cells and to insert into a model erythrocyte membrane system, as indicated by their capacity to reduce the rotational diffusion of band 3 protein (Dufton et al, 1984).

In the light of these observations, it was important to try and establish whether the region within the human IgE CH4 domain of which the mast cell triggering peptide is representative is likely to be accessible in the native immunoglobulin molecule. Unfortunately, no X-ray crystallographic data are available yet on IgE. But, by assuming that the 3-dimensional conformation of the human $C_\varepsilon 4$ domain resembles that of the $C_\varepsilon 3$ domain, it has been possible by use of computer graphics to throw some light on this question. This approach reveals that a considerable portion of the ε-chain sequence 497-506, and particularly the N terminal cationic region, is likely to be accessible in the free monomeric IgE molecules (Stanworth, 1984). But, of course, it is possible that the bridging of mast cell bound IgE antibody molecules by allergen would result in changes in their conformation, rendering this part of the $C_\varepsilon 4$ domains even more accessible. Moreover, it is not inconceivable that such a peptide would be selectively cleaved out of the IgE molecules' Fc regions by a mast cell membrane ectoprotease, activated as a result of bridging by allergen.

2. Characterisation of binding sites within the IgE molecule

As mentioned in the Introduction, the availability of the firstly discovered myeloma form of human IgE enabled us to perform both PK and PCA inhibition studies with proteolytic and chemical cleavage fragments. Of these, only whole Fc fragment (injected 24 hours prior to the sensitising serum) brought about completed inhibition of the subsequent binding of reaginic antibodies to the normal recipients' skin mast cells (Stanworth et al, 1968). But, as was speculated at that time, if we had succeeded in showing that a smaller Fc sub-fragment was likewise inhibitory, it would have been possible that a synthetic peptide of similar amino acid sequence could be developed as a potentially new form of anti-allergy compound.

It was, therefore, surprising to find some years later that Hamburger (1975) claimed to have accomplished this, in producing a synthetic peptide representative of a human CH2 domain sequence (Asp-Ser-Asp-Pro-Arg) which was capable of inhibiting the binding of IgE to human skin mast cells in vitro and to human basophils in vitro. But, although our own laboratory succeeded in confirming the in vitro inhibition results, and in demonstrating similar inhibition of IgE mediated PCA reactions in baboons (Stanworth et al, 1978), using a pentapeptide synthesised independently in Birmingham, we felt that the partial blocking observed (by injecting relatively high doses of peptide into the normal recipients' skin 4 hours prior to the sensitising serum) was attributable to a non-specific effect. This interpretation of the apparent ability of the pentapeptide to block the binding of IgE to Fc receptors on mast cells is now widely accepted. Yet, Hamburger has gone on to organise chemical trials of the efficacy of the pentapeptide in the treatment of hayfever and has recently reported data from one such double blind placebo-controlled trial in 96 allergic rhinitis patients (Dennis et al, 1986) which purport to provide evidence that six weeks' treatment with the pentapeptide alleviates the patients' stuffy nose symptom.

We have adopted a more systematic approach in using synthetic ε-chain peptides in an attempt to define precisely the structural basis of the mast cell Fc(ε)R binding sites within the IgE molecule. Initially, we have been focussing our attention on rat IgE, using purified rat peritoneal mast cells as targets in IgE binding-inhibition studies. Moreover, as studies undertaken in several laboratories based on enzymatic cleavage (Dorrington and Bennich, 1978) and the use of other procedures (Perez-Montfort and Metzger, 1982; Holowka and Baird, 1983) suggest that the mast cell Fc(ε)R binding site(s) is located in the CH3 and/or CH4 domains of IgE, we have synthesised peptides composed of certain continuous amino acid sequences within these regions of the rat (and, more recently, human) IgE molecule. We have also been producing antibodies, both polyclonal and monoclonal, against these peptides, to serve as additional structural probes.

The sequences were chosen from the primary structure of rat IgE heavy chain, which had been deduced from the nucleotide sequence of the mRNA coding for this immunoglobulin (reported by Hellman et al, 1982). The basic criterion for their selection was that they should be well exposed on the surface of the intact Fc dimer. Consequently, sequences incorporating a high number of polar amino acids likely to be accessible to aqueous solvent molecules were synthesised by the solid phase procedure using t-Boc amino acid derivatives. Moreover, as the precise tertiary structures of the rat IgE domains are not yet known, here too it was necessary to extrapolate from the known 3-dimensional structure of human λIgG1 (revealed by the X-ray crystallographic studies of Deisenhofer, 1981) in predicting the likely spatial configurations of hydrophobic sequences within the rat Cε4 and Cε3 domains. Another criterion for their selection which we adopted was the avoidance of sequences involved in lateral CH4-CH4 domain contact.

Seven different rat IgE sequences (listed in Table 1) have thus been selected and synthesised, and antisera have been raised to them in rabbits following their coupling to carrier KLH by use of glutaraldehyde (as described in Burt et al, 1986). The specificities of the antisera, and their reactivities with rat IgE, have been confirmed by indirect and inhibition ELISA. Each rabbit immunised with peptide-KLH conjugate produced antisera which reacted specifically with the immunising peptide down to very high dilutions (ie. titres of >1/62,500), but not with other synthetic rat ε-chain peptides of similar length. Both the synthetic peptides themselves, and the anti-peptide antisera, have been used to delineate the extent of that region in the rat IgE molecule which binds to Fc(ε)R on mast cells by determining, for instance, their ability to compete with the binding of radio-labelled rat IgE to purified serosal mast cells. Whilst the antisera have also been tested for an ability to elicit the release of histamine from IgE sensitised mast cells (by mimicking the cross-linking stimulus of specific antigen).

Four out of the seven synthetic ε-chain peptides tested (representative of sequences Ser414-Arg428 in the CH3 domain and Tyr459-Arg472, Leu491-Ser503 and His542-Lys557 in the CH4 domain) proved capable of inhibiting significantly the binding of I^{125}-IgE to mast cells in vitro. Intriguingly, these are representative of those same sequences which become more accessible to reaction with the corresponding anti-peptide

Table 1. Rat ε-chain sequences which have been synthesised and used to produce specific anti-peptide antibodies.

Peptide No	Domain	Sequence
130	CH_3	NH_2-Glu-Ser-Glu-Asn-Ile-Thr-Val-Thr-Trp-Val-Arg-Glu-Arg-Lys-Lys-Ser-Ile-Gly-NH_2
129	CH_3	NH_2-Tyr-Ser-Ile-Leu-Pro-Val-Asp-Ala-Lys-Asp-Trp-Ile-Glu-Gly-Glu-Gly-NH_2
124	CH_4	NH_2-Tyr-Val-Phe-Leu-Pro-Pro-Glu-Glu-Glu-Glu-Lys-Asp-Lys-Arg-NH_2
128	CH_4	NH_2-Try-Leu-Gln-Asp-Ser-Lys-Leu-Ile-Pro-Lys-Ser-Glu-His-Ser-NH_2
122	CH_4	NH_2-Try-Arg-Leu-Glu-Val-Thr-Lys-Ala-Leu-Trp-Thr-Gln-Thr-Lys-Gln-NH_2
123	CH_4	NH_2-His-Glu-Ala-Leu-Arg-Lys-Glu-Pro-Arg-Lys-Leu-Glu-Arg-Thr-Ile-Ser-Lys-NH_2
131	CH_4	NH_2-Gly-Asn-Thr-Ser-Leu-Arg-Pro-Ser-Glu-Ala-Ser-Met-NH_2

antisera as a result of heating the IgE in solution at 56°C for one hour (see Table 2); treatment which is known to abrogate the cytophilic activity of IgE for mast cells (Stanworth and Kuhns, 1965). The implication of these findings (reported in Stanworth and Burt, 1985) is that the ε-chain sequences in question contribute to the Fc(ε)R binding activity of the immunoglobulin molecule; a conclusion consistent with our finding that the same peptides themselves are capable of inhibiting the binding of IgE to mast cells.

Yet, in apparent contradiction to this conclusion are our findings (Table 3) that antibodies directed against sequences 378-396 in the $C_\varepsilon 3$ domain and against three sequences in the $C_\varepsilon 4$ domain (ie. 459-472, 522-535 and 542-557) are reactive with receptor-occupied IgE molecules; as reflected by their ability to cross-link them and thereby initiate histamine release, because this finding suggests that most of the surface residues, including two of the "heat-sensitive" sequences referred to above, are accessible even when the IgE molecule is already bound to Fc(ε)R on mast cells. What is the explanation of this paradox? We have turned again to computer graphics to provide a possible answer.

Again, the computer graphics model of the CH2 and CH3 domains of human IgG1, based on the X-ray crystallographic coordinates published by Deisenhofer (1981) referred to earlier, has been adapted in that the 3-dimensional structures of the framework regions have been adjusted to resemble those of the CH3 and CH4 domains of rat IgE, by substituting the

Table 2. Ability of rat IgE and rat IgE heated at 56°C for 1 hour (rat IgE 56°C) to inhibit binding of antipeptide sera to solid - phase rat IgE. Dilutions of anti-peptide sera or rabbit anti-rat IgE (Fc) giving OD492 values of approximately 1 in absence of inhibitor were pre-incubated overnight at 4°C with 1.52 g/ml affinity-purified native rat IgE or IgE heated at 56°C for 1 hour prior to additon to microtitre-place wells coated with 1 μg/ml rat IgE.

Antiserum Specificity	% Inhibition + SEM (n=3)	
	RAT IgE	RAT IgE (56°C)
CH3-domain		
Gly 378 - Gly 396	30.5 + 3.3	28.6 + 2.3
Ser 414 - Gly 428	3.4 + 3.9	13.5 + 2.5
CH4-domain		
Tyr 459 - Arg 472	37.1 + 2.4	78.9 + 1
Leu 491 - Ser 503	0	39.5 + 5.5
Arg 522 - Glu 535	33 + 5.4	42.4 + 4
His 542 - Lys 557	47.0 + 1.8	90.4 + 0.7
Gly 560 - Met 571	39.8 + 3.9	42.7 + 3.8
Rat IgE (Fc)	77.9 + 0.3	30.8 + 1.6*

*0.08 μg/ml rat IgE inhibitor.

Table 3. Ability of anti-peptide sera to release histamine from rat mast cells. Rat serosal mast cells were incubated at 37°C for 30 minutes in the presence of various dilutions of anti-peptide sera. Results are expressed as percentage of total histamine released into supernatant for each test. Percentage histamine release in presence of buffer alone was 2.9 + 0.3%.

Antiserum Specificity	% Histamine Release ± SEM (n=3) Serum Dilution					
	1/2	1/4	1/8	1/16	1/100	1/1000
Pre-immune	3.1+0.3	2.2+0.06	2.2+0.03	1.4+0.1		
Glu378-Gly396	11.1+0.6	8.5+0.3	5.6+0.3	3.6+0.2	-	-
Ser414-Gly428	5.1+0.1	3.8+0.2	2.9+0.3	3.4+0.1	-	-
Tyr459-Arg472	11.6+0.7	8.6+0.03	4.8+0.2	4.3+0.4	-	-
Leu491-Ser503	4.9+0.3	3.8+0.07	2.8+0.2	2.0+0.1	-	-
Arg522-Glu535	20.3+0.9	17.0+0.2	12.7+0.5	9.0+0.2	-	-
His542-Lys557	13.0+0.5	7.9+0.3	6.9+0.3	5.0+0.4	-	-
Gly560-Met571	60.1+0.6	60.1+0.08	51.8+0.9	37.2+0.6	-	-
Rat IgE (Fc)	-	-	-	-	79.4	58.8

Table 4. Most continuous surface: A B D' E (D' being from other ε-chain).

Peptide	Domain	ε-Sequence	γ_1-Chain equivalent
A	$C_\varepsilon 3$	414-428	304-318
B	$C_\varepsilon 4$	542-557	429-443
D'	$C_\varepsilon 4$	459-472	349-363
E	$C_\varepsilon 4$	491-503	382-394

heterologous amino acids in the former (as described in Sutton et al, 1986). The objective was to ascertain whether the sequences represented by the four peptides which (for the reasons outlined above) appeared to be implicated in the binding of IgE to mast cells (ie. those listed in Table 4) formed a continuous part of the IgE molecular surface, which could constitute a lateral Fc(ε)R binding site. Intriguingly, three of the four peptides (A, B and E in Table 4) within one of the pair of ε-chains and one (D′) from the other do meet such a requirement! If, indeed, the IgE antibody molecule does bind to Fc(ε)R on mast cells in this manner, it would leave the corresponding sequences in the other ε-chain free and therefore available for interaction with the anti-peptide antibodies (thus explaining our apparently paradoxical histamine release data).

CONCLUDING COMMENTS

An insight has been provided into the scope of using both synthetic ε-chain peptides and anti-peptide antibodies as probes in attempts to elucidate completely the structural basis of IgE antibody activity. The work is now being extended to the synthesis and functional characterisation of the corresponding (and other) sequences of human IgE; and monoclonal, as well as polyclonal, antibodies are being produced against these. Nevertheless, even at this stage, it is hoped that sufficient evidence has been provided to illustrate the power and the potential of this approach, which could well find application to the study of the role of membrane as well as cytophilic immunoglobulins (and related macromolecular structures) in other types of cell-ligand interaction.

We are now aiming to exploit our own findings in the development of potentially new forms of anti-allergy compound as has been recently discussed elsewhere (Stanworth et al, 1986). Included amongst these are synthetic ε-chain peptides representative of those Fc sequences involved in the binding of IgE antibody molecules to mast cells, as well as specific antibodies against these, which are readily reactive with the parent immunoglobulin molecules (irrespective of the location of the antigenic sequences within the 3-dimensional structure). But, in the light of our finding of the conformational complexity of the Fc(ε)R binding site, the former (ie. the peptides themselves) would seem to be the less promising as potential therapeutic agents. In this same vein, we are also in the process of producing specific antibodies against the putative mast cell triggering IgE sequence (the characterisation of which was described in the previous section), which will hopefully prove to be valuable reagents, too, in our studies aimed at obtaining more direct evidence that the Fc(ε)R-bound IgE molecules provide a triggering signal to the mast cells following their cross-linking by allergen, rather than merely playing a passive role in this process.

REFERENCES

Bennich, H, and Hahr-Lindstrom, H Von (1978). Structure of immunoglobulin E. Prog. Immun. II, 1, 49-58.

Burt, D S, Hastings, G Z, and Stanworth, D R (1986). Localisation of binding site(s) on IgE for a specific receptor on mast cells. Protides of the Biol. Fluids 34th Colloq. 243-246. Ed. H Peeters (Pergamon Press).

Coleman, J W, Helm, B, Stanworth, D R, and Gould, H (1985). Inhibition of IgE effector function by a dimeric human ε-chain fragment in E. coli.

Deisenhofer, J (1981). Crystallographic refinement and atomic models of a human Fc fragment and its complex with fragment B of protein A from Staphylococcus aureus at 2.9-2.8A resolution. Biochemistry 20, 2361-2370.

Dennis, S et al (1986). Hepp (IgE pentapeptide) in allergic rhinitis. J. Allergy Clin. Immunol. 77, 213 (Abstr.).

Dorrington, K J, and Bennich, H (1978). Structure-function relationships in human immunoglobulin E. Immun. Rev. 41, 13-25.

Dufton, M J, Cherry, R J, Coleman, J W, and Stanworth, D R (1984). The capacity of basic peptides to trigger exocytosis from mast cells correlates with their capacity to immobilize band 3 proteins in erythrocyte membranes. Biochem. J. 223, 67-71.

Hamburger, R N (1975). Peptide inhibition of Prausnitz-Küstner reaction. Science 189, 389-390.

Hellman, L, Petterson, U, Ensstrom, A, Karsson, I, and Bennich, H (1982). Structure and evolution of the heavy chain from rat immunoglobulin E. Nucl. Acid. Res. 10, 6041-6049.

Holowka, D, and Baird, B (1983). Structural studies on the membrane-bound immunoglobulin E-receptor complex. 2. Mapping of distances between sites on IgE and the membrane surface. Biochemistry 22, 3475-3484.

Ishizaka, T, and Ishizaka, K (1978). Triggering of histamine release from rat mast cells by divalent antibodies against IgE receptors. J. Immunol. 120, 800-805.

Jasani, B, Kreil, G, Mackler, B F, and Stanworth, D R (1973). Studies on mast cell triggering action of certain artificial histamine liberators. Int. Archs. Allergy Appl. Immun. 45, 74-81.

Jasani, B, Kreil, G, Mackler, B F, and Stanworth, D R (1979). Further studies on the structural requirements for polypeptide - mediated histamine release from rat mast cells. Biochem. J. 181, 623-632.

Merrifield, R B (1963). Solid phase peptide synthesis and the syntheis of a tetrapeptide. J. Am. Chem. Soc. 85, 2149-2154.

Perez-Montfort, R, and Metzger, H (1982). Proteolysis of soluble IgE-receptor complexes: localisation of sites on IgE which interact with the Fc receptor. Molec. Immunol. 19, 113-125.

Roy, P D, Moran, D M, Bryant, V, Stevenson, R, and Stanworth, D R (1980). Further studies on histamine release from rat mast cells in vitro induced by peptides. Biochem. J. 191, 233-237.

Stanworth, D R (1971). Immunoglobulin E (reagin) and allergy. Nature Lond. 233, 310-316.

Stanworth, D R (1973). Immediate hypersensitivity: the molecular basis of the allergic response. "Frontiers of Biology" Series (North Holland, Amsterdam).

Stanworth, D R (1984). The role of non-antigen receptors in mast cell triggering processes. Molec. Immunol. 21, 1183-1190.

Stanworth, D R, and Kuhns, W J (1965). Quantitative studies on the assay of human skin-sensitizing antibodies (reagins). Immunology 8, 323-344.

Stanworth, D R, and Burt, D S (1986). Anti-ε-chain antibodies as probes in the study of mast cell triggering. Molec. Immunol. 23, 1231-1235.

Stanworth, D R, Coleman, J W, and Khan, Z (1984). Essential structural requirements for triggering of mast cells by a synthetic peptide comprising a sequence in the $C_{\varepsilon}4$ domain of human IgE. Molec. Immunol. 21, 243-247.

Stanworth, D R, King, S M, Roy, P D, and Moran, D M (1978). Investigation of the reputed inhibition of the Prausnitz-Küstner reaction by the pentapeptide Asp-Ser-Asp-Pro-Arg. Int. Archs. Allergy Appl. Immun. 56, 409-415.

Stanworth, D R, Burt, D S, and Hastings, G Z (1986). The use of synthetic peptides in the delineation of immunoglobulin antigenic epitopes and Fc effector functions. Ciba Found. Symp. 119, 226-244.

Stanworth, D R, Humphrey, J H, Bennich, H, and Johansson, S G O (1968). Inhibition of Prausnitz-Küstner reaction by proteolytic-cleavage fragments of human myeloma protein of immunoglobulin class E. Lancet ii, 17-18.

Stanworth, D R, King, S M, Roy, P D, Moran, J M, and Moran, D M (1979). Synthetic peptides comprising sequences of the human immunoglobulin E heavy chain capable of releasing histamine. Biochem. J. 180, 665-668.

Sutton, B J, Burt, D S, Hastings, G Z, and Stanworth, D R (1987). Modelling of the mast cell Fc (ε) R combining sites of rat IgE. In preparation.

STRUCTURE AND EXPRESSION OF GENES INVOLVED IN T

LYMPHOCYTE RECOGNITION AND ACTIVATION

M.J. Owen[+], M.J. Crumpton[o], J. Dunne[+], G. Krissansen[o], J. Lamb* and W. Sewell[o]

[+]Imperial Cancer Research Fund, Tumour Immunology Unit
Dept. of Zoology, University College London, Gower Street
London WC1E 6BT, UK

[o]Imperial Cancer Research Fund, Lincoln's Inn Fields
London WC2A 3PX, UK

*MRC Tuberculosis and Related Infections Unit, Hammersmith
Hospital, Du Cane Rd, London W12 OHS, UK

INTRODUCTION

Human T lymphocytes can be activated by two apparently distinct pathways. The first pathway is mediated through the T cell receptor (TcR) complex following corecognition of antigen and major histocompatibility complex (MHC) gene products (Reinherz et. al., 1982). The TcR complex comprises an αβ heterodimer (Ti) which is linked non-covalently to a non-polymorphic glycoprotein, the CD3 antigen (see Kronenberg et al., 1986 for a review). The CD3 antigen in turn comprises at least three polypeptide chains, γ, δ and ε (Borst et al., 1983; Kanellopoulos et al., 1983). The αβ heterodimer is sufficient to confer clonal variability in the recognition of antigen/MHC to a T cell (Dembic et al., 1986). The CD3 antigen, which is obligatorily expressed with the αβ heterodimer (or with TcR γ chains: see Brenner et al., 1986; Bank et al., 1986) has been implicated in the signal transfer process consequent to specific binding of a T cell to a target cell or antigen presenting cell. Several events have been implicated in the signal transfer process, including phosphorylation of the CD3 γ chain, increased phosphatidyl inositol bis phosphate turnover and downregulation of the TcR complex from the cell surface (Weiss et al., 1984; Cantrell et al., 1985; Davies et al., 1985; Imboden et al., 1985).

The CD2 antigen (T11; E-rosette receptor; LFA 2) is a glycoprotein of apparent molecular weight about 50,000 and is expressed on virtually all thymocytes and peripheral T cells. T cell proliferation is initiated by certain combinations of anti-CD2 monoclonal antibodies apparently in a macrophage-independent fashion (Meuer et al., 1984). The function of CD2 is obscure, not least because a candidate for the natural ligand for CD2 has only recently existed. Thus, CD2 on the T cell is now thought to bind to LFA3 on the target cell, an event which may be important in initiating cellular interaction prior to specific association of the TcR complex with antigen/MHC (Shaw et al., 1986).

That the CD2 antigen may be more than simply an adhesion molecule is suggested by experiments that demonstrate intercommunication between the CD2 receptor and TcR complex. Thus, antibodies against one receptor have been reported to exert inhibitory effects towards activation via the other receptor pathway (see, for example, Meuer et al., 1984). This intercommunication may be important in the regulation of the T cell response to antigen/MHC or in proliferative events associated with the generation of MHC restriction and self-tolerance within the thymus (Reinherz, 1985).

A complete understanding of the functions of these two receptors requires a knowledge of their structures and of the regulation of their expression during ontogeny and maturation. Here, we describe firstly the structure and expression of the T3 γ component of the T cell receptor complex (deduced from cDNA sequence) and the implications of the structural predictions for T3 function. Secondly, the structure of the CD2 glycoprotein is described. Thirdly, experiments that extend our knowledge of the interaction of these two activation pathways are presented.

STRUCTURE OF HUMAN AND MURINE T3γ CHAIN

Recently, cDNA clones encoding the human CD3 γ chain have been isolated by immunoscreening of a λgt11 library prepared using RNA from the human T leukaemic line Jurkat (Krissansen et al., 1986). The murine homologue was subsequently isolated by cross-hybridisation using the human probe (Krissansen et al., 1987). Both the murine and human probes revealed easily detectable CD3γ transcripts, as assessed by Northern hybridisation analysis, in all T cells studied regardless of phenotypic state of maturity (Fig 1). Since CD3 δ and ε transcription has also been shown to be an early event in T cell maturation (Van den Elsen et al., 1984; Gold et al., 1986), the T3γ, δ and ε genes may be coordinately expressed very early in thymocytedevelopment. The genomic structure of T3γ is currently being elucidicated in order to investigate possible regulatory elements that might mediate such coordinate expression. The human T3γ probe revealed two transcripts, of about 0.8 and 3.5kb, which varied in relative amount in RNA from different T cell lines (Fig 1). These transcripts most probably arise as a result of differential usage of polyadenylation signals at the 3' end of the T3γ gene.

The cDNA sequence has been used to predict the structures of the human and murine γ chains. Each chain possesses a 22 amino acid signal sequence followed by a 79 residue hydrophilic region which contains 2 potential N-glycosylation sites (N-X-S/T) in the human and/in the mouse. Because both human and murine T3γ chains are known to be glycosylated, the N-terminal segment is presumably situated at the external face of the bilayer as no precedent exists for glycosylation within the cytoplasm. The external hydrophilic domain is followed by a 27 residue predominantly hydrophobic segment that is postulated to span the lipid bilayer. A characteristic feature of the human and murine γ transmembrane segments is that they contain a centrally placed glutamic acid residue. The presence of an acidic residue in this region is a characteristic of T3 chains, although the δ and ε chains have an aspartate rather than glutamate residue. The hydrophilic intracellular domain (residues 117-160) is large relative to the total size of the polypeptide and incorporates a candidate site, containing two serine residues, for phosphorylation by protein kinase C.

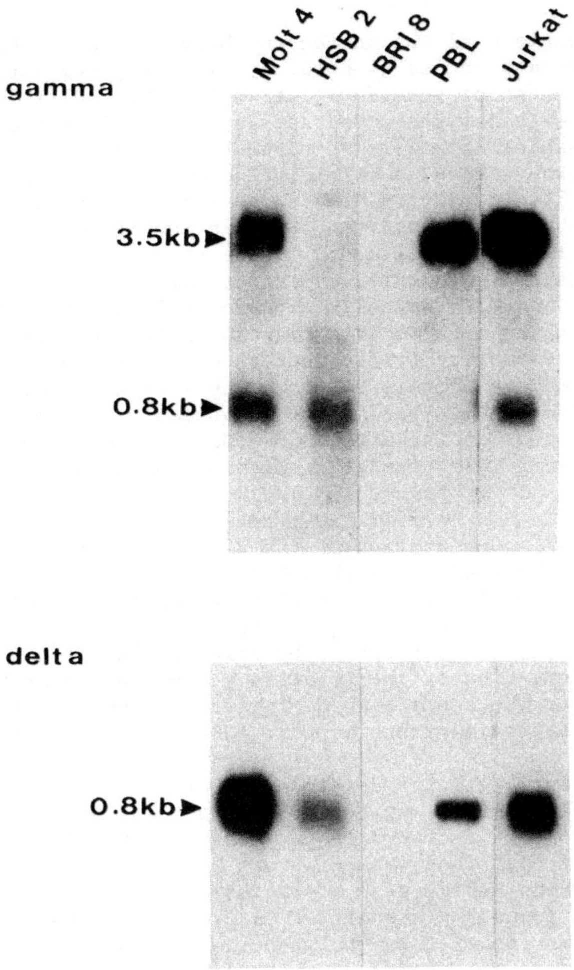

Fig 1. Northern hybridisation analysis of T cell mRNA. T cell lines of various phenotypic stages, both immature (HSB2: $T3^-T4^-T8^-$) and mature (Molt 4 and Jurkat:$T3^+T4^+T8^+$) are represented, together with peripheral blood lymphocytes (PBL) and a B cell line (BR18). The blot was probed sequentially with a CD3 γ and δ probe (Van den Elsen et al., 1985).

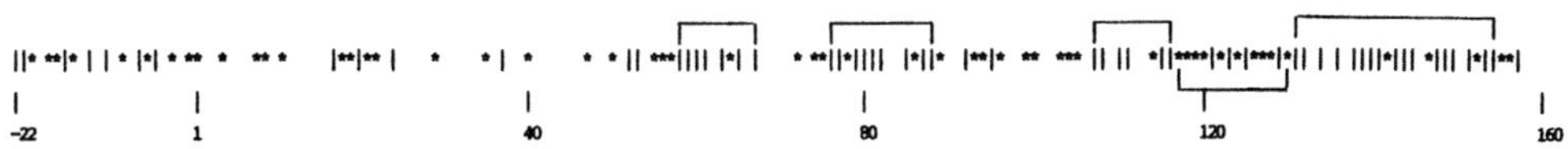

Fig 2. Scheme for homology of human and murine CD3 γ and δ chains. A vertical bar represents an identical amino acid for all four chains and a star depicts identity only between γ chains. Brackets refer to regions of γ-δ or γ-γ homology along the polypeptide chain.

Sequence comparison of the murine and human γ and δ chains has revealed a high overall degree of homology, strongly suggesting that they arose by a process of gene duplication (Fig 2). Division of the chains into extracellular, transmembrane and intracellular domains reveals that the weakest homology is shown by the external and transmembrane domains whereas the internal domain shows a high degree of homology (Fig 2). In particular, it was necessary to insert a gap equivalent to nine residues into the δ chain immediately following the signal peptide to increase alignment. These extra residues in the γ chain are predominantly encoded by a discrete exon in the CD3γ gene (S-T Wah, GWK, MJC and MJO, unpublished observation). Comparison of the mouse and human γ chains reveals that their intracellular domains are almost totally conserved (>90%) whereas murine and human δ chains share about 80% homology in this region. One site that has been completely conserved between the murine and human γ chains is a segment (residues 117-130) that contains the potential serine phosphorylation site at position 126. This site is an alanine in the human and mouse . chains.

The high overall conservation of the γ and δ intracellular regions, including the putative γ phosphorylation site indicates that this region of the T3 molecule may be vitally important in its function, either directly in the signal transduction process or in autoregulation of the T cell response by down-regulation of the TcR complex. The conservation of the putative γ protein kinase C phosphorylation site which has been implicated in several systems in receptor downregulation is strong support for the latter role.

Although the extracellular domain of the T3γ and δ chains are much less conserved, limited regions of strong homology are evident. In particular, sequences in two regions whish together incorporate 3 of the 4 extracellular cysteines showed strong homology between murine and human γ chains. These residues may form intrachain disulphide bridges and thus represent important structural determinants required for the appropriate conformation of the γ polypeptides and/or for its association with other components of the CD3/Ti complex. It is worth noting that the weak overall primary sequence homology between the external regions of the CD3 γ and δ chains does not necessarily imply that they adopt a substantially different tertiary conformation. Thus, although β_2-microglobulin and an Ig constant region domain share only limited sequence homology (about 30% for a C_H3 domain) X-ray crystallographic studies have demonstrated that both molecules strongly resemble each other in their 3-dimensional structures (Becker and Reeke, 1985).

STRUCTURE OF THE CD2 ANTIGEN

Human cDNA clones encoding the CD2 antigen have been isolated using the same "expression cloning" approach as was employed for the human T3γ gene (Sewell et al., 1986). Northern blotting analysis revealed two transcripts, of about 1.7 and 1.3 kb, which were present in peripheral blood T cells but not in B cells (Fig 3). Although >95% of T cells and thymocytes are phenotypically CD2 positive, many long-term T leukaemic cell lines of both mature and immature phenotype were surface CD2-negative and expressed low or undetectable levels of CD2 transcripts. The reason for this apparent high rate of CD2 gene inactivation is unknown.

The CD2 DNA sequence contained an open reading frame encoding 360

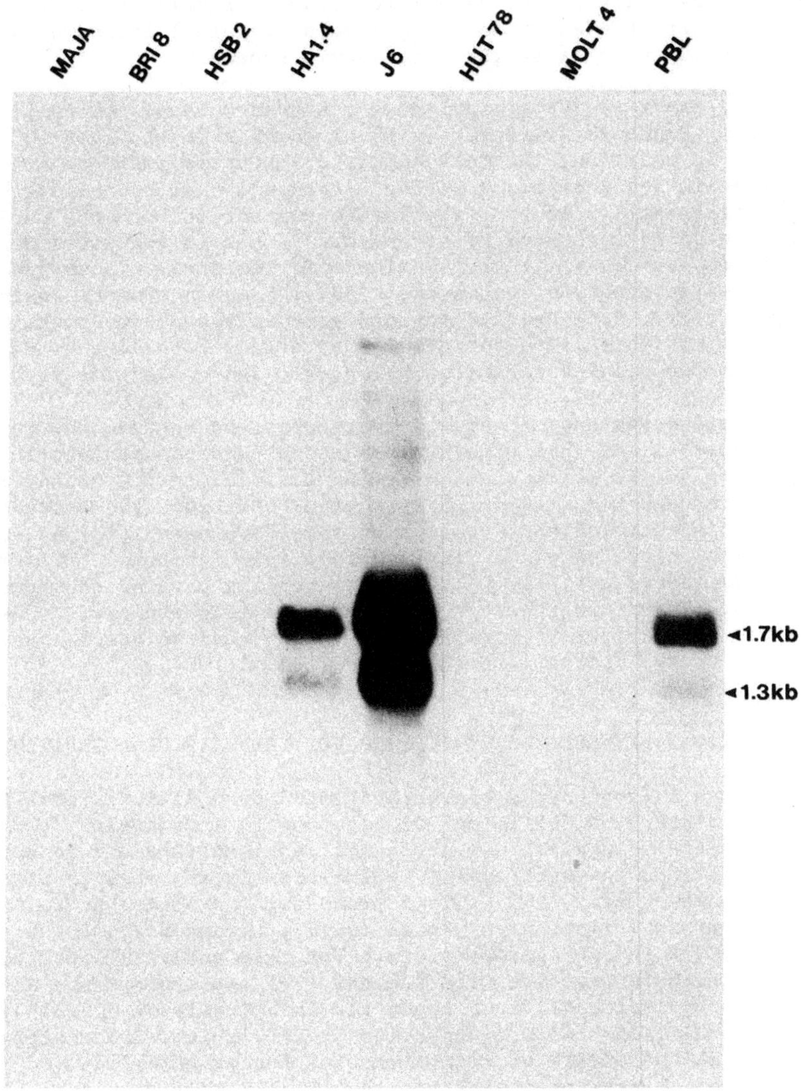

Fig 3. Northern hybridisation analysis of T cell mRNA. The T lineage leukaemic lines HSB2, J6 (a Jurkat subline) HUT78, MOLT4 together with the functional helper T cell clone HA1.4, peripheral blood T cells (PBL) and the B lymphoblastoid cell lines MAJA and BR18 are represented. The probe used is described in Sewell et al., (1986).

amino acids. The signal peptide which comprised the N-terminal 24 residues was followed by an extracellular region of 185 predominantly hydrophilic amino acids containing three potential N-linked glycosylation sites. This region precedes a hydrophobic segment of 26 amino acids which possesses all the characteristics of a transbilayer peptide (with the exception of a glycine triplet) including a cluster of basic amino acids at the cytoplasmic boundary.

The predicted C-terminal domain has an unusual composition with 27 prolines, 23 basic residues and 13 glutamines in the last 100 amino acids. In addition, the only acidic or aromatic residues in the cytoplasmic sequence occur in the C-terminal 6 amino acids. There is a repetitive pattern in the cytoplasmic segment in both the nucleotide and amino acid sequences, most obviously seen in two stretches which are homologous in 9 out of 14 amino acid residues. These particular sequences incorporate continuous runs of 5 and 4 proline residues, respectively. Proline-rich regions generally separate protein domains. If this is so for the CD2 cytoplasmic tail, this region may exist as two domains separated by an extended connecting peptide.

Limited regions of homology were observed between the CD2 amino acid sequence and that of other members of the immunoglobulin superfamily. In particular, a region surrounding a cysteine residue midway through the extracellular region (position 122) showed substantial homology to a region of a V_K domain containing the N-terminal cysteine of the intrachain disulphide bond. This region in CD2 also showed homology to the corresponding part of the human CD4 antigen. Based upon these homologies, CD2 is postulated to be a number of the Ig superfamily (Sewell et al., 1986) and to resemble a truncated version of the CD4 antigen (Williams et al., 1987).

INTERACTIONS BETWEEN THE CD3/Ti AND CD2 PATHWAYS OF ACTIVATION

Human T lymphocytes can be activated by positive signalling through either the CD3/Ti or CD2 receptors. In addition, a negative growth signal can also be generated if antigen is added in supraoptimal concentrations to functional T cell clones in the absence of accessory cells (Lamb et al., 1983). This observation prompted us to investigate whether a similar negative signal could be transduced to the antigen receptor via the CD2 glycoprotein. For this analysis the T cell clone HA1.7, which is reactive with the carboxyl terminus of the HA-1 molecule of influenza virus haemagglutinin (residues 306-319), was used (Lamb et al., 1982). Preincubation of HA1.7 with either supraoptimal concentrations of p14 or with a combination of anti-$T11_2$ and $T11_3$ antibodies in the absence of accessory cells abolished the ability of these cells to respond to an immunogenic challenge of p14 (i.e. in the presence of presenting cells). In contrast, the response to IL2 was enhanced as compared to the medium control (Table 1). In the presence of accessory cells, however, HA1.7 proliferated in response to anti-$T11_2$ and $T11_3$.

Collectively, these results suggest that the CD2 protein requires accessory cells to activate HA1.7 and that, in the absence of accessory cells, it can deliver a negative signal that is functionally identical to that of supraoptimal antigen.

Preincubation of HA1.7 with anti-$T11_2$ and $T11_3$ resulted in profound phenotypic changes. In particular, subsequent staining with anti-CD3 revealed that CD3/Ti was substantially downregulated to about

Table 1. Anti-CD2 antibody-induced antigen specific T-cell unresponsiveness

Preincubation		Response (cpm ± %sem)		
T cells	Antigen/Antibody	APC	APC + p14	IL2
-	-	107 ± 9	85 ± 9	-
+	-	99 ± 27	15410 ± 2	20771 ± 17
+	p14	155 ± 13	117 ± 11	37639 ± 3
+	anti-$T11_2$+$T11_3$	80 ± 19	141 ± 10	33710 ± 12

HA1.7 cloned helper T cells were preincubated for 16 hr in the absence of accessory cells with the HA peptide p14 (50μg/ml) or with the anti-CD2 antibodies $T11_2$ and $T11_3$. After washing, the cells were cultured with irradiated peripheral blood mononuclear cells ± p14 (0.3 μg/ml) or with IL2 alone. Following 60 hr incubation, proliferation was assessed by [^{3}H]-thymidine incorporation. The results are expressed as mean cpm ± %sem of triplicate cultures.

10% of its control levels. A similar effect was observed on tolerance induction with p14 when CD3-Ti surface levels were reduced to about 5% of the control. CD2 levels were also downregulated (about 50%) by tolerogenic anti-$T11_2$+$T11_3$ preincubation but upregulated by tolerogenic p14 preincubation. IL2-receptor levels were increased by 2-3 fold with both tolerogenic stimuli. These phenotypic changes were in part mirrored by changes in steady-state mRNA levels. Thus, when compared with the levels of actin mRNA, Tiβ and CD3 δ mRNAs were downregulated, whereas Tiα levels were unchanged when anti-$T11_2$ and $T11_3$ was used as a tolerogenic signal. In contrast, after preincubation with p14, α, β and δ mRNA levels were unaltered. CD2 mRNA levels were marginally increased after preincubation with p14 but were about 2-fold downregulated by anti-$T11_2$ and $T11_3$ treatment. In both instances IL2-receptor mRNA levels were increased by at least 10-20 fold. These observations suggest that the phenotypic changes observed are the result of a combination of transcriptional and post-transcriptional regulation of receptor gene expression.

The present studies are in contrast with some previous observations (Meuer et al., 1984) in that they suggest a monocyte requirement for anti-$T11_2$+$T11_3$ activation of HA1.7. The reason for this discrepancy is unclear. Possible explanations include the failure in previous studies completely to remove presenting cells or a differential requirement for monocytes depending on the T cell clone or subset. The apparent requirement for monocytes (at least in this system) is presumably related to a need for receptor crosslinking for activation. The more efficient the CD2 system is as an activation pathway, the less crosslinking, and therefore the fewer monocytes, would be required.

The interaction between the CD2 and CD3/Ti pathways may be of importance in the autoregulation of T cell activation. Although the ligand for CD2 has not been identified unequivocally, the LFA3 glycoprotein has been proposed as a candidate (Shaw et al., 1986). It has been suggested that LFA3-CD2 interactions are partially responsible for initial non-specific interactions between cytotoxic T cells and target cells prior to interaction between CD3/Ti and antigen/MHC. If this is the case, it is possible that both positive and negative signals, such as those described here, may minimise the possibility of inappropriate activation of T cells in which the CD3/Ti receptor is unoccupied.

The mechanism of CD2-CD3/Ti "crosstalk" is unknown but presumably involves common second messenger systems such as the polyphosphoinositol pathway or intracellular G proteins. The structures of the two receptors described here, in particular those of the cytoplasmic domains, will be of immense value in elucidating these mechanisms.

REFERENCES

Bank, I., De Pinho, R. A., Brenner, M. B., Cassimeris, J., Alt, F. W. and Chess, L. A., 1986, Nature, 322:179.

Becker, J. W., and Reeke, G. N., 1985, Proc.Natl.Acad.Sci.USA,82:4225.

Borst, J., Prendiville, M., and Terhorst, C., 1983, Eur. J. Immunol., 13:576.

Brenner, M. B., McLean, J., Dialynas, D. P., Strominger, J. L., Smith, J. A., Owen, F. L., Seidman, J. G., Ip, S., Rosen, F., and Krangel, M. S., 1986, Nature, 322:145.

Cantrell, D. A., Davies, A. A., and Crumpton, M. J., 1985, Proc. Natl. Acad. Sci. USA, 82:8158.

Davies, A. A., Cantrell, D. A., and Crumpton, M. J., 1985, Biosci. Rep., 5:867.

Dembic, Z., Haas, W., Weiss, S., McCubrey, J., Kiefer, H., and von Boehmer, H., 1986, Nature, 320:232.

Gold, D. P., Puck, J. M., Pettey, C. L., Cho, M., Coligan, J., Woody, J. N., and Terhorst, C., 1986, Nature, 321:431.

Imboden, J. B., Weiss, A. and Stobo, J.D., 1985, Immunology Today, 6:328.

Kanellopoulos, J. M., Wigglesworth, N. M., Owen, M. J., and Crumpton, M. J., 1983, EMBO Journal, 2:1807.

Krissansen, G. W., Owen, M. J., Fink, P. J., and Crumpton, M. J., 1987, J. Immunol., In Press.

Krissansen, G. W., Owen, M. J., Verbi, W., and Crumpton, M. J., 1986, EMBO Journal, 5:1799.

Kronenberg, M., Siu, G., Hood, L. E., and Shastri, N., 1986, Ann. Rev. Immunol., 4:529.

Lamb, J. R., Eckels, D. D., Lake, P., Woody, J. N., and Green, N., 1982, Nature, 300:66.

Lamb, J. R., Skidmore, B. J., Green, N., Chiller, J. M., and Feldmann, M. F., 1983, J. Exp. Med., 157:1434.

Meuer, S. C., Hussey, R. E., Fabbi, M., Fox, D., Acuto, O., Fitzgerald, K. A., Hodgdon, J. C., Protentis, J. P., Schlossman, S. F., and Reinherz, E.L., 1984, Cell, 36:897.

Reinherz, E. L., 1985, Immunology Today, 6:75.

Reinherz, E. L., Meuer, S. C., Fitzgerald, K. A., Hussey, R. E., Levine, H., and Schlossman, S. F., 1982, Cell, 30:735.

Shaw, S., Ginther Luce, G. E., Quinones, R., Gress, R. E., Springer, T. A., and Sanders, M. E., 1986, Nature, 323:262.

Sewell, W. A., Brown, M., Dunne, M. J., Owen, M. J., and Crumpton, M. J., 1986, Proc. Natl. Acad. Sci. USA, In Press.
Van den Elsen, P., Shepley, B.-A., Cho, M., and Terhorst, C., 1985, Nature, 314:542.
Weiss, A., Imboden, J., Shoback, D., and Stobo, J., 1984, Proc. Natl. Acad. Sci. USA, 81:4169.
Williams, A. F., Barclay, A. N., Clark, S. J., Paterson, D. J., and Willis, A. C., 1987, J. Exp. Med., In Press.

T-CELL RECOGNITION OF PRE-S REGIONS OF HBsAg CAN BYPASS NONRESPONSE TO THE S REGION

David R. Milich*, Alan McLachlan*, and George B. Thornton**

*Department of Basic and Clinical Research
Scripps Clinic and Research Foundation, La Jolla, CA;
**Johnson and Johnson Biotechnology Center, Inc., San Diego, CA

INTRODUCTION

The specific serologic marker of hepatitis B virus (HBV) infection is the hepatitis B surface antigen (HBsAg), which is present both in the intact virion and as free circulating filamentous and spherical 22-nm particles. The HBsAg is composed of a major polypeptide, p25, and its glycosylated form, gp28. However, additional polypeptides of higher m.w. (p39/gp42 and gp33/gp36) have been identified associated preferentially with the intact virion and the filamentous form of 22-nm particles (1). The p25 polypeptide is encoded by the S gene beginning from the third possible translational initiation site of a larger open reading frame (ORF) and is preceded in phase by 174 codons (*adw* subtype) designated the pre-S region (2). The large ORF for HBsAg terminates in a single stop codon but can initiate at three possible translational start codons, which define the pre-S(1), pre-S(2), and S regions, yielding p39, p33, and p25, respectively. All three polypeptides share the 226 amino acid residues of the S region (p25); p33 consists of the p25 sequence plus an amino-terminal 55 residues [pre-S(2)] (3) and p39 consists of the p33 sequence plus an amino-terminal 119 residues [pre-S(1)] (1) (see Fig. 1). Therefore, three different envelope polypeptides are expressed by the variable use of initiation codons in one ORF, and HBsAg-containing virions or particles may vary in composition relative to these three polypeptides. Herein, we designate purified HBsAg particle preparations by virtue of the highest m.w. polypeptide present (i.e. HBsAg/p39, HBsAg/p33, and HBsAg/p25).

RESULTS AND DISCUSSION

<u>Influence of H-2 phenotype on antibody response to HBsAg particles composed of p25 alone or p25 plus pre-S containing polypeptides</u>. The secondary responses after HBsAg/p39 immunization were directly compared with the secondary responses after HBsAg/p25 and HBsAg/p33 immunization in a panel of H-2 congenic mice (Table I). Immunization with HBsAg/p25 elicits anti-S region responses in all strains except B10.S and B10.M Immunization with HBsAg/p33 elicits anti-pre-S(2) responses in all strains except the B10.M strain, and note that it also elicits an anti-S response in the S region nonresponder, B10.S strain (boxed number in Table I). The availability of a nonresponder strain to both S and pre-S(2) region determinants (B10.M) allowed us to determine if the pre-S(1) region would

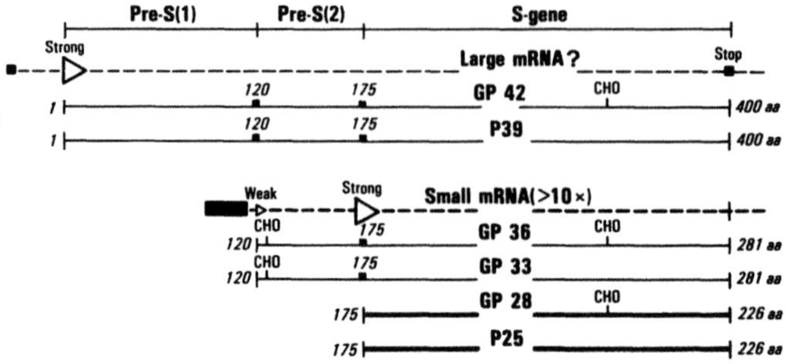

Figure 1. Representation of the translation of the 3 coterminal envelope polypeptides of HBsAg (p39, GP33 and p25). The p39 polypeptide is translated from a putative large mRNA, and GP33 and p25 are derived from shorter, more abundant mRNAs. Amino acid positions are depicted from the NH_2- terminus (1) to the COOH-terminus (400). Adapted from Heermann, et al. (1).

provide alternative T-cell recognitiion sites that the B10.M strain may be able to recognize, and if so, would recognition of pre-S(1) at the T-cell level influence the B10.M antibody response to the pre-S(2) and S regions? HBsAg/p39 immunization elicited anti-pre-S(1)-specific responses in all strains, and furthermore, elicited anti-S and anti-pre-S(2) responses in all strains, including an S-specific response in the "nonresponder" B10.S strain, and S and pre-S(2)-specific responses in the "nonresponder" B10.M strain (boxed numbers in Table I). This result suggests that the B10.M strain possesses pre-S(1)-specific T-cells that are capable of helping B-cell clones specific for S and pre-S(2) region determinants as well as pre-S(1)-specific B-cell clones.

Summary of T-cell proliferative responses to S and pre-S region antigens. The T-cell proliferative responses after immunization with HBsAg/p25, HBsAg/p33 and HBsAg/p39 also were examined, and the results for three representative strains (B10.D2, B10.S and B10.M) are summarized in Figures 2-4. These H-2 haplotypes were chosen because they represented three distinct patterns of antibody production in terms of specificity (See Table I). The B10.D2 strain was the only responder to immunization with HBsAg/p25 at the T cell level, which provided T-cell help (Th) for anti-S antibody production (Fig. 2). The B10.D2 strain also exhibited T-

TABLE 1

Influence of H-2 Genotype on the Humoral Response to HBsAg Particles of Varied Composition

Immunogen	Strain	H-2	Specific Antibody Titer (1/dilution)		
			S	pre-S(2)	pre-S(1)
HBsAg/p25	B10.D2	d	81,920	0	0
	B10	b	20,480	0	0
	B10.BR	k	5,120	0	0
	B10.S	s	0	0	0
	B10.M	f	0	0	0
HBsAg/p33	B10.D2		40,960	10,240	0
	B10		10,240	40,960	0
	B10.BR		1,280	2,560	0
	B10.S		640[a]	10,240	0
	B10.M		0	0	0
HBsAg/p39	B10.D2		81,920	5,120	640
	B10		20,480	40,960	10,240
	B10.BR		5,120	1,280	2,560
	B10.S		5,120	10,240	1,280
	B10.M		10,240	1,280	10,240

[a]The boxed numbers represent an antibody response to a specific region of HBsAg which is not observed when the strain is immunized with that same antigen (i.e. B10.S is nonresponsive to the S region when immunized with HBsAg/p25). Table is from Milich et al. (15).

Figure 2. Summary of T cell proliferative response (T) and in vivo antibody production (B) of H-2 congenic, murine strains immunized with HBsAg/p25. A plus in the T column represents significant, dose-dependent, T cell proliferation and IL-2 production by HBsAg/p25-primed, draining lymph node cells (LNC) challenged in vitro with HBsAg/p25. A plus in the B column represents significant antibody production after secondary immunization with HBsAg/p25.

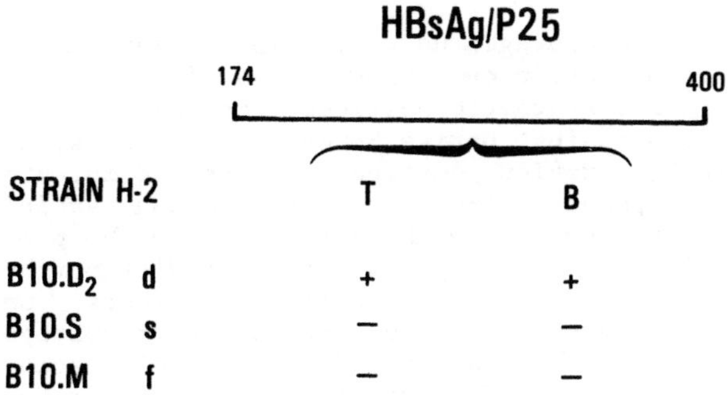

Figure 3. Summary of T cell proliferative responses (T) and in vivo antibody production (B) of H-2 congenic, murine strains immunized with HBsAg/gp33.

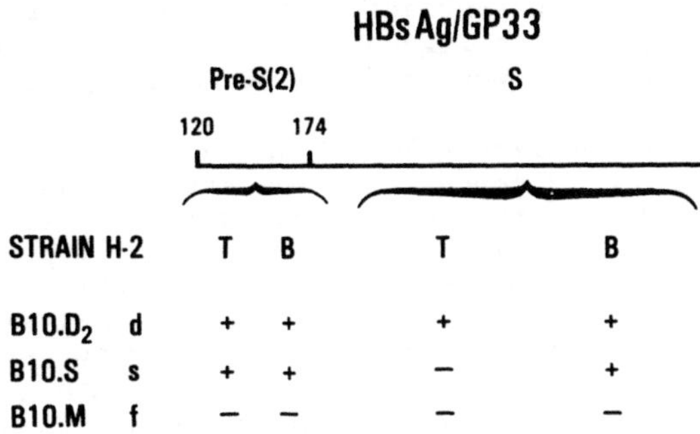

Figure 4. Summary of T cell proliferative responses (T) and in vivo antibody production (B) of H-2 congenic, murine strains immunized with HBsAg/p39.

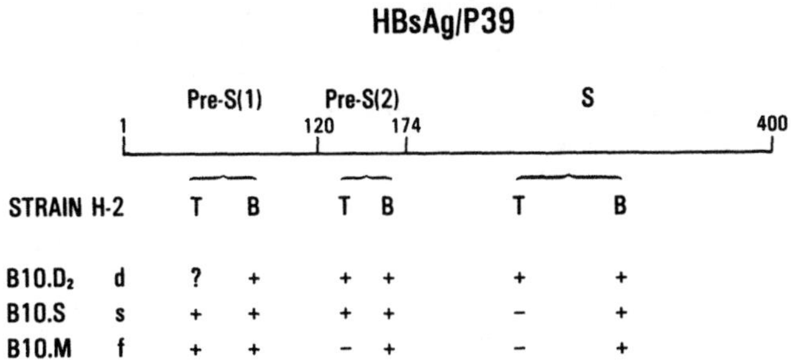

cell sensitization to the pre-S(2) region, as well as the S region, after HBsAg/p33 immunization (Fig. 3). In contrast, the S region nonresponding B10.S strain only demonstrated a T-cell response to the pre-S(2) region, which correlated with anti-pre-S(2) and anti-S region antibody synthesis. Therefore, Th cells specific for the pre-S(2) region can provide functional help for both pre-S(2) and S region-specific B-cell clones. The B10.M strain was nonresponsive at the T-cell level to both the S and pre-S(2) regions, and subsequently produced no anti-HBs. However, the B10.M strain was capable of responding at the T-cell level to the pre-S(1) region after HBsAg/p39 immunization (Fig. 4). Notably, pre-S(1)-specific Th cell(s) could provide functional help for pre-S(2) and S specific B-cell clones, as well as for pre-S(1)-specific B-cells since antibodies to all regions were produced. The B10.S strain also recognized the pre-S(1) region at the T-cell level in addition to the pre-S(2) region, and produced antibodies to all three regions.

Fine specificity of antibody binding sites within the pre-S regions. The resistance of native pre-S(2) antigen to reduction and denaturation are consistent with the presence of continuous as opposed to conformation-dependent determinants in the pre-S(2) region (4,5). This is in contrast to the major group and subtype-specific determinants of the S region, which are highly dependent on intact disulfide bonds (6,7). Substantial preliminary data and the conformation-independent nature of the pre-S(2) region encouraged us to attempt to map antibody binding sites on the native protein by employing a series of truncated group- and subtype-specific synthetic peptides. Monoclonal and murine polyclonal antisera raised against native HBsAg/p33 particles, the isolated p33, or synthetic pre-S(2) region peptides were assayed for binding activity on a series of solid-phase peptides and native HBsAg particles. The results indicate that the murine antibody response to the pre-S (2) region is focused on residues 133 through 143, and two distinct but overlapping epitopes were identified within 11 continuous residues. One epitope, defined by p133-139, is group specific, and the other epitope defined by p137-143, is influenced by a subtype-dependent amino acid substitution at residue 141. However, the influence of residue 141 was "covert" in that it was only detected when synthetic antigens of 19 amino acids or smaller were used as the solid-phase ligand. The minimum size of both epitopes (p133-139 and p137 and 143) was seven amino acids (Fig. 5).

To localize relevant antibody epitopes within the pre-S(1) region, a panel of H-2 congenic murine strains was immunized with HBsAg/p39 particles of the *adw* subtype and secondary antisera were analyzed for IgG antibody reactivity with a series of synthetic peptides representing the majority of the pre-S(1) region of the adw and ayw subtypes. Immunization with native HBsAg/p39 particles did not elicit antibodies reactive to the NH_2-terminal 32 residues. Anti-HBs/p39 sera from 3 of the five strains bound the 32-53/d sequence, and the B10 strain antiserum bound the y subtype equivalently to the d subtype sequence (Table 2). The B10 antiserum also bound p41-53/d, and since the 41-47 sequence is conserved between subtypes this is the likely group-specific site recognized by the B10 strain. The B10.BR and B10.M strains recognized a subtype-specific site within the 32-53 sequence, therefore, at least 2 distinct antibody binding sites exist within the 32-53 sequence, one is group-specific (p41-53) and the other subtype-specific. The 53-73/d and 74-89/d sequences did not represent antibody binding sites recognized by any of the antisera. In contrast, the 94-117 *d* sequence represented the dominant antibody binding site for all strains (Table 2). Furthermore, all strains produced antibody reactive to the y subtype 94-117 sequence as well. This may be explained by the fact that the conserved 94-105 sequence also represented an efficient antibody binding site for all strains. However, only 3 strains recognized the 106-117/d sequence, and this antibody binding site was subtype-specific since the 106-117/y peptide was marginally to nonreactive. Therefore, at least 2 distinct antibody binding sites exist within the p94-117 sequence, one is group-specific (p94-105) and the other is subtype-specific (106-117). Although immunization with native HBsAg/p39 particles did not elicit a p12-32-specific antibody response, we were able to induce antibody by immunizing SJL/J mice with the uncoupled synthetic peptide. This antiserum did not bind either the NH_2-terminal fragment (p12-21) or the COOH-terminal fragment (p22-32), but did bind an overlapping sequence (p16-27). Cumulatively, this analysis defined 5 distinct antibody binding sites within the pre-S(1) region of HBsAg/p39;

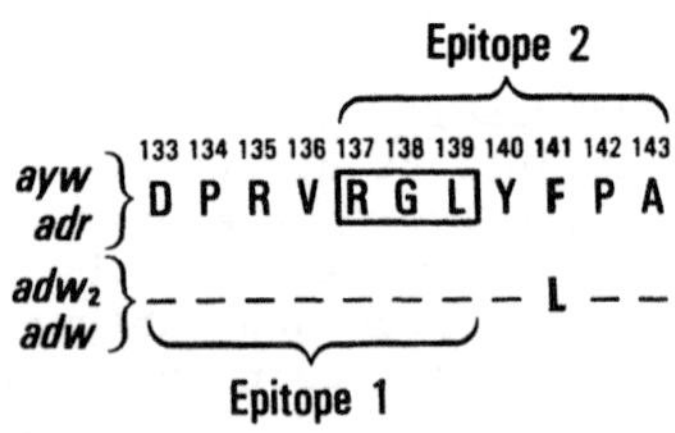

Figure 5. Amino acid sequence of two distinct and overlapping antibody binding sites within the pre-S(2) region. Epitope 1 (p133-139) is conserved in the ayw, adr, adw, and adw_2 subtypes. Epitope 2 (p137-143) contains a subtype-dependent amino acid substitution at residue 141 (phenylalanine [ayw, adr]; leucine [adw, adw_2]). The three-amino acid overlap between epitopes 1 and 2 is depicted. Figure from Milich, et al. (16).

T-cell populations to provide functional T cell help for a series of B-cell specificities on HBsAg. Two pre-S(1)-specific T-cell determinants were chosen (i.e. p12-32, p94-117), which induced only minimal antibody responses. This allowed us to prime T-cell helper cells with peptides and determine in vivo antibody production after challenge with a suboptimal dose of HBsAg/p39 in the same animal as opposed to performing transfer experiments. This approach requires the memory T-cells primed by immunization with peptide to be recalled by challenge with native particles indicating the relevance of the synthetic T-cell sites to the native molecule. Using this protocol it was demonstrated that priming with a single synthetic peptide, p12-32, elicited T cell helper function resulting in in vivo antibody production to p16-27, p133-140, p135-145 in the pre-S region and group and subtype-specific determinants in the S region (Fig. 7). Similarly, priming with p94-117 elicited T-cell helper function resulting in in vivo antibody production specific for p32-53, p94-105, p106-117, p133-140, p135-145 in the pre-S region, but did not prime antibody production to S region determinants (Fig. 7). These results indicate that T cells primed to a single determinant are sufficient to provide functional help to multiple B-cell clones, which recognize unique epitopes on a complex, particulate antigen.

Note that the pre-S(1)-specific, T-cell recognition sites, p12-32 and p94-117, primed antibody production specific for unique as well as common B cell determinants. For example, p94-117 primed an anti-p32-53 response, whereas, p12-32 did not. This data provides strong evidence that the fine specificity of the T helper cell can influence the fine specificity of the antibody produced, and is consistent with the variable anti-p32-53 and anti-p106-117 responses amongst H-2 congenic strains immunized with HBsAg/p39 particles. Previous studies in the HBsAg system suggested the presence of subtype-specific T cells, which selectively cooperated with subtype-specific B cell clones (9,10). The molecular mechanism whereby T-cells can provide differential help for B cell clones with different specificities on the same polypeptide is difficult to explain in the context of T-cell-B cell interaction models, however, this phenomenon has been previously observed in other antigen systems (11-13).

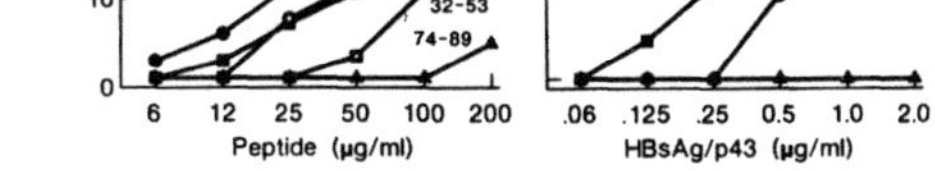

Figure 6. Localization of pre-S(1) specific T cell determinants. A group of 5 SJL/J mice was immunized with 4 µg of HBsAg/p39 and T cell proliferative responses specific for the indicated peptides were determined (a). In the reciprocal experiment, groups of 5 SJL/J mice were immunized with 100 µg of the synthetic peptides: P12-32 (■); p94-117 (○); p32-53 (□); or p74-89 (▲), and T cell proliferative resonses specific for HBsAg/p39 were determined (b).

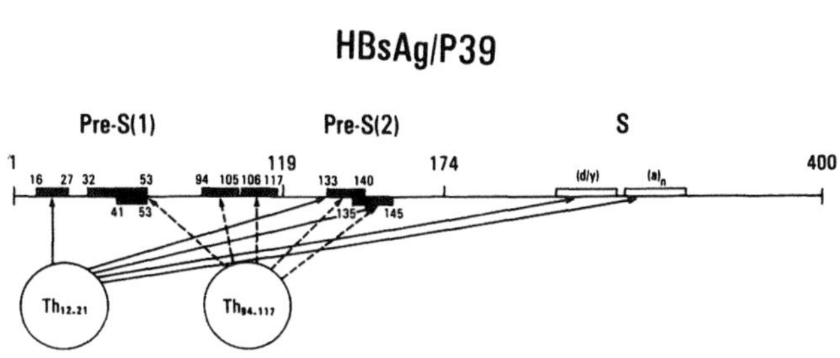

Figure 7. Summary of T and B cell recognition of HBsAg/p39. Defined antibody binding sites are represented by solid boxes, and the NH_2 and COOH-terminal coordinates are depicted. Serologically determined antibody binding sites [i.e., S region group (a) and subtype (d/y-specific)] for which there are no consensus sequences are represented by open boxes. T cell helper (Th) activity and the antibody specificities elicited are represented by the arrows. The specificities of the Th cells are depicted.

TABLE 2

Localization of antibody binding sites within the pre-S(1) region

Strains	Peptide Antigens Antibody Titer (1/dilution)								
	32-53/d	32-53/y	41-53/d	53-73/d	74-89/d	94-117/d	94-105/d	106-117/d	106-117/y
B10	2,560	2,560	1,280	0	0	10,240	10,240	10,240	80
B10.BR	320	40	0	0	0	2,560	640	0	0
B10.M	640	40	40	0	0	10,240	1,280	0	0
B10.S	0	0	0	0	0	2,560	1,280	1,280	0
B10.D2	0	0	0	0	0	1,280	10,240	5,120	80

p16-27, p32-53, p41-53, p94-105, and p106-117. Similarly, 2 distinct antibody binding sites within the pre-S(2) region were identified; p133-139, and p137-143 (operationally p133-140 and p135-145 were utilized to represent these epitopes in solid-phase antibody assays).

Identification of T-cell recognition sites within the pre-S regions of HBsAg. Analysis of T-cell recognition of a pre-S(2) region sequence, p120-145, revealed nonoverlapping T and B-cell recognition sites. Whereas antibody binds to 2 sites within the COOH-terminus the recognition by T-cells is focused on the NH_2-terminal p120-132 sequence (8). However, p120-132-primed T-cells did not recognize this sequence on the native HBsAg particle. Therefore, identification of a peptide sequence which elicits significant T-cell activation does not guarantee that the resulting T-cell population(s) will recognize the same sequence in the native protein. In contrast, pre-S(1)-specific T-cell recognition sites were defined which are relevant to both the peptide sequence and native HBsAg/p39. Mice of the SJL/J strain were primed with HBsAg/p39 and draining popliteal lymph node (PLN) cells were challenged in vitro with a panel of synthetic peptides derived from the pre-S(1) sequence and the T-cell proliferative responses determined. As shown in Figure 6a, peptides 1-21, 12-32 and 94-117 elicited significant, dose-dependent T-cell proliferative responses, whereas, peptides 32-53 and 74-89 were minimally to nonreactive. These results indicate that the overlapping sequence between p1-21 and p12-32 (i.e. 12-21), and 94-117 represent sites recognized by T cells primed to the native pre-S(1) region. The reciprocal experiment of priming with the p12-32 and p94-117 peptides and challenging in vitro with HBsAg/p39 (Fig. 6b) confirms localization of T-cell determinants within these sequences. Note that p32-53 and p74-89-primed T cells did not proliferate upon challenge with HBsAg/p39.

A single synthetic T cell determinant can prime T-cell helper function for anti-HBs production to multiple epitopes on HBsAg. The variable antibody responses to the p32-53 and p106-117 sequences after immunization of a panel of H-2 congenic strains with HBsAg/p39 suggested the influence of H-2-linked genes on antibody fine specificity. Since these strains share the same B10 genetic background and presumably the same B-cell repertoires, these results indicated that the fine specificity of T-cell recognition may influence antibody fine specificity. Identification of a number of T-cell and B-cell recognition sites within the pre-S(1) and pre-S(2) regions of HBsAg permitted us to directly address this question by examining the ability of distinct peptide-primed

Berzofsky (14) has proposed a T-cell-B cell reciprocity circuit in which B-cell immunoglobulin receptor-antigen-Ia interactions may limit T-cell specificity, which in turn limits B-cell specificity. In the context of this hypothesis, the B-cell clone specific for the p32-53 epitope may present the p39 polypeptide in the context of Ia in such a way as to be recognized by the T cell clone(s) specific for p94-117, but not by the p12-32-specific T cell clone(s), and therefore will not receive the necessary T cell helper signals from p12-32-primed T cells.

SUMMARY

The objective of the studies reported herein was to identify and characterize T cell and B cell recognition sites within the pre-S regions of HBsAg/p39, and to analyze functional T-cell-B cell interactions at the level of in vivo antibody production. The results indicate: (1) several peptides within the pre-S(1) region of HBsAg were identified which can induce and elicit HBsAg/p39-specific T-cell proliferation; (2) a 10 amino acid peptide, p12-21, and the 94-117 sequence define pre-S(1)-specific T-cell recognition sites; (3) five distinct, pre-S(1)-specific antibody binding sites and 2 pre-S(2)-specific antibody binding sites were identified; (4) synthetic pre-S(1) region T-cell determinants can prime in vivo antibody production to multiple B-cell epitopes within the pre-S(2) and S regions, as well as within the pre-S(1) region; and (5) specificity of the primed T cell population can influence the specificity of the B-cell response.

ACKNOWLEDGEMENTS

We thank Drs. Pierre Tiollais, Robert Louie and John Gerin for providing the HBsAg particles, Mr. Kenway Hoey, and Ms. Janice Hughes for technical assistance, and Ms. Jane Verenini for preparation of the manuscript. This is publication No. 4649BCR from the Scripps Clinic and Research Foundation. This work was supported by Grants AI20720 and AI00585 from the NIH and by a grant from the Johnson & Johnson Co.

REFERENCES

1. Heermann, K.H., Goldman, U., Schwartz, W., Seyffarth, T., Baumgarten, J., and Gerlich, W.H. 1984. J. Virol. 52:396.
2. Tiollais, P., Charnay, P., and Vyas, G.N. 1981. Science 213:406.
3. Stibbe, W., and Gerlich, W.H. 1983. J. Virol. 46:626.
4. Neurath, A.R., Kent, S.B.H., and Strick, N. 1984. Science 224:392.
5. Milich, D.R., Thornton, G.B., Neurath, A., Kent, S., Michel, M., Tiollais, P., and Chisari, F.V. 1985. Science 228:1195.
6. Vyas, G.N., Rao, K.R., and Ibrahim, A.B. 1972. Science 178:1300.
7. Dreesman, G.R., Hollinger, F.B., McCombs, R.M., and Melnick, J.L. 1973. J. Gen. Virol. 19:129.
8. Milich, D.R., McLachlan, A., Chisari, F.V., and Thornton, G.B. 1986. J. Exp. Med. 164:532.
9. Milich, D.R., Leroux-Roels, G.G., Louie, R.E., and Chisari, F.V. 1984. J. Exp. Med. 159:41-56.
10. Milich, D.R., Peterson, D.L., Leroux-Roels, G.G., Lerner, R.A., and Chisari, F.V. 1985. J. Immunol. 134:4203.
11. Checka, J.M., Stratton, J.A., Miller, A., and Sercarz, E. 1976. Eur. J. Immunol. 6:639.
12. Berzofsky, J.A., Richman, L.K., and Killon, D.J. 1979. Proc. Natl. Acad. Sci. USA 76:4046.
13. Compos-Neto, A., Levine, H., and Schlossman, S.F. 1982. Cell. Immunol. 69:128.
14. Bersofsky, J.A. 1983. T-B reciprocity. Surv. Immunol. Res. 2:223.
15. Milich, D.R., McLachlan, A., Chisari, F.V., Kent, S.B.H., and Thornton, G.B. 1986. J. Immunol. 137: 315.
16. Milich, D.R., McLachlan, A., Chisari, F.V., Nakamura, T., and Thornton, G.B. 1986. J. Immunol. 137:2703.

ANALYSIS OF T-CELL RECEPTOR GAMMA CHAIN EXPRESSION IN THE THYMUS

D. M. Pardoll+, A. M. Lew*, W.L. Maloy*, B.J. Fowlkes§, A. Kruisbeek¶, J.A. Bluestone†, R.H. Schwartz+ and J.E. Coligan*

+Laboratory of Immunology, *Laboratory of Immunogenetics §Laboratory of Microbial Immunity, National Institute of Allergy and Infectious Diseases and †Transplantation Biology Section, Immunology Branch and ¶Biological Response Modifiers Section, National Cancer Institute, National Institutes of Health, Bethesda, Maryland 20892

SUMMARY

While much is known about the structure and function of the T-cell receptor (TCR) αβ heterodimer, information has just begun to emerge about the γ protein, the product of a third rearranging T-cell receptor gene. We describe the use of antiserum to a carboxy-terminal peptide common to several of the murine gamma chain constant regions and a monoclonal antibody to the murine T3 complex to identify products of this T-cell receptor gene family in a subpopulation of $Lyt2^-$, $L3T4^-$ thymocytes. The gamma chain has a molecular weight of 35kD, is disulfide bonded to a 45kD partner termed delta (δ) and is associated with the T3 complex. The cells that bear this second T-cell receptor appear to represent a distinct lineage differentiating within the thymus.

INTRODUCTION

Antigen-specific, MHC-restricted recognition by mature T-cells is mediated by the clonotypic αβ heterodimeric receptor (Allison, McIntyre & Bloch, 1982; Meuer et al., 1983; Haskins et al., 1983; Kaye et al., 1983; Samelson, Germain & Schwartz, 1983; Marrack & Kappler, 1986; Dembic et al., 1986). A search for the genes encoding the α and β proteins revealed a third T cell receptor-like gene, termed γ, which rearranges in cells of the T lineage (Saito et al., 1984). A clue to the possible function of the TCRγ product came from the finding that γ mRNA is expressed at high levels in early murine fetal thymocytes and analogous $Lyt2^-$, $L3T4^-$ cells from adult thymus (Raulet et al., 1985; Snodgrass et al., 1985). Using an antipeptide serum and a monoclonal hamster antibody to the murine T3 complex, we have shown that a subset of adult $Lyt2^-$, $L3T4^-$ thymocytes express γ chain on their surface in association with the T3 complex.

RESULTS

The murine γ gene family has been extensively characterized at the DNA level (Garman, Doherty & Raulet, 1986; Hayday et al., 1985). To investigate γ expression at the protein level, we generated a rabbit antiserum against the KLH-conjugated heptapeptide (CGNEKKS) that corresponds to the carboxy terminus of C1, C2 and C3. This antiserum (anti-γ) has the potential to recognize the majority of products of the known γ genes.

Because γ mRNA levels are high in immature thymocytes, studies were initially carried out on these subpopulations. About 3-4% of adult thymocytes express low levels of Ly1 and no Lyt2 or L3T4. Immunofluorescent staining of Lyt2⁻, L3T4⁻ cells with the anti-T3 revealed that a portion (≧5%) express high levels of T3 (Fig. 1A). In mature phenotype T cells, there is a requirement for coordinate expression of T3 with an αβ heterodimer (Weiss et al., 1986). Because of the absence of TCRα mRNA and the elevated levels of TCRγ mRNA in the Lyt2⁻, L3T4⁻ subpopulation (Raulet et al., 1985), we sought to determine whether the T3 molecules expressed on these cells were associated with a TCRγ protein.

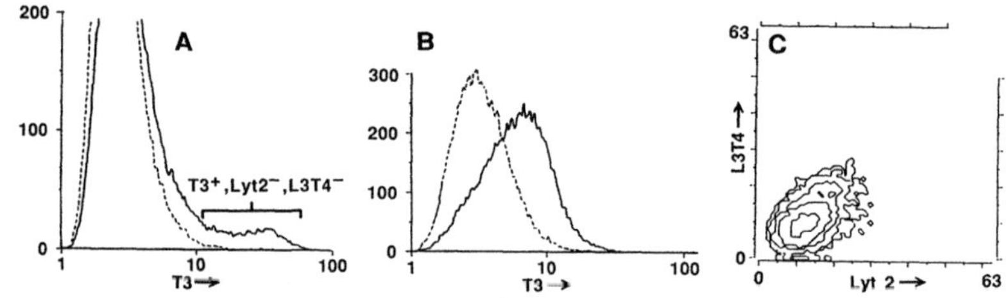

Fig. 1. Surface T3 expression of freshly isolated and cultured Lyt2⁻, L3T4⁻ thymocytes. (a) Lyt2⁻, L3T4⁻ cells isolated from fresh adult B6 mouse thymus by cytotoxic elimination with a monoclonal antibody to Lyt2, anti-L3T4 and anti-Ly1.2 were stained with the monoclonal antibody to T3, 145-2C11, followed by a FITC-labeled mouse antibody to hamster immunoglobulin (Ig) (——) or with the mouse antibody to hamster Ig (----). (b) Lyt2⁻, L3T4⁻ cells cultured 4 days in recombinant IL-1, recombinant IL-2, WEHI-3 conditioned medium and supernatant from Con A stimulated rat spleen cells were stained as above with anti-T3 followed by FITC-labeled mouse antibody to hamster Ig (——) or with FITC-labeled mouse antibody to hamster alone (----). (c) Two color analysis of Lyt2⁻, L3T4⁻ cells cultured 4 days as above.

Immunoprecipitation of surface radioiodinated, unfractionated adult mouse thymocytes with the anti-γ did not reveal any evidence of gamma protein (Fig. 2A). Immunoprecipitation with the anti-T3 showed the expected αβ components in addition to T3 components (Fig. 2A). However, both the anti-γ and anti-T3 immunoprecipitated a protein with a molecular weight of 35kD from freshly isolated Lyt2⁻, L3T4⁻ cells (Fig. 2B). By contrast, the size of the α and β chains is 38kD to 43kD. When excess γ peptide was present during the anti-γ immunoprecipitation, the 35kD band was eliminated (first lane), implying that this protein is specifically immunoprecipitated by the anti-γ (second lane). Immunoprecipitation with anti-T3 clearly revealed an additional 45kD protein (third lane) not easily seen with the anti-γ because of the effect of the immunoglobulin front which caused background bands to merge in this region. Both the anti-γ and anti-T3 immunoprecipitated a 80kD proteins under nonreducing conditions (Fig. 2C), indicating that the 35kD and 45kD proteins exist as a disulfide linked heterodimer.

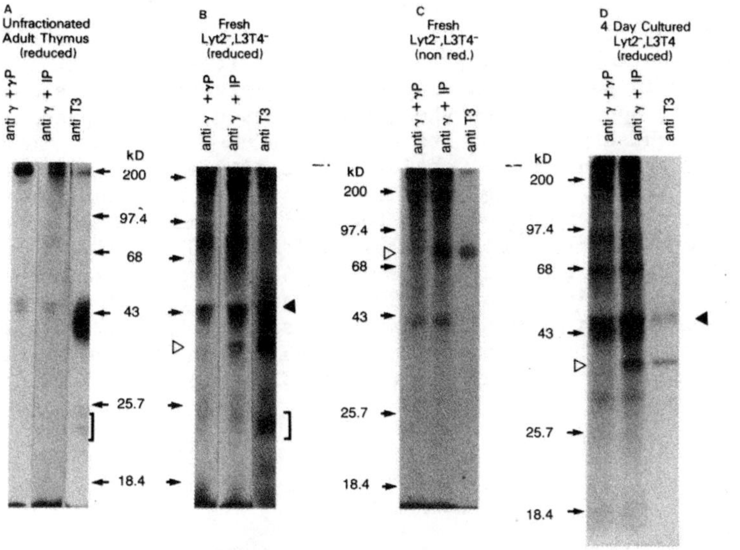

Fig. 2. Immunoprecipitation of unfractionated thymocytes and freshly isolated Lyt2$^-$, L3T4$^-$ thymocytes with anti-γ and anti-T3 antibody. (A) Unfractionated thymocytes, (B, C) fresh Lyt2$^-$, L3T4$^-$ cells and (D) 4 day cultured (majority T3$^+$) Lyt2$^-$, L3T4$^-$ cells were ^{125}I-surface labeled, lysed with NP-40 (for anti-γ) or digitonin (for anti-T3) and immunoprecipitated with the anti-γ + γ peptide (γP) (lane 1, each panel), anti-γ + irrelevant peptide (IP) (lane 2 each panel), or the anti-T3 (lane 3 each panel). All samples were run on SDS-PAGE gels under reducing conditions except for C which was run under nonreducing conditions.

Further biochemical characterization of the γ receptor complex was facilitated by a procedure that enabled us to selectively grow out T3$^+$, Lyt2$^-$, L3T4$^-$ thymocytes. When these cells were cultured in a combination of IL-1, IL-2, rat Con A supernatant and WEHI-3 conditioned medium (as a source of IL-3), T3$^+$ cells proliferated. After 4 days of culture, the majority of live cells were T3$^+$ while retaining the Lyt2$^-$, L3T4$^-$ phenotype (Fig. 1B,C). The pattern seen on one dimensional reducing SDS-PAGE gels of anti-γ and anti-T3 immunoprecipitates of the 4 day cultured cells is virtually identical to freshly isolated Lyt2$^-$, L3T4$^-$ cells (Fig. 2D), suggesting that, at the biochemical level, they are representative of the *in vivo* T3$^+$, Lyt2$^-$, L3T4$^-$ population. Figure 3 shows the results of diagonal gels (1st dimension under nonreducing conditions, 2nd dimension under reducing conditions) from anti-γ and anti-T3 immunoprecipitations of these 4 day cultured cells. A 35kD and a 45kD protein are clearly seen below the diagonal in both cases. These two spots were completely absent when excess γ peptide was added to the anti-γ immunoprecipitation. This experiment proves that the receptor on these cells is a disulfide-linked heterodimer.

In order to determine which of the T3-associated proteins reacts with the anti-γ, digitonin lysates were first immunoprecipitated anti anti-T3. After elution with SDS, the disulfide bond between the two chains of the heterodimer was broken by reduction with dithiothreitol, followed by alkylation with iodoacetamide. The noncovalently linked chains of the T3-associated heterodimer were then immunoprecipitated with the anti-γ and run on an SDS-PAGE gel. Under these conditions, only the 35kD protein is seen (Fig. 4A), indicating that this molecule is the γ chain. This experiment also confirms that the γ protein is T3-associated.

To gain information on Vγ expression in these cells, we utilized the enzyme N-glycosidase F, which removes N-linked carbohydrate groups. This analysis is informative for the murine γ proteins because the Vγ1.2-Cγ2 chain has no N-linked carbohydrate acceptor sites (Saito et al., 1984). Both the γ chain and its 45kD partner are N-glycosidase F sensitive (Fig. 4B). It appeared that the γ chain reduced to the predicted core molecular weight of 32kD and its partner reduced to 35kD. To confirm that all of the γ protein is N-glycosidase F sensitive, anti-γ immunoprecipitates were treated with N-glycosidase F followed by reduction and alkylation and then reprecipitated with the anti-γ. Under these conditions, all the 35kD material reduced to 32kD and no 35kD material is present in the N-glycosidase F treated sample (Fig. 4C). Taken together, these results indicate that all of the 35kD γ chain is N-glycosylated. The important conclusion from this analysis is that, in this thymic subpopulation, there is not detectable expression of the Vγ1.2-Cγ2 gene, which should have a native molecular weight of 32kD and be N-glycosidase resistant.

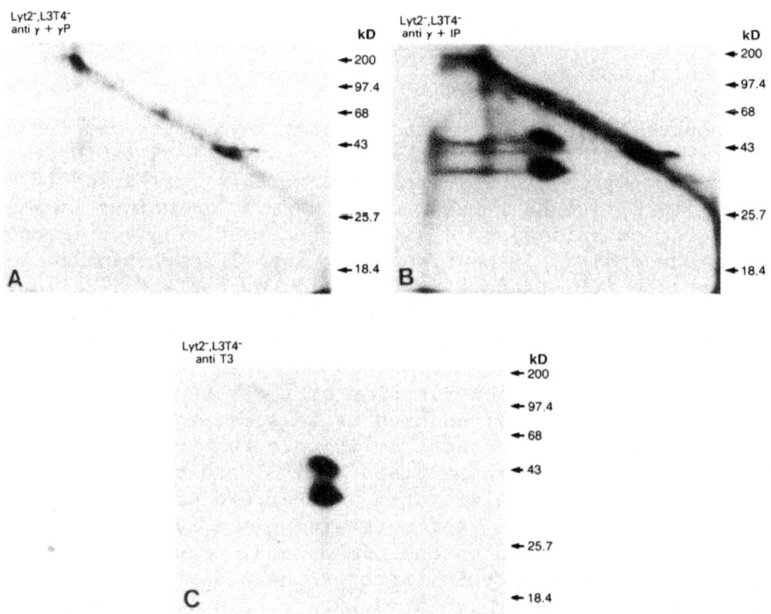

Fig. 3. Diagonal gels of anti-γ and anti-T3 immunoprecipitates of 4 day cultured Lyt2$^-$, L3T4$^-$ cells. Four day cultured cells were surface radioiodinated and lysates prepared as in Fig. 3. Immunoprecipitates with (A) anti-γ + γ peptide (γP), (B) anti-γ + irrelevant peptide (IP) and (C) anti-T3, were run without reduction in the first dimension and then under reducing conditions in the second dimension.

It is difficult to reconcile these findings with models that directly link γ expression on thymic precursors to MHC restriction of αβ bearing T cells, either due to developmental selection of γβ heterodimers (Raulet et al., 1985; Snodgrass et al., 1985) or reexpression of selected γδ receptors on mature T cells (Langman, 1978). Either of these models would predict that the same γ chain would be expressed in developing thymocytes as in mature αβ bearing T cells (i.e. Cγ2-Cγ1.2). The predominant expression of the glycosylated γ species (derived for Cγ1) in C57BL/6 thymus instead suggests that the γδ receptor may define a separate T-cell lineage whose intrathymic development precedes that of classic αβ T-cells (Fig. 5). The presence of γ gene rearrangements in mature cells with the αβ receptor (Saito et al., 1984) as well as partial β gene rearrangements in cells that bear the γδ receptor (data not shown) indicates that both lineages may derive from a common precursor. Recent evidence suggests that immature thymocytes begin to rearrange their TCR genes synchronously (Born et al., 1986). However, the γ (and possibly δ) locus complete a V-J-C rearrangement in most thymocytes at a time when most β locus rearrangements are incomplete (D-J-C). Therefore, the γδ heterodimer would be the first T cell receptor to appear in the developing thymus. Since

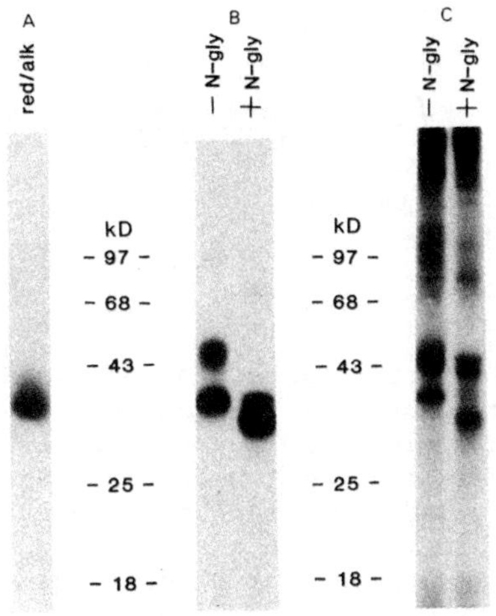

Fig. 4. Reduction-alkylation and N-glycosidase F treatment of 4 day cultured Lyt2⁻, L3T4⁻ thymocytes. (A) A digitonin lysate of surface radioiodinated 4 d cultured Lyt2⁻, L3T4⁻ cells was immunoprecipitated with anti-T3 followed by elution with SDS, reduction with dithiothreitol, alkylation with iodoacetamide, and immunoprecipitation with anti-γ. The immunoprecipitate was run on a 10% reducing SDS-PAGE gel. (B) Cells were immunoprecipitated with anti-T3 and eluted as above. Half the sample was treated with N-glycosidase F (lane 2) and half was not (lane 1). After treatment, samples were run on a 10% reducing SDS-PAGE gel. (C) Cells were immunoprecipitated with anti-γ followed by treatment with N-glycosidase as in B, and then reduced and alkylated as in A. They were then reimmunoprecipitated with anti-γ and run on a 10% reducing SDS-PAGE gel. All the bands in the 40-45kD region represented background which was not γ-peptide inhibitable (data not shown).

thymocytes with the γδ heterodimer predominantly express 1.0 kb β mRNA (data not shown), which is the product of an incomplete D-J rearrangement, it is likely that once the product of a productively rearranged γ and δ gene is synthesized, further rearrangement of β (and α) genes does not occur. If the rearrangement of γ or δ is nonproductive, no full length protein is produced and the cell continues to rearrange its β and α genes in an attempt to produce an αβ heterodimer.

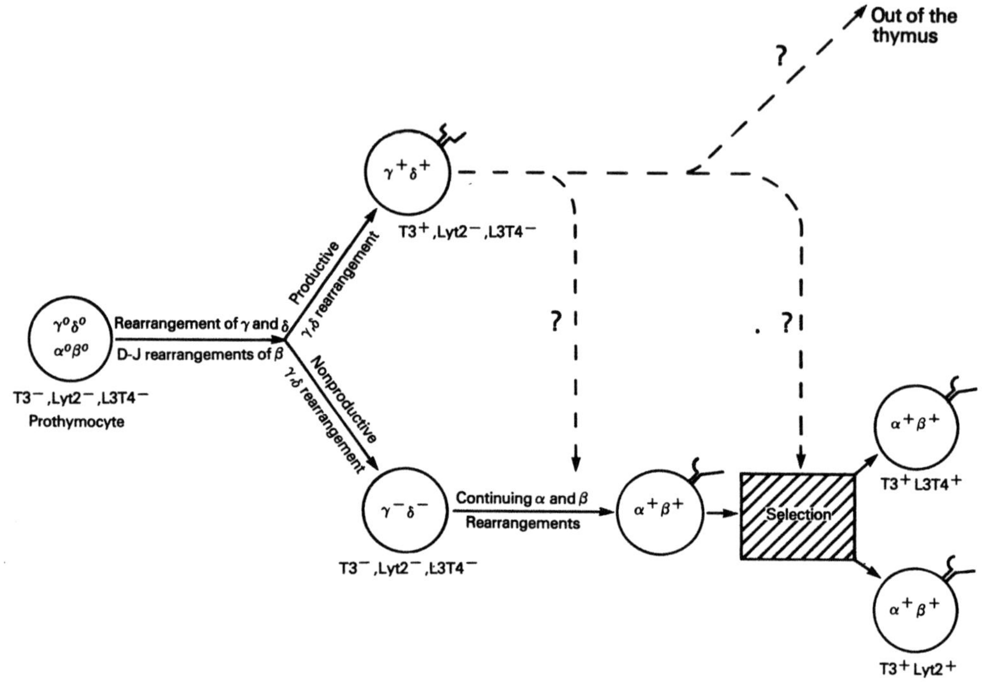

Fig. 5. Model for developmental expression of two distinct T-cell receptors. Synchronous rearrangement of TCR genes is envisioned to occur in prothymocytes upon entry into the thymus. Completed rearrangements occur in the γ and δ genes at a point when rearrangements of β (and α) are partial. If productive γ and δ rearrangements occur, a T3-γδ receptor is produced halting further rearrangements of β and α, committing the cell to this lineage. If a nonproductive γ or δ rearrangement occurs, the cell continues to rearrange its α and β genes and can become a T3-αβ bearing cell subject to intrathymic selection mechanisms.

REFERENCES

Allison, J., McIntyre, B., and Bloch, D., 1982, J. Immunol. 129:2293.

Born, W., Rathbun, G., Tucker, P., Marrack, P., and Kappler, J., 1986, Science 234:479.

Dembic, Z., Haas, W., Seigried, W., von Boehmer, H., and Steinmetz, M., 1986, Nature 320:232.

Garman, R.D., Doherty, P.J. and Raulet, D.H., 1986, Cell 45:733.

Haskins, K., Kubo, R., White, J., Piegeon, M., Kappler, J., and Marrack, P., 1983, J. Exp. Med. 157:1149.

Hayday, A.C., Saito, H., Gillies, S.D., Kranz, D.M., Tanigawa, G., Eisen, H.N. and Tonegawa, S., 1985, Cell 40:259.

Kaye, J., Procelli, S., Tite, J., Jones, B., and Janeway, C.A., 1983, J. Exp. Med. 158:836.

Langman, R.E., 1978, Rev. Physiol. Biochem. Pharmacol. 81: 1.

Marrack, P. and Kappler, J., 1986, Adv. Immunol. 38:1.

Meuer, S., Fitzgerald, K., Hussey, R., Hodgdon, J., Schlossman, S., and Reinherz, E., 1983, J. Exp. Med. 157:705-719 (1983).

Raulet, D.H., Garman, R.D., Saito, H., and Tonegawa, S., 1985, Nature 314:103.

Saito, H., Kranz, D.M., Takagaki, Y., Hayday, A.C., Eisen, H.N., and Tonegawa, S., 1984, Nature 309:757.

Samelson, L., Germain, R., and Schwartz, R. 1983, PNAS USA 80:6972.

Snodgrass, H.R., Dembic, A., Steinmetz, M., and von Boehmer, H., 1985, Nature 315:232.

Weiss, A. and Stobo, J.D., 1984, J. Exp. Med. 160:1284.

PRODUCTION OF SUPPRESSOR FACTOR BY T-CELLS FROM MICE IMMUNIZED WITH PNEUMOCOCCAL POLYSACCHARIDE

Christopher E. Taylor and Rani Bright

The Medical College of Pennsylvania

Department of Microbiology and Immunology
3300 Henry Avenue, Philadelphia, PA 19129

ABSTRACT

Factor(s) derived from plate purified T-cell cultures obtained from mice 16 hr after immunization with Type III pneumococcal polysaccharide (SSS-III), suppressed the antibody response to SSS-III. Such suppression was antigen specific. Adsorption of the suppressor factor (SF) with SSS-III covalently bound to Sepharose 4B column did not alter the ability of SF to suppress the antibody response. However, adsorption of SF with Ig^{+}(B) cells taken from mice 48 hr after immunization with an immunogenic dose (0.5 ug) of SSS-III, completely removed the suppressive activity. Suppression of the antibody response was observed only when SF was administered 24 hr before to 24 hr after immunization with SSS-III. These results suggest that antigen specific suppressor T cells release soluble factor(s) which acts directly on antigen-stimulated B cells or may inhibit the induction of amplifier T-cells.

INTRODUCTION

A number of studies have shown that suppressor T-cells regulate the antibody response to Type III pneumococcal polysaccharide in an antigen specific manner (1-4). It has also been demonstrated that these suppressor T-cells function early during the course of a normal antibody response, suggesting that suppressor cells act mainly to restrict the expansion of B-cells from the precursor cell pool (3). However, the exact mechanisms by which the antibody response is downregulated remains to be elucidated. Studies by other investigators demonstrate that suppressor T-cells function by inhibiting the activity of helper cells via the release of cell free products (5-6). Some of these cell free products bind antigen while others bind idiotypic determinants (ID). In the antibody response to SSS-III only a single suppressor T-cell has been described. This suppressor cell can be activated by ID on antigen stimulated B-cells (7). This may suggest that any putative suppressor factors produced may be directed at antigen stimulated B-cells. This study was conducted to characterize soluble factors released from antigen specific suppressor T cells.

METHODS

Mice. Female BALB/cByJ mice (8 to 10 wk of age), obtained from The Jackson Laboratory, Bar Harbor, ME, were used throughout this work.

Immunologic methods. Numbers of antibody-producing plaque-forming cells (PFC) specific for SSS-III or dextran B1355 were detected by a slide version of the technique of localized hemolysis-in-gel by using indicator SRBC coated with polysaccharide by the $CrCl_3$ method, as described (1-4).

Student's t-test was used to assess the significance of the differences observed. Differences were considered to be significant when probability (p) values of <0.05 were obtained.

Isolation of spleen cells by plate-separation procedure. The method used for the recovery of nonimmunoglobulin-bearing (Ig^-) cells from spleen cell suspensions has been described in detail (7). Briefly, affinity-purified goat anti-mouse Ig antibody (GAMIg) was diluted in 0.05 M Tris, pH 9.5, and 10 ml of the resulting solution were poured onto plastic petri plates. Spleen cell suspensions (treated to remove erythrocytes) were added to plates coated with GAMIg antibody. After appropriate incubation the unattached cells were decanted.

The purity of the cell suspensions recovered by the plate-separation procedure was assessed by fluorescence-activated cell sorter analysis (FACS-II System: Becton Dickinson, Mountain View, CA) (7). In the experiments to be described the nonadherent cell suspension used was found to contain <2% Ig^+ and 96% Thy-1.2$^+$ cells; the adherent cell suspensions contained >97% Ig^+ cells.

Preparation of soluble factor. Spleens were harvested from mice 16 hr after immunization with 0.5 ug of SSS-III. Spleen cell suspensions were prepared, and spleen cells were cultured at a density of 5 x 10^7 cells/ml for 24 hr in a mixture of 50% Iscove's medium (GIBCO) and 50% Ham's nutrient F-12 medium (GIBCO) supplemented with 10,000 U of penicillin and streptomycin, 50mM L-glutamine, 20nM sodium bicarbonate (7.5%), 0.1 M insulin, and 0.1 M transferrin. Cell free supernantant fluid was obtained from spleen cell cultures by centrifugation (1500 rpm for 20 min), filtered by passage through 0.45-um Millipore filters (Millipore Corp., Bedford, MA), and stored at -70°C until used. Unless stated otherwise, the suppressor factor (SF) was given 3 hr before immunization with 0.5 ug SSS-III.

RESULTS

Effect of SF on the Magnitude of the antibody response to SSS-III. In this experiment SF was obtained by culturing plate purified Ig^- (T) cells taken from immunized mice for 24 hr. The SF obtained was given to recipient animals 3 hr before immunization with 0.5 ug SSS-III. The results show that the injection of SF resulted in significant suppression (71%) of the PFC response to SSS-III ($p < 0.05$). The suppression produced was similar to that noted when SF was obtained from whole spleen cell cultures (63%; $p < 0.05$). No suppression was observed when mice were injected with SF derived from cultures of B cells (Ig^+ cells) or plastic adherent cells (not shown).

Table 1. Effect of SF on the antibody response to SSS-III

Pretreatment[a]	SSS-III Specific PFC/Spleen[b]	Mean % Suppression
None	4.12 ± 0.07 (13,060)	
SF-Ig^-	3.58 ± 0.25 (3,814)	71
SF-whole	3.69 ± 0.14 (4,920)	63

[a] Donor mice were injected with 0.5 ug SSS-III; 16 hr later spleen cell suspensions were prepared and cultured for 24 hr. A portion (0.4 ml) of SF, obtained from cell culture of whole spleen cells (SF-whole) or Ig^- cells derived from immunized donors (SF-Ig^-) was given i.v. to naive recipients 3 hr before immunization.

[b] Log_{10} PFC per spleen ± SEM for groups of 10 mice 5 days after immunization with SSS-III; geometric means are in parentheses.

The ability of SF to cause suppression after adsorption with SSS-III-Sepharose-4B. We tested the hypothesis that the suppressive factor (SF) may be SSS-III specific antibody which can alter the antibody response of recipient mice via antibody-mediated feedback mechanism. The adsorbed and unadsorbed portions of the same pool of SF were injected (i.v.) into recipient mice, 3 hr before immunization with 0.5 ug SSS-III. The results are shown below in Table 2. SF adsorbed with SSS-III immobilized on a column (Sepharose 4B) caused a 62% suppression of the antibody response to SSS-III ($p < 0.05$); the degree of suppression paralleled that noted for animals receiving unadsorbed SF (66%; p 0.05). These findings show that SF does not bind to the antigen and suggest that SF is not SSS-III specific antibody. Studies reported elsewhere (8) show that SF can be prepared from donor mice given a subimmunogenic dose (0.005 ug) of SSS-III. Because the dose of 0.005 ug SSS-III does not result in any detectable serum antibody or PFC within 6 days after antigen is given, the latter findings support the statement that the suppression observed (due to SF) is not mediated by SSS-III specific antibody.

Table 2. Ability of SF to cause suppression after adsorption with SSS-III Sepharose 4B

Treatment[a]	SSS-III-Specific PFC/Spleen[b]	Mean % Suppression
None	4.22 ± 0.07 (16.677)	-
SF before adsp.	3.76 ± 0.11 (5.751)	66
SF after adsp.	3.81 ± 0.12 (6.393)	62

[a] SF was adsorbed with a Sepharose 4B column (coated with SSS-III) before the injection (i.v.) of 0.4 ml SF into recipient mice.

[b] Log_{10} PFC per spleen ± SEM for groups of 10 mice 5 days after immunization with 0.5 ug SSS-III; geometric means are in parentheses.

Antigen specificity of the suppression induced by SF. We also examined whether the suppresion, of antibody response to SSS-III is antigen specific (7). Besides SSS-III, two other antigens were used: SRBC, and dextran (8). In this experiment mice were injected with SF or culture medium and three hours later immunized with 0.5 ug SSS-III, 5 x 10^8 SRBC or 100 ug dextran B-1355. The antibody responses in all cases were assessed 5 days following immunization. Table 3 depicts the results. The administration of SF produced significant ($p < 0.05$) suppression of the antibody response (71% and 65%). No significant ($p > 0.05$) alteration of antibody response to SRBC or dextran was noted after SF was given. These findings suggest that the suppression mediated by SF is antigen specific.

Table 3. Antigen specificity of soluble factor

Treatment[a]	SSS-III PFC/Spleen[b]	SRBC PFC/Spleen[b]	Dextran PFC/Spleen[b]
Medium	4.26 ± 0.05 (18.370)	5.33 ± 0.048 (215,200)	4.89 ± 0.07 (76,980)
SF	3.73 ± 0.045 (5,321)	5.32 ± 0.04 (206,900)	5.04 ± 0.11 (110,200)
(% Supp)	(71)	(3)	(0)

[a] Culture medium or SF was given (i.v.) 3 hr before immunization with 0.5 ug SSS III or 5 x 10^8 SRBC or 100 ug dextran B-1355.

[b] Log_{10} PFC per spleen ± SEM for groups of eight mice 5 days after SSS-III, SRBC or dextran B-1355; geometric means are in parentheses.

Adsorption of SF with immune B cells. The results of previous studies showed that antigen specific suppressor T-cells can be activated by the infusion of immune B cells (7). The development of suppressor T-cells can be inhibited by pretreating the immune B cells with anti-IgM, anti-IgD or anti-ID antibody (unpublished observations). Therefore, we tested the possibility that SF released from suppressor T-cells are directed against ID on B-cells. Here, SF was adsorbed with Ig^+ cells obtained 48 hr after immunization with 0.5 ug SSS-III or 100 ug dextran B1355. SF was also adsorbed with Ig^+ cells from naive animals. Adsorption was done for 30 min at 4°C. Recipient animals were injected with adsorbed and unadsorbed portions of SF 3 hr before immunization. The results (Table IV) show that SF adsorbed with naive B cells or B-cells obtained from donors immunized with dextran caused a significant suppression ($p < 0.05$) of antibody response to SSS-III (56% and 64% respectively). No suppression was observed when SF was adsorbed with B-cells from mice immunized with SSS-III. The data suggest that SF is directed at a restricted clone of antigen stimulated B cells.

Table IV. Effect of adsorption with immune B-cells on the capacity of SF to suppress the antibody response to SSS-III

Treatment[a]	SSS-III-Specific PFC/Spleen[b]	Mean Suppression
a) None	4.17 ± 0.03 (14,770)	
b) SF (unadsorbed)	3.73 ± 0.09 (5,338)	64
c) SF (SSS-III B cell-ads.)	4.29 ± 0.03 (19,440)	0
d) SF (dextran B cell-ads.)	3.73 ± 0.12 (5,360)	64
e) SF (naive B cell-ads.)	3.82 ± 0.10 (6,528)	56

[a] SF was adsorbed with B-cells from mice immunized with 0.5 ug SSS-III (c), or 100 ug dextran B1355 (d), or naive B-cells (e). Adsorption was done at 4°C for 30 min. Later, adsorbed or unadsorbed portions of SF were injected into recipients 3 hr before immunization with 0.5 ug SSS-III.

[b] Log_{10} PFC per spleen ± SEM for groups of eight mice 5 days after immunization with SSS-III; geometric means are in parentheses.

Effect of time lapse between the injections of SF and immunization with SSS-III. The foregoing experiment suggest that SF acts directly on antigen stimulated B-cells. However, it is conceivable that SF may act on amplifier T-cells (9) or on other suppressor cells. Here, SF was given to groups of mice at various intervals before or after immunization with SSS-III. The results, published elsewhere (8), show that when SF was given 24 hr prior to immunization or 24 hr after immunization with SSS-III there was no significant suppression (p 0.05) of antibody response. Substantial suppression was seen only when SF was given 24 hr or less prior to immunization, at the time of immunization, or 24 hr post immunization. These findings indicate that SF acts early in the course of the antibody response either directly on B-cells or by inducing another suppressor T-cell that alters amplifier T-cell activity.

DISCUSSION

Communication between cells of the immune system occurs invariably by means of biologically active factors. The results of the present study demonstrate that cell free products released from cultures of T cells from immunized animals can suppress the antibody response to SSS-III. Indeed, soluble factors have been described, for a number of systems, that are active in vivo or in vitro. Some of these factors have been extensively characterized with respect to dependence on accessory cells for induction, ability to bind antigen, idiotype or MHC gene products, and the involvement of single or multiple factors (10,11).

In this report, the degree of suppression obtained using the suppressive factor (SF) was similar to that noted in previous studies in which suppression was transferred with intact T-cells (3). The results show that substantial suppression of antibody response to SSS-III was seen when SF was given around the time of immunization of the recipient animals (8). This observation is consistent with earlier reports that antigen-specific suppressor T-cells, generated in response to SSS-III, act early during the course of the antibody response. The results suggest that SF presumably binds to and limits clonal expansion of antigen reactive B-cells. However, we also considered the hypothesis that SF induces another suppressor T cell which acts by inhibiting amplifier T-cell activity (9). The latter line of reasoning stems from the observation that amplifier T cell activity peaks at 48 hr after immunization with SSS-III (9). Nonetheless, the fact that SF can be adsorbed with immune B-cells, makes the antigen stimulated B-cells a more likely target. Studies have shown that immune B-cells treated to remove any residual antigen are capable of activating suppressor T-cells (12). The results presented in this study (Table 2) show that SF does not bind to antigen. These findings strongly suggest that SF binds to ID on antigen stimulated B-cells. This hypothesis is supported by the observation in these studies, that the suppression observed when SF is administered is antigen specific.

References

1. Baker, P.J., P.W. Stashak, D.F. Amsbaugh, and B. Prescott. 1971. Characterization of the antibody response to Type III pneumococcal polysaccharide at the cellular level. I. Dose-respone studies of the effect of prior immunization on the magnitude of the antibody response. Immunology 20:469.
2. Baker, P.J., P.W. Stashak, D.F. Amsbaugh, and B. Prescott. 1974. Regulation of the antibody response to Type III pneumococcal polysaccharide. IV. Role of suppressor T cells in the development of low-dose paralysis. J. Immunol. 112:2020.
3. Baker, P.J., D.F. Amsbaugh, P.W. Stashak. G. Caldes, and B. Prescott. 1982. Direct evidence for the involvement of T suppressor cells in the expression of low-dose paralysis to Type III pneumococcal polysaccharide. J. Immunol. 128:1059.
4. Baker, P.J., D.F. Amsbaugh, P.W. Stashak, G. Caldes, and B. Prescott. 1981. Regulation of antibody response to pneumococcal polysaccharide by thymus derived cells. Rev. Infect. Dis. 3:332.
5. Kapp, J.A., C.M. Sorensen, and C.W. Pierce. 1983. Antigen-specific suppressor T cell interactions. II. Characterization of two different types of suppressor T cell factors specific for L-glutamic acid^{50}-L-tyrosine^{50} (GT) and L-glutamic acid^{60}-L-alanine^{30}-L-tyrosine^{10} (GAT). J. Exp. Med. 158:1962.
6. Fresno, M., L. McVay-Boudreau, G. Nabel, and H. Cantor. 1981. Antigen-specific suppressive protein synthesized by cloned T cells. J. Exp. Med. 153:1260.
7. Taylor, C.E., P.W. Stashak, G. Caldes, B. Prescott, T.E. Chused. A. Books, and P.J. Baker. 1983. Activation of antigen specific suppressor T cells by B cells from mice immunized with Type III pneumococcal polysaccharide. J. Exp. Med. 158:703.
8. Taylor, C.E., and P.J. Baker. 1985. Production of soluble suppressor factor by spleen cells from mice immunized with Type III pneumococcal polysaccharide. J. Immunol. 135:2551.
9. Taylor, C.E., P.W. Stashak, J. Chiang, W.M. Leiserson, G. Caldes, B. Prescott, and P.J. Baker. 1984. Characteristics of amplifier T cells involved in the antibody response to the capsular polysaccharide of Type III Streptococcus pneumoniae. J. Immunol. 132:3103.
10. Dorf, M.E. and B. Benacerraf. 1984. Suppressor-cell interactions. Annu. Rev. Immunol. 2:126.
11. Tada T., and K. Okumura. 1980. The role of antigen specific T cell factors in the immune response. Adv. Immunol. 28:1.
12. Baker, P.J., C. Taylor, M.B. Fauntleroy, P.W. Stashak, and B. Prescott. 1985. The role of antigen in the activation of regulatory T cells by immune B cells. Cell. Immunol. 96:376.

"AUTO-REACTIVE" T-CELL HYBRIDOMAS AND THE ROLE OF FOETAL CALF SERUM

Ann M. Pullen and Alan J. Munro

Department of Pathology
Cambridge University
Cambridge, UK.

SUMMARY

A panel of "auto-reactive" T-cell hybridomas has been generated by fusing Sendai virus-primed, Peyer's patch T cells from CBA mice with BW 5147. The hybridomas produce Il-2 in response to stimulation by Class II-positive syngeneic cells in the absence of added Sendai virus. The stimulator genes for two hybridoma clones have been mapped using recombinant mouse strains and the restriction has been confirmed by inhibition with monoclonal anti-Class II antibodies.

Hybridomas grown in serum-free medium do not respond to syngeneic cells in the absence of foetal calf serum (FCS) and the response is restored by the addition of FCS, but not bovine serum albumin (BSA), normal mouse serum or Sendai virus. The component of FCS which is required for stimulation of the hybridomas has been partially purified and characterised. Its mode of action has been investigated and it acts on the stimulator cells and not on the hybridomas.

INTRODUCTION

In recent years several groups have reported the generation of putative auto-reactive T-cell clones and hybridomas during attempts to produce T-cell populations specific for a wide variety of exogenous antigens (Endres, Marrack and Kappler, 1983; Rock and Benacerraf, 1983; Faherty, Johnson and Zauderer, 1985; Muller and Kaufmann, 1985; Julius and Heusser, 1986; Saito et al., 1986). It has been postulated that the ease with which these auto-reactive T cells are isolated suggests that they occur at high frequencies in vivo and are important in immunoregulation (Kawanishi, Ozato and Strober, 1985; Saito et al., 1986). However there is still debate over whether these auto-reactive T cells are truly self-reactive and recognise self-MHC antigens alone, or whether they are merely in vitro artefacts, responding to non-polymorphic antigens present in the cultures in a self-restricted fashion. This matter has recently been discussed by Bretscher (1986) who questioned the significance of auto-reactive T cells. The role of xenogeneic or allogeneic sera in culture medium is particularly controversial (reviewed by Denizot and Golstein, 1982) and the experiments reported here address this issue.

MATERIALS AND METHODS

Mice

Inbred mice were obtained from our own animal house in the Department of Pathology, Cambridge University. The strains used in this work include: CBA, AKR, C3H/He (all $H-2^k$), C57Bl ($H-2^b$), BALB/c ($H-2^d$), DBA-1 ($H-2^q$) and SJL ($H-2^s$). H-2 recombinant mice obtained from Olac Ltd included B10.A(4R), B10.A(5R), A.TL and B10.AQR.

Media and reagents

Serum-free medium: RPMI-1640 basal medium supplemented with human albumin (fraction V) and transferrin to a total protein concentration of 730ug/ml (NEN Research Products). Complete medium: Standard RPMI-1640 (Gibco) supplemented with 10% heat-inactivated foetal calf serum (Gibco). Both media were supplemented with 100 i.u./ml benzyl penicillin, 100 i.u./ml streptomycin, 0.1mg/ml gentamycin, 1mM sodium pyruvate, 2mM L-glutamine (all Gibco) and $2x10^{-5}$ M 2-mercaptoethanol (Sigma). Sendai virus vaccine was supplied by MA Bioproducts, Dyna Sciences Corp. and pure Sendai virus preparation by Abtek Biologicals. Monoclonal anti-$I-A^k$ (Ia.2) and anti-$I-E^k$ (Ia.7) antibodies were obtained from Sera-lab. Recombinant IL-2 was kindly supplied by Cetus Corp.

Generation of Peyer's patch T cell hybridomas

8-12 week old CBA mice were immunised intra-Peyer's patch with Sendai vaccine. The gut was exposed and about 10ul vaccine injected into each patch. 7 days later the mice were killed and the Peyer's patches (PP) removed and a single cell suspension prepared by protease digestion according to the method of Frangakis et al. (1982). Viable cells were separated on Ficoll-paque and were enriched for T-cells by passing down nylon wool columns. PP T-cells were cultured at 10^6/ml along with $2x10^5$/ml irradiated (3000 rads), syngeneic plastic-adherent PP cells to act as antigen presenting cells. The cultures were in complete medium with pure Sendai virus included at a 1/25,000 dilution. After culture for 6 days at 37°C in a humidified atmosphere of 5% CO_2/95% air, the viable cells were fused with BW 5147 at a ratio of 5:1, using polyethylene glycol 1500. Hybridomas were selected by culture in HAT medium.

Culture conditions

Irradiated peritoneal wash-out cells or spleen cells (3000 rads) were used as stimulator cells. 200ul cultures in flat-bottomed, 96 well plates generally contained 10^6 spleen cells which were cultured for 24h prior to the addition of $2x10^4$ hybridoma cells. After 2 further days in culture supernatants were collected and stored at -20°C prior to assay for IL-2 activity.

Supernatants were tested for their ability to support the growth of the IL-2 dependent cell line, CTL-D. Test cultures contained 100ul supernatant and 100ul CTL-D at 10^5/ml in complete medium. Cultures were incubated for 24h, and 6h before the termination of culture, cells were pulsed with 1uCi titrated thymidine (Amersham International). The cells were harvested on to glass filter papers and were dried before the assessment of tritiated thymidine incorporation was made by liquid scintillation counting. Results are expressed as cpm tritiated thymidine incorporation and are the means for triplicate cultures. Duncan's range test was used for the statistical analysis of the data, and values underlined are significantly greater than the BW alone controls.

Table 1. Stimulation of hybridomas by syngeneic cells and Sendai virus

		Hybridoma				
Stimulators	Medium	BW	33	53	57	89
None	355	249	272	270	280	226
Spleen cells	242	211	14264	7610	239	11215
Virus alone	225	311	308	302	235	270
Spleen cells + virus	261	337	11077	9974	473	13386

RESULTS

When the hybridomas were tested for any antigen specificity by assessing their ability to respond to pure Sendai virus in the presence of syngeneic antigen presenting cells, several hybridomas were found to respond to syngeneic cells in the absence of added virus (Table 1). This apparent "auto-reactivity" was not due to viral contamination of the animal stocks since spleen cells from isolator-reared mice gave similar results. The ability of the T cell hybridomas to respond was unstable and it was therefore essential to clone the hybridoma lines to stabilise their activity. Hybridoma clones 89.2 and 33.11 were used in the subsequent experiments and BW was always included to provide a negative control.

The hybridoma clones were stimulated by cells from mice of the k haplotype and not from mice of the b,d,q or s haplotypes. Recombinant mice were used to map the $H\text{-}2^k$ stimulator gene (Table 2). It was shown using A.TL and B10.AQR that the gene whose product stimulated the hybridomas was in the I region of the MHC. To further characterise the stimulator gene the recombinant congenic mouse strains B10.A(4R) and B10.A(5R) were used. The stimulator gene for hybridoma 89.2 was mapped to $I\text{-}A^k$, since B10.A(4R) was a stimulator whilst B10.A(5R) was not. Since hybridoma 33.11 responds to A.TL and B10.AQR but not B10.A(4R) or B10.A(5R) the crucial gene for stimulating hybridoma 33.11 must be E^k_β. The determinant responsible for stimulating hybridoma 33.11 may be on E^k_β or may be formed by the association of E^k_β with E^k_α or A^k_α. The restriction patterns have been confirmed by inhibition by monoclonal anti-Class II antibodies. Anti-$I\text{-}A^k$ but not anti-E^k, inhibits the stimulation of hybridoma 89.2. Both reagents inhibit the stimulation of hybridoma 33.11, this is of interest since it suggests that the determinant responsible for stimulating this hybridoma may indeed be formed by the trans-isotypic association of E^k_β with A^k_α.

The hybridomas were adapted to grow in serum-free medium and were subsequently tested for their ability to respond to stimulation by syngeneic cells in the absence of serum (Table 3). Under these conditions the hybridomas did not respond and the addition of FCS, but not BSA, normal mouse serum or Sendai virus, restored the response. It was decided to investigate which component of FCS is responsible for stimulating the hybridomas.

Table 2. Mapping of the MHC determinant recognised by hybridomas

	MHC				Hybridoma	
Stimulators	K	I-A	I-E	D	89.2	33.11
A.TL	s	k	k	d	+	+
B10.AQR	q	k	k	d	+	+
B10.A(4R)	k	k	b*	b	+	-
B10.A(5R)	b	b	k	d	-	-

* E^k_β is only found cytoplasmically since E^b_α is non-functional.

Table 3. Lack of stimulation of hybridomas under serum-free conditions

		Hybridoma			
Stimulators	Medium	Medium	BW	89.2	33.11
Peritoneal cells	serum-free	38	60	112	166
	complete	88	120	22359	6393
Spleen cells	serum-free	94	59	189	265
	complete	138	324	41259	9193

Several batches of FCS were tested for their ability to support the stimulation of the hybridomas and the batch which showed maximum activity was used in subsequent experiments. Upon heat-inactivation of this batch of FCS its ability to stimulate the hybridomas increased. Indeed the FCS retained its stimulating activity after heating at 100°C for 15 min.

Since the major protein component of FCS, BSA (fraction V), did not stimulate the hybridomas to produce IL-2, attempts were made to fractionate the stimulating activity. Fractionation of FCS was carried out by HPLC on a TSK G4000SW gel filtration column, the fractions were subsequently tested for their ability to support the stimulation of the hybridomas and the stimulating activity accompanied the major protein peaks.

Separation of the FCS by HPLC on a TSK DEAE-5PW ion exchange column with elution by a sodium chloride gradient buffered with 8mM sodium phosphate, pH7.2, provided a more useful purification step. 5% of the stimulating activity accompanied the main protein peak eluted by 0.12M NaCl, while at least 50% of the activity was eluted from the column by 0.3M NaCl. This suggests that the material is highly acidic or is bound strongly by hydrophobic interactions. Attempts to recover activity after fractionation on a hydrophobic column have been unsuccessful. The activity of the material eluted by 0.3M NaCl from the ion exchange column is trypsin-sensitive. The material is labile at 4°C and is unstable to freezing and thawing and this has hampered its further purification.

There are a number of possible explanations for the FCS requirement for stimulation of the hybridomas: the FCS component maybe (i) the antigen which is recognised by the hybridomas in an MHC-restricted fashion, or it may (ii) induce the expression of an auto-antigen on the stimulator cells, or alternatively it may be (iii) essential for the secretion of Il-2 by the hybridomas. Possiblity (iii) can be excluded since the hybridomas respond by IL-2 secretion to stimulation by Con A under serum-free conditions.

The mode of action of the FCS component has been investigated by FCS-pulsing either the stimulators or the hybridomas prior to culture (Table 4). The component acts on the stimulator cells and not on the hybridomas. Incubation of FCS with the stimulators for at least 2h at 37°C is necessary for the subsequent stimulation of the hybridomas. Moreover, FCS is required at the initiation of the cultures, since its late addition does not lead to the stimulation of significant IL-2 production by the hybridomas.

DISCUSSION

The data reported above suggests that the T cell hybridomas generated during attempts to produce Sendai virus-specific hybridomas do not recognise a self-antigen alone, but rather that they recognise a component

Table 4. Exposure of spleen cells or hybridomas to FCS prior to culture

		Hybridoma		
	Medium	BW	89.2	33.11
Treatment of spleen cells				
None	1591	1980	1970	2239
FCS 10'	1916	2166	2455	1831
FCS 30'	1709	2351	2531	1828
FCS 150'	1836	2561	4319	1981
FCS 240'	1770	2388	7658	2360
FCS Overnight	2269	3235	35305	13542
Treatment of hybridoma cells				
None	1626	2232	1948	2029
FCS 10'	1998	2227	2933	1776
FCS 30'	1839	2278	2650	1966
FCS 150'	1625	2302	2617	2092
FCS 240'	1768	2326	2621	1834
FCS in culture on day 0	1804	2741	17271	6149
FCS in culture on day 1	1636	1773	2717	2037

of FCS with MHC-restriction. However, the possibility that the FCS induces or enhances the expression of an auto-antigen which subsequently stimulates the hybridomas has not been formally excluded.

Attempts to purify the component of FCS responsible for stimulating the hybridomas have been hampered by its instability, both during storage at 4°C and to freezing and thawing. Inclusion of carrier-BSA in samples has not alleviated this problem. The component is trypsin-sensitive and sticks to other major protein constituents of serum. However, it binds to DEAE-ion exchange resin and can be dissociated from it by 0.3M NaCl, suggesting that it is acidic or is bound by hydrophobic interactions.

The mode of action of the FCS component was investigated. It was shown that the component is not required for IL-2 secretion by the hybridomas, since they produce IL-2 in response to Con A in serum-free medium. Pulsing experiments demonstrated that the component acted on the stimulators and not on the hybridomas. Incubation of the stimulators for at least 2h at 37°C with FCS was necessary for their subsequent ability to stimulate the hybridomas in serum-free medium. Addition of FCS to the cultures along with the hybridomas did not stimulate IL-2 production, showing that the FCS is required at the initiation of culture. It is possible that when cultured in serum-free medium the stimulator cells loose their ability to process or present the FCS component as antigen.

The Peyer's patch T-cell hybridomas reported here were initially thought to be "auto-reactive" but have subsequently been demonstrated to be responding to a component of FCS in a self-restricted fashion. It is important to elucidate whether putative auto-reactive T-cells reported by others are truly self-reactive or whether they too respond to nominal antigens they are exposed to *in vitro*. Even if the possibility of the T-cells responding to a component of xenogeneic or allogeneic serum can be excluded, it is still feasible that the T cells may be responding to antigens encountered during preparation (Huber et al., 1982) or other medium components such as antibiotics.

REFERENCES

Bretscher, P.A., 1986, How significant are "autoreactive" T cells?, Immunol. Today, 7:301.

Denizot, F. and Golstein, P., 1982, The functional effects of foetal calf serum on mouse lymphocytes in culture, Bull. Inst. Pasteur, 80:247.

Endres, R.O., Marrack, P. and Kappler, J.W., 1983, An IL-2 secreting T cell hybridoma that responds to a self class I histocompatibility antigen in the H-2D region, J. Immunol., 131:1656.

Faherty, D.A., Johnson, D.R. and Zauderer, M., 1985, Origin and specificity of autoreactive T cells in antigen-induced populations, J. Exp. Med., 161:1293.

Frangakis, M.V., Koopman, W.J., Kiyono, H., Michalek, S.M., and McGhee, J.R., 1982, An enzymatic method for preparation of dissociated murine Peyer's patch cells enriched for macrophages, J. Immunol. Methods, 48:33.

Huber, C., Merkenschlager, M., Gattringer, C., Royston, I., Fink, U., and Braunsteiner, H., 1982, Human autologous mixed lymphocyte reactivity is primarily specific for xenoprotein determinants absorbed to antigen-presenting cells during rosette formation with sheep erythrocytes, J. Exp. Med., 155:1222.

Julius, M.H. and Heusser, C.H., 1986, Autoreactive or self-restricted?, Eur. J. Immunol., 16:867.

Kawanishi, H., Ozato, K. and Strober, W., 1985, The proliferative response of cloned Peyer's patch switch T cells to syngeneic and allogeneic stimuli, J. Immunol., 134:3586.

Muller, I., and Kaufmann, S.H.E., 1985, Antigen-reactivity pattern of T-cell hybridomas from Mycobacterium bovis BCG-infected mice, Infect. Immun. 49:838.

Rock, K.L. and Benacerraf, B., 1983, The role of Ia molecules in the activation of T lymphocytes. III. Antigen-specific, Ia-restricted interleukin 2-producing T cell hybridomas with detectable affinity for the restricting I-A molecule, J. Exp. Med. 157:359.

Saito, K., Tamura, A., Narimatsu, H., Tadakuma, T., and Nagashima, M., 1986, Cloned auto-Ia-reactive T cells elicit lichen planus-like lesion in the skin of syngeneic mice, J. Immunol., 137:2485.

CELL ANOMALIES ASSOCIATED WITH SPACEFLIGHT CONDITIONS

Gerald R. Taylor

Medical Sciences Space Station Office (SD12)
NASA Lyndon B. Johnson Space Center
Houston, TX 77058

INTRODUCTION

In this paper is presented an abbreviated historical review of previous spaceflight studies which relate to an understanding of the infectious disease process in flight. The offensive components, that is the causative agents, have been extensively studied. Intercrew transfer of microorganisms, "simplification" of the autoflora, and contamination of the cabin's internal environment are well understood. Considerably less well understood is the defensive component of the infectious process. For a variety of reasons, the study of inflight human immune dysfunction has been uncoordinated, fragmented, and sometimes contradictory. However, we have been able to assemble enough data to: (1) demonstrate that the human immune system is altered during spaceflight and (2) develop a plan whereby the nature, degree, and significance of immune dysfunction can be studied in a manner which could allow the mechanism(s) of action to be elucidated. This paper, which presents the historical background and the NASA objectives for future tests, does not discuss the possible mechanisms involved. This latter subject is presented by the paper entitled "Human Mononuclear Cell In Vitro Activation in Microgravity and Post-space Flight," by Richard Meehan, also presented at this Conference. The two papers are intended as companions, both of which are required to complete the spaceflight human immune dysfunction story.

SPACEFLIGHT MICROBIOLOGY STUDIES

Survival of Microorganisms in the Spaceflight Environment

Investigations of microbiological specimens in space were initiated in 1935 with the stratospheric flight of the American high altitude balloon, Explorer 2 (Stevens, 1936), during which seven species of fungi survived exposure at 25 km for 4 hr. In the six years from 1954 to 1960, various species of *Neurospora* were carried on no less than 30 balloon and sounding rocket flights at altitudes of up to 150 km (Beischer and Fregly, 1962). These pre-spaceflight tests were important in that they established the fact that certain species could survive high altitude flight and therefore must be taken seriously in the impending development of space travel technology (Jenkins, 1968; Parfenov and Lukin, 1973).

Studies in Earth-orbital flight were initiated with the launch of the Russian craft, Sputnik 2, in 1958 (Antipov et al., 1962). In the first decade of orbital flight, Russian scientists evaluated 56 different species and preparations of biological materials including viruses, bacteria, yeasts, fungi, plants, animals, and tissue cultures, whereas the United States evaluated 35 different species and cellular preparations (Jenkins, 1968). Early studies conducted by Russian investigators included an evaluation of microbial growth on Sputnik 5 and other nonrecovered satellites with the aid of an automated device known as "Bioelements." This device was designed to measure the rate of gas production in actively growing Clostridium butyricum cultures, and to relay these data to Earth. Major growth rate differences were not obtained between flight samples and the ground control group (Zhukov-Verezhnikov, 1962). Clostridium sporogenes, flown aboard the American Discoverer 17 satellite, remained viable, although there was some degree of labilization which could be correlated with the measured irradiation from an intense solar flare that occurred during the flight (Bulban, 1961). No changes in the number of viable phage particles, plaque morphology, or reproduction rate were detected with Aerobacter aerogenes 1321 bacteriophage and T-2 coliphage, also carried aboard the 24-hour flight of the Sputnik 5 satellite (Zhukov-Verezhnikov, 1962). Actinomycetes (Streptomyces spp.) were tested on Sputnik 5, with the growth of returned inflight colonies being accelerated sixfold when compared with analogous laboratory controls (Antipov et al., 1962). No changes in postflight growth were detected with A. aerogenes 1321, Escherichia coli B, Staphylococcus aureus 0.15, and C. butyricum spores either for the 108 minute flight of Vostok 1 or the 1518 minute flight of Vostok 2 (Zhukov-Verezhnikov, 1962).

Microbial Genetic Stability In Flight

The E. coli K-12 (lambda) phage and host system was carried aboard most of the flights of the Sputnik series, all six of the manned flights of the Vostok series, Voskhod 1 and 2, the unmanned biosatellite Cosmos 110, and the lunar flights Zond 5 and 7 (Zhukov-Verezhnikov, 1965). This system was used as a radiation dosimeter because increases in phage production could be stimulated by as little as 0.3 rad of gamma radiation as well as by comparatively small doses of protons and rapid neutrons. Because the method of phage induction consists of injury to the genetic apparatus, the lysogenic bacteria system could also provide information about the potential mutagenic activity of cosmic radiation. The Sputnik flights demonstrated that the test system could remain intact and viable during space flight. Although the results from the first two Vostok flights, which were 2 and 25 hours long respectively, demonstrated no detectable effect on the elementary and poorly compensated genetic process, as reflected in the production of phage by lysogenic bacteria. However, later studies conducted throughout the remainder of the Vostok series demonstrated that the number of resulting phage in the spaceflight samples exceeded that in the ground controls. This was interpreted as indicative that spaceflight factors had an inducing effect on the lysogenic bacteria (Zhukov-Verezhnikov, 1963). Further, it was reported that the spaceflight effect, measured in terms of increased phage production, as compared with the magnitude of spontaneous phage production in the ground controls, increased with mission duration throughout the Vostok series (Parfenov and Lukin, 1973). This effect was not considered to be entirely due to the galactic radiation received because there was not a linear relationship between excessive phage production and length of time in orbit, and the resultant effect was much greater than would be expected from measurements of incoming radiation (Zhukov-Verezhnikov, 1965). Laboratory studies conducted in conjunction with the Vostok 1 through 4 missions demonstrated that simulated launch vibration followed by exposure to cobalt gamma-radiation resulted in an increase in mutation rate, as measured by phage production, which was somewhat higher than that obtained by the same level of gamma-radiation alone. Simulated launch vibration alone, or following radiation had no effect on the measured parameter. These results engendered the speculation that the launch vibrations produced by the Vostok rocket increased the sensitivity of the lysogenic bacteria to subsequent galactic radiation, thus accounting for the excessive phage production (Zhukov-Verezhnikov, 1965).

Tests were conducted on Voskhod 1 and 2 to determine the effectiveness of the radiation protecting substances, Beta-mercaptopropylamine and 5-methoxytryptamine, while at the same time evaluating the contribution space radiation actually plays in genetic disturbances in the *E. coli* K-12 (lambda) bacteriophage system (Antipov et al., 1967). Although phage production was reduced as expected, there also was a reduction in the incidence of spontaneous phage production. This indicated that some mechanism in addition to, or in place of, radiation protection was influencing the test. The investigators concluded that the radiation protectors were effective in space but they were unable to separately evaluate the effect of galactic radiation on the microbial genetic apparatus.

Salmonella typhimurium, and *E. coli* bacteriophage induction systems were tested as part of the 45-hour Earth-orbital flight of the American Biosatellite II (Mattoni, 1968). During the flight, different aliquots of cells were exposed to a total dose of from 265 to 1648 rad of strontium gamma-radiation with the resulting radiation response curves being compared with appropriate ground control curves. The space-flown *S. typhimurium* cells were more resistant to gamma-radiation, as indicated by a decrease in phage production (Mattoni et al., 1971). Efforts to reproduce these results with acceleration, vibration, and clinostat tests were unsuccessful. This decrease in phage induction supports the results reported for the *E. coli* system flown on Cosmos 110 but is counter to the results reported for all of the other Russian coliphage studies. This apparent contradiction is not surprising in view of the greatly different test conditions involved. The fact remains that the total spaceflight environment has been shown to exert an influence on the bacteriophage induction system, and that the degree of the effect is dependent upon the combination of environmental factors which have yet to be studied in detail.

American genetic studies designed to measure the effect of ionizing radiation, in combination with reduced gravity, on *Neurospora crassa* conidia were initiated on Gemini XI (phosphorus-Beta exposure) and Biosatellite II (strontium-gamma exposure). Flight cells suspended in agar and exposed to radiation demonstrated higher levels of survival and lower frequencies of mutation induction, as compared to ground controls, indicating that the space flight affected a protective influence (de Serres, 1969). On the basis of these experiments, and reports of alterations among space-flown plant and animal systems, de Serres concluded that positive effects are due to the temporary influence of weightlessness on fundamental metabolic processes, with induction and recovery phenomena being more drastically altered in rapidly metabolizing systems than in relatively inert systems such as resting spores.

Microbial Alteration In Flight

During the Apollo 16 flight to the Moon, ten microbial strains were placed outside the command module so that they could be exposed to solar ultraviolet and space vacuum (Taylor et al., 1974). The use of various combinations of optical filters to provide exposure to varying amounts of solar irradiation at peak wavelengths of 254, 280, and 300 nm, allowed for a different dose-response curve at each of these three wavelengths

(Chassay and Taylor, 1973). T-7 bacteriophage preparations of E. coli which were exposed to inflight irradiation, were found to be more sensitive to UV light than were irradiated ground-based controls (Spizizen, 1971). There was no significant difference between the mean of inflight survivors and any of the appropriate ground-based controls for spores of three strains or Bacillus subtilis and one strain of Bacillus thuringiensis. B. thuringiensis was also evaluated in terms of the production rate of a lipolytic Alpha-exotoxin, a deforming Beta-exotoxin, and a crystalline delta-endotoxin, all of which have well established biological behavior. Statistically significant differences in the capability of the postflight isolates to produce toxins were not found among the treatment groups (Wrenn et al., 1973). The combined action of space vacuum and solar UV irradiation at a peak wavelength of 254 nm resulted in greater loss of viability of B. Subtilis strain 168 spores than was observed in irradiated ground-based controls. This was interpreted as a synergistic effect in which the spores were sensitized to solar UV by the space vacuum (Bucker, et al., 1973). B. Subtilis strains HA 101 and HA 101(59)F both contain multiple genetic markers whereas strain HA 101(59)F is also defective in the ability to repair radiation damage and is therefore highly susceptible to the damaging effects of ultraviolet irradiation. Survival rates for these space-flown spores did not differ significantly from analogous ground controls (Spizizen and Isherwood, 1973). Aeromonas proteolytica cells, used as a model system to evaluate the effect of space flight and solar UV on the production of an endopeptidase which can cause intracutaneous hemorrhage and a hemolysin which is active against human erythrocytes, demonstrated no difference between survival rates, enzyme production, or UV sensitivity of space-flown cells when compared with appropriate ground-based controls (Foster, 1973). There were no significant differences between postflight survival rates of non-irradiated cells when compared with appropriate ground-based controls of the yeasts Rhodotorula rubra and Saccharomyces cerevisiae and the filamentous fungi Trichophyton terrestre and Chaetomium globosum, (Volz, 1973).

Crew Medical Microbiology Studies

Detailed medical microbiological evaluations of American astronauts were initiated with the Apollo series of space flights. Illness events of microbial origin were not uncommon in the first three missions with crewmembers experiencing upper respiratory problems, influenza, viral gastroenteritis, rhinitis, pharyngitis, or mild dermatologic problems (Wooley, 1972). Following each of the Apollo 7 through Apollo 11 missions, the number of crewmembers from whom a particular pathogen could be recovered was generally higher than before launch, indicating transfer of pathogenic species between individuals during space flight. Also, postflight increases in the number of body sites from which these species were isolated were observed, with S. aureus and the Beta-hemolytic streptococci most consistently displaying postflight increases (Berry, 1970). Similar increases in staphylococci, accompanied by increases in antibiotic resistance, have been reported to occur following Russian flights (Zaloguyev, 1970).

Several authors have warned, as summarized by Shilov (1970), that returning space travelers may experience a microbial shock and may respond negatively to renewed contact with potentially pathogenic microorganisms which are absent in the spaceflight environment. This warning is based on the assumption that contact with potential pathogens during space flight would be very limited, resulting in a reduction of immunocompetence. However, data from actual space flights show that there is usually an increase in the distribution of pathogens (Taylor, 1974). Therefore, any reduction in immunocompetence is not likely to be in response to decreased contact with pathogenic components of the autoflora. Extensive quarantine preventive measures, initiated with the Apollo 14 mission, were designed to allow the autoflora to equilibrate at a level consistent with confinement and to allow contracted infectious agents to demonstrate themselves before flight (Wooley, 1972). It is likely that this contributed to the complete lack of microbial problems during, or immediately following, subsequent Apollo flights (Taylor, 1974).

An inflight malfunction of the Apollo 13 Service Module provided an opportunity to evaluate the effect of a crippled life support system on the infectious disease process. Following several days in a cold, damp, habitat in an extremely stressful situation, one of the astronauts developed a severe urinary tract infection from which Pseudomonas aeruginosa was eventually isolated in high numbers. This situation required inflight antibiotic therapy, which was ineffective until the crewmember could be returned to Earth where bacterial isolation and antibiotic sensitivity tests could be performed (Taylor, 1974). Several investigators, as summarized by Zaloguyev et al. (1971), have demonstrated a reduction in body resistance and increases in microbial toxigenic activity, virulence, or pathogenicity following stressful confinement of the human host in space-simulation studies. Combined evaluation of these reports proved the requirement for an inflight clinical sample analysis capability to be included on spaceflight missions. This is especially important for long-duration or deep space missions in which it would be either inconvenient or impossible for crewmembers to quickly return to Earth for diagnosis and treatment.

In addition to the more obvious exogeneous diseases which may afflict crewmembers, the importance of endogenous infections has been identified by several authors and is reviewed by Chukhlovin et al. (1971). Concern for infections involving endogenous microorganisms is based upon the recognition that the unusual environment offered by the space ship may so influence the indigenous microflora that previously innocuous microorganisms may become noxious. An example of this potential problem may be found with the potentially pathogenic yeast Candida albicans which was recovered from the oral cavity of a large number of astronauts throughout the Apollo series (Taylor, 1972). Although it is not uncommon to find this species in the mouth of healthy adults, its subsequent behavior during space flight is of medical importance. Russian investigators have reported a 30-fold increase in incidence of C. albicans in the pharnyx of subjects who had been confined to a closed test chamber for one month. These investigators concluded that the confinement normalized the bacterial flora, resulting in reduced microbial competition, with subsequent overgrowth of this potentially pathogenic yeast (Zaloguyev et al., 1971). Such a normalization of bacterial species has not been demonstrated in samples collected from Apollo crewmembers, although C. albicans is often the only fungal species recoverable from Apollo crewmember samples collected immediately after termination of a mission (Taylor et al., 1973). It has been observed that this resistance of C. albicans populations to space flight could become quite important if long-term inflight antibiotic therapy was required, providing the opportunity for a loss of competing species and eventual overgrowth of this organism (Ginsberg, 1971). The above observations tend to support the view, proposed by several authors, and reviewed by Fox (1971), that microflora changes may occur in the spacecraft environment and that these changes may not be compatible with man's health and welfare on extended duration missions.

Postflight increases have been reported in the oral autoflora of Russian cosmonauts accompanied by dysbacteriosis in which the normal throat flora are almost entirely crowded out by Gram-negative, non-hemolytic diplococci. Extensive microbial evaluations, performed on the crew following the 18-day Soyuz 9 space flight, revealed a large quantity of Gram-positive, nonsporogenous bacteria on the skin and nasal passages which was not there preflight (Zaloguyev et al., 1970). It was also reported that this dysbacteriotic change in the skin and nasal automicroflora was accompanied by variations of some unnamed characteristics of natural immunity.

Detailed studies were continued with the joint US/USSR Apollo-Soyuz Test Project flight in which 3 American astronauts and 2 Russian cosmonauts shared a small orbiting living volume. Although various potential pathogens were recovered from each of the 5 crewmembers before and after flight, no inflight disease events were reported. Interpersonnel transfer of pathogens were demonstrated within crews but not between crews. Significantly, inflight simplificaton of, and dysbacteriotic changes in, the population of medically important microorganisms did not occur (Taylor and Zaloguyev, 1977).

The long-duration (30, 60, and 89 days) U.S. Skylab stays provided an opportunity to better evaluate the medical implications of previously-noted microbial alterations. Gross microbial contamination of the Skylab environment, intercrew transfer of pathogens, and numerous inflight disease events, presumably of microbial origin, were demonstrated. Evaluation of major microbial population groups tended to support the theory of microbial simplification for anaerobic bacteria, but not for other microbes (Taylor, et al., 1977).

SUMMARY HISTORY OF IMMUNOLOGY STUDIES

Although cellular immune responses of American astronauts and Soviet cosmonauts have been studied by various methods for two decades, there remains a paucity of reliable information upon which to draw conclusions. Analyses after the 11 flights of the American Apollo Program failed to show consistent postflight alterations in RNA or DNA sythesis in response to Phytohemagglutinin (PHA) exposure, although a postflight lymphocytosis was reported for a majority of the 33 crewmembers (Kimzey, et al., 1975). The technique used for lymphocyte isolation during the Apollo series has been shown to selectively remove "B" lymphocytes and a subset of "T" lymphocytes prior to culture (Miller, 1977) and may have contributed to the inability of the researchers to demonstrate alterations. Similarly, following the three American Skylab visits, the postflight functional capacity of crew lymphocytes, measured in terms of DNA synthesis in response to PHA, was unchanged. However, postflight RNA synthesis was reported to have been depressed concomitant with an increase in leukocyte absolute count (Kimzey, 1977). Among the total of 9 astronauts in Skylab, the mean scores for gingival inflammation and dental calculus approximately doubled over preflight values during their 30 to 59 days in space although in no case was there a noted dental or oral disability. It is noteworthy that these responses occurred during a time when careful oral hygiene was maintained by the affected astronauts (Brown, et al., 1977). Following the joint US-USSR Apollo-Soyuz Test Project (ASTP) flight, variable lymphocyte responses to a variety of mitogens, as well as absolute leukocytoses, were reported (Criswell and Cobb, 1977). However, because the astronauts were exposed to toxic levels of nitrogen tetroxide upon landing, it was not possible to attach any spaceflight-related importance to the resulting data.

Alterations in the in vitro response of cosmonaut lymphocytes were reported following the flights of Soyuz 6, 7, 8, and 9 (Kanstantinova et al., 1973). Tritiated uridine uptake was estimated by photographic film exposure with variable results. These analyses gave an early indication that lymphocyte activity may be depressed following space flight. Comparative numerical measurements of preflight and postflight peripheral lymphocytes and leukocytes were taken for the above missions, for the Soyuz 11 visit to the Salyut 1 Space Station, and for the two Soyuz visits to the Salyut 4 Space Station. Although results were variable, they imply a postflight leukocytosis concurrent with a postflight lymphocytopenia (Konstantinova et al., 1978). In addition, "diminished postflight reactivity of T lymphocytes" was reported after both the 30-day and the 63-day visits to Salyut 4 (Konstantinova et al., 1978). Following the flights of Soyuz 24, Salyut 5, Soyuz 26, and Soyuz 27, and the 96-day Soyuz 28/Salyut 6 mission, there was an increase of both the spontaneous lymphocyte activity and the maximum PHA-induced blastogenic response. However, a decrease in T lymphocyte number and blast transformation was again reported following the 140-day mission to Salyut 6 (Lesnyak and Tashpulatov, 1981).

Up to the beginning of the Shuttle Era, there was sufficient reason to speculate that in vitro stimulability of lymphocytes was altered by space flight. However, previous methods, which included single incubation times and an inadequate range of mitogen concentrations, rendered detailed appraisal impossible. For this reason a highly sensitive modification of the Apollo and Skylab methodology was used for the first time with the Space Shuttle crewmember lymphocyte samples. This method allowed for a direct correlation of tritiated thymidine uptake to both incubation time and to mitogen concentration (Taylor and Dardano, 1983), and accurate estimations of the maximum PHA response under optimal conditions. As a result, it was demonstrated that the in vitro blastogenic responsiveness of crew peripheral blood lymphocytes were significantly reduced following each of the first four U.S. Shuttle flights (Taylor, 1983).

Additional data collected before and after 11 of the first 12 U.S. Space Shuttle flights show that absolute lymphocyte numbers, lymphocyte blastogenic capability, and eosinophils present in the peripheral blood of crewmembers are generally reduced postflight (Taylor et al., 1985). As these responses also resemble those associated with physical and emotional stress, it is unknown if they were directly related to space flight per se. Data from Space Shuttle flights 41B and 41D, involving 11 crewmembers, indicate a postflight decrease in circulating monocytes and lymphocytes identified as "B" cells, using monoclonal antibodies against cell surface phenotype antigens. Furthermore, the reduced "T" lymphocyte blastogenesis was shown to correlate with the decreased monocyte count (Correlation coefficient = 0.697). Since monocytes serve a critical role during lymphocyte activation as potent immunoregulator cells through release of cytokines, these findings suggest a possible mechanism of blunted in vitro mitogen induced blastogenesis (Taylor et al., 1985).

Serum complement levels have been measured with postflight values changing variously when compared to preflight means. C3 levels were significantly higher following the 16, 18, and 49-day Salyut flights, whereas C4 levels were generally unchanged postflight (Cogoli and Tschopp, 1985). The notable exception to this was the 49-day Salyut 5 flight for which significantly higher postflight C4 values, as well as a large increase in serum IgA, IgG, and IgM levels were reported (Talas et al., 1983).

In vitro alpha interferon production has been studied with lymphocytes taken from cosmonauts before and after space flight (Talas et al., 1983). UV-inactivated Newcastle Disease virus was used as the inducer.

In two samples, the production of interferon was significantly lower after flight, but in the other two it remained unaltered. The induction of interferon production correlated fairly well with the natural killer activity of lymphocytes. The same authors also determined the synthesis of interferon by lymphocytes from noncrewmember donors cultured in space in the presence of four different inducers. In microgravity, production of interferon was almost five times higher than that in the ground controls.

In contrast to these results, analysis of adult rats flown aboard the U.S. Shuttle Spacelab 3 showed that only one of the ten rats that had flown in space produced marginal levels of circulating interferon, and that nine of the ten flown rats produced no interferon (as compared to good production by seven of the ten ground control animals). These results were interpreted by the investigators to indicate that the in vivo production of gamma interferon was severely inhibited in rats subjected to space flight and the attendant periods of weightlessness (Gould et al., 1985).

Cogoli et al. (1984) have reported interesting results with various cell cultures exposed to hypergravity and hypogravity. The proliferation of chicken embryo fibroblasts, Hela cells, Sarcoma Galliera cells, Friend leukemia virus-transformed cells, and mitogen-stimulated lymphoblasts was enhanced by up to 30 % under hypergravity conditions and depressed in a ground-based rotating clinostat model which partially simulated hypogravity. In an experiment conducted aboard the U.S. Spacelab 1, the response of inflight cultured lymphocytes to Concanavalin A was reported to be only 3 % of that obtained with simultaneous ground control cultures. More recently, Cogoli et al. (unpublished report) have repeated these studies on the 1985 German D1 Shuttle payload. In this experiment, fresh-drawn human lymphocytes, as well as cultures of lymphocytes collected before flight, produced inflight growth less than 10 % of the ground controls. In an effort to sort out the effect of the ambient microgravity, cells were also cultured, in flight, in a one-g simulating centrifuge incubator. In this case the loss of growth was approximately 60 % when compared to ground controls.

FUTURE IMMUNOLOGY INVESTIGATIONS IN SPACE

The Federation of American Societies of Experimental Biology (FASEB) has been under contract to the NASA to provide scientific assessments of topics in the biomedical sciences and to make recommendations for future inflight studies, if appropriate. In 1985 the Federation convened an ad hoc working group to review previous inflight immunological studies. They subsequently reported their review to the NASA (Beisel and Talbot, 1985). This independent analysis was combined with NASA goals to establish the NASA philosophy, as outlined below, for near-term spaceflight immunology research activities.

The NASA considers inflight interpersonal transfer if microorganisms, the efficacy of preflight isolation, and inflight "simplification" of autoflora to have been thoroughly studied. Whereas these factors materially affect planning for future long-duration spaceflight missions, the parameters are well enough understood that preventive measures can be built into the mission planning activity. For example, microbial contamination of air and onboard potable water supplies is a recognized potential source of illness. This becomes especially important in extended space stays, such as would be required for Lunar base occupation or Mars exploration, where recycling of waste water will be an operational necessity.

The NASA considers it significant that, whereas no consistent alterations in humoral immune function have been reported, neutrophilia, relative lymphopenia, and impaired blastogenic responsiveness of "T" lymphocytes have been demonstrated repeatedly in postflight blood samples from space crews. Other important space-related alterations of human immune function include postflight eosinopenia, monocytopenia, reduced percentage of "B" lymphocytes and monocytes, decreased natural killer cell activity, and decreased production of alpha-interferon by lymphocytes.

Currently, a paucity of reliable data on the effects of space flight on immunocompetence prevents a firm scientific conclusion about the potential operational and clinical significance of reported changes. However, the FASEB ad hoc committee was able to independently arrive at conclusions which supported the overall thrust of the NASA immunology program (Beisel and Talbot, 1985). They identified the central issue to be to determine whether the known changes to, and as yet unstudied changes in, the immune system and the microflora of space crews represent a significant, potential health problem for space crews. For example, the altered blastogenic responsiveness of lymphocytes from postflight blood specimens is an important change that needs precise explanation. Such an explanation might be an inability of "T" lymphocytes to generate growth factors and growth factor receptors, suggesting marked dysfunction with implications for serious impairment of immunocompetence. Another examples is the mild gingivitis experienced by Skylab astronauts. This phenomenon could indicate a neutrophilic dysfunction such as impairment of cell surface adhesion reactions. However, whether neutrophil function remains normal in flight and during the first few days postflight remains unknown. This analysis has led to a recommendation by the FASEB of the following studies to be conducted in the near term.

1. Determine inflight immune responses of space crewmembers including antibody production and delayed type hypersensitivity reactions to common antigens.

2. Study the capacity of activated T-lymphocytes obtained postflight from space crews to make lymphokines such as interleukin-2, interleukin-3, and gamma-interferon and to generate lymphokine receptor such as that for interleukin-2. For T-lymphocyte transformations, PHA and ConA are appropriate nonspecific mitogens; PPD, mumps, streptokinase-streptodornase, tetanus toxoid, and *Candida albicans* are useful specific antigens.

3. Examine recruitment of human neutrophils and mononuclear cells and the release of their lysosomal contents inflight as well as postflight by means of in vivo induction of localized skin inflammation. The resulting minor skin lesions offer a means of observing wound healing as well.

4. Examining mouth washings for neutrophils as another means of acquiring some data on the inflammatory response as it relates to gingivitis or other oral lesions.

5. Determine the temporal pattern of changes in key human immunologic parameters such as white blood cell count, differential count, and blastogenic responsiveness of T-lymphocytes. Possibly related variables should also be measured in the blood specimens for this study including

epinephrine, cortisol, acute phase reactants (C-reactive protein, haptoglobin, ceruloplasmin, orosomucoid, alpha-1-antitrypsin) as well as plasma zinc, iron, and copper.

6. Determine the following functional capacities of peripheral blood neutrophils and monocytes obtained from specimens from space crew personnel at selected times postflight: chemotactic response, adherence, locomotion, phagocytosis, degranulation, bactericidal activity, oxidative metabolism, and respiratory burst.

7. Conduct preflight and postflight studies to evaluate the uptake of complement-altered red blood cells by the reticuloendothelial system.

8. Measure in vivo macrophage phagocytosis using the uptake of chromium-tagged, antibody-coated red blood cells by the splenic macrophages and the hepatic Kupfer cells.

As a result of an analysis of what is not known, as well as what is know regarding human immune dysfunction during space flight, these short-term goals have been accepted by the NASA. It is hoped that meaningful inflight experiments will be conducted within the next decade which will result in real progress towards the goal of understanding spaceflight immunoincompetence.

REFERENCES

Antipov, V. V., Bayerskiy, R. M., Gazenko, O. G., Genin, A. M., Gyurdzhian, A. A., Zhukov-Verezhnikov, N. N., Zhuravlev, B. A., Karpova, L. I., Parfenov, G. P., Seryapin, A. D., Shepelev, E. Ya, and Yazdovskiy, V. I., 1962, Some results of medical and biological investigations in the second and third satellites, Probl. Space Biol., 3:295-313.

Antipov, V. V., Kozlov, V. A., Parfenov, G. P., and Saksonov, P. P., 1967, The results of biological studies made on board the Voskhod and Voskhod 2 spaceships, Life Sci. Space Res., 5:119-21.

Beischer, D. E., and Fregly, A. R., 1962, Animals and man in space through the year 1960, USNSAM, Monograph 5.

Beisel, W. R., and Talbot, J. M., 1985, "Research Opportunities on Immunocompetence in Space," FASEB, Bethesda.

Berry, C. A., 1970, Summary of medical experience in the Apollo 7 through 11 manned space flights, Aerosp. Med., 41:500-19.

Brown, L. R., Frome, W. J., Handler, S., Wheatcroft, M. G., Reider, L. J., 1977, Skylab oral health studies, in: Biomedical Results of Skylab," R. S. Johnston and L. F. Dietlein, eds., National Aeronautics and Space Administration SP-377, pp. 35-44, Washington.

Bucker, H., Horneck, G., Wollenhaupt, H., Schwager, M., and Taylor, G.R., 1973, Viability of Bacillus subtilis spores exposed to space environment in the M-191 experiment system aboard Apollo 16, Presented XVI COSPAR Conference, Konstanz, FRG.

Bulban, E. J., 1961, Anti-radiation shielding may be reduced, Aviat. Res., 74:40-41.

Chassay, C. E., and Taylor, G. R., 1973, Description of the microbial ecology evaluation device, in: "Proceedings of the Microbial Response to Space Environment Symposium," G. R. Taylor, ed., National Aeronautics and Space Administration Publication TMX-58103 pp. 21-39.

Chukhlovin, A. B., Ostroumov, P. B., and Ivanova, S. P., 1971, Development of staphlococcal infection in human subjects under the influence of some spaceflight factors, Kosmi. Biol. Med., 5:61-65.

Cogoli, A., and Tschopp, A., 1985, Lymphocyte reactivity during space flight, Immun. Today, 6:1-4.

Cogoli, A., Tschopp, A., and Fuchs-Bislin, P., 1984, Cell sensitivity to gravity, Science 225:228-230.

Criswell, B. S., and Cobb, K., 1977, Cellular immune response: Experiment MA-031, in: "Apollo-Soyuz Test Project Summary Science Report," National Aeronautics and Space Administration SP-142, pp. 257-262.

de Serres, F. J., 1969, Effects of radiation during spaceflight on microorganisms and plants on the Biosatellite II and Gemini XI missions, Life Sci. Space Res., 7:62-66.

Foster, B. G., 1973, Effects of solar irradiation on extracellular enzymes of Aeromonas proteolytica, in: "Proceedings of the Microbial Response to Space Environment Symposium," G. R. Taylor, ed., National Aeronautics and Space Administration Publication TMX-58103, pp. 137-51.

Fox, L., 1971, The ecology of microorganisms in a closed environment, Life Sci. Space Res., 9:69-74.

Ginsberg, H. S., 1971, Immune states in long-duration space flights, Life Sci. Space Res., 9:1-9.

Gould, C. L., Williams, J. A., Mandel, A. D., and Sonnenfeld, G., 1985, Effect of flight in mission SL-3 on interferon gamma production by rats, In Press, The Physiologist.

Jenkins, D. W., 1968, USSR and US bioscience, BioScience, 18:543-49.

Kimzey, S. L. , Fisher, C. L., Johnson, P. C., Ritzman, S. E., and Mengel, C. E., 1975, Hematology and immunology studies, in: "Biomedical Results of Apollo," National Aeronautics and Space Administration SP-368, pp. 213-222.

Kimzey, S. L., 1977, Hematology and immunology studies, in: "Biomedical Results from Skylab," National Aeronautics and Space Administration SP-377 pp. 249-282.

Konstantinova, I. V., Antropova, Ye. N., Legen'kov, V. I., and Zazhirey, V. D., 1973, Study of reactivity of blood lymphoid cells in crew members of the Soyuz-6, Soyuz-7, and Soyuz-8 spaceships before and after flight, Kosmicheskaya Biologiya i Meditsina, 7:35-40.

Konstantinova, I. V., Nefedov, Yu. G., Yeremin, A. V., Drozdova, V. I., Skryabin, A. S., Guseva, O. A., and Mukhina, N. N., 1978, Immunological reactivity and prediction of allergic complications in the crew of the second expedition of Salyut 4, Kosmicheskaya Biologiya i Avikosmicheskaya Meditsina, 12:15-29.

Lesnyak, A. E., and Tashpulatov, R. Yu., 1981, Effects of space flights on lymphocyte blast transformation in cosmonauts' peripheral blood Kosmicheskaya Biologiya i Aviakosmicheskaya Meditsina 15:32-34.

Mattoni, R. H. T., 1968, Spaceflight effects and gamma radiation interaction on growth and induction of lysogenic bacteria, Bioscience, 18:602-8.

Mattoni, R. H. T., Keller, E. C., Jr., Ebersold, W. T., Eiserling, F. A., and Romig, W. R., 1971, Induction of lysogenic bacteria in the space environment, in: "The Experiments of Biosatellite II,"J. Saunders, ed., National Aeronautics and Space Administration Document SP-204, pp. 309-24.

Miller, R. G., 1977, Physical separation of lymphocytes, in: "The Lymphocyte," Part 1, Chapter 5, pp. 205-223, Marcel Dekker, Inc., New York.

Parfenov, G. P., Lukin, A. A., 1973, Results and prospects of microbial studies in outer space, Space Life Sci., 4:160-79.

Shilov, V., 1970, Microbes and space flight, Aerosp. Med., 41:1353.

Spizizen, J., 1971, Microbiological problems of manned space flight, Life

Sci. Space Res. 9:65-68.
Spizizen, J., Isherwood, J. E., 1973, Effects of space environment on T-7 bacteriophage and spores of Bacillus subtilis 168, "Proceedings of the Microbial Response to Space Environment Symposium, "G. R. Taylor, ed., National Aeronautics and Space Administration Publication TMX-58103, pp. 65-68.
Stevens, A., 1936, 1971, Nat. Geogr. Mag., 69:693-712
Talas, M., Batkai, L., Stoger, I., Nagy, K., Hiros, L., Konstantinova, I., Rykova, M., Mozgovava, I., Guseva, O., and Kozharinov, V., 1983, Results of space experiment program "Interferon," Acta Microbiologica Hungarica, 30:53-61.
Taylor, G. R., 1972, "Apollo 14 Microbial Analysis," National Aeronautics and Space Administration Publication TMX-58094.
Taylor, G. R., Henney, M. R., and Ellis, W. L., 1973, Change in the autoflora of Apollo astronauts, Appl. Microbiol. 26:804-813.
Taylor, G. R., 1974, Recovery of medically important microorganisms from Apollo Astronauts, Aerospace Med. 45:824-828.
Taylor, G. R., Spizizen, J., Foster, B. G., Volz, P. A., Bucker, H., Simmonds, R. C., Heimpel, A. M., and Benton, E. V., 1974, A descriptive analysis of the Apollo 16 microbial response to space environment experiment, Bioscience, 24:505-511.
Taylor, G. R., and Zaloguyev, S. N., 1977, Medically important microorganisms recovered from Apollo-Soyuz Test Project (ASTP) crewmembers, Life Sci. Space Res., 15:207-121.
Taylor, G. R., Graves, R. C., Brockett, R. M., Ferguson, J. K., and Mieszkuc, B. J., 1977, Skylab environmental and crew microbiology studies, in: "Biomedical Results from Skylab," National Aeronautics and Space Administration SP-377, pp.53-63.
Taylor, G. R., 1983, Hematological and immunological analysis, in: Shuttle OFT Medical Report, National Aeronautics and Space Administration TMX-58252,. pp. 35-48.
Taylor, G. R., and Dardano, J. R., 1983, Human cellular immune responsiveness following space flight, Aviat. Space Environ. Med. 54(Suppl. 1):S55-S59.
Taylor, G. R., Neale, L. S., and Dardano, J. R., 1985, Immunological analyses of U.S. Space Shuttle Crewmembers, Avia. Space Environ. Med., 57:213-217.
Volz, P. A., 1973, Mycological studies housed in the Apollo 16 microbial ecology evaluation device, in: "Proceedings of the Microbial Response to Space Environment Symposium," G. R. Taylor, ed., National Aeronautics and Space Administration Publication TMX-58103 pp. 121-135.
Wooley, B. C. 1972, "Apollo Experience Report: Protection of Life and Health," National Aeronautics and Space Administration Publication MSC-04748.
Wrenn, R. T., Simmonds R. C., and Heimpel, A. M., 1973, Postflight analysis of Bacillus thuringiensis organisms exposed to spaceflight conditions, "Proceedings of the Microbial Response to Space Environment Symposium," G. R. Taylor, ed., National Aeronautics and Space Administration Publication TMX-58103, pp. 105-120.
Zaloguyev, S. N., Shinkareva, M. M., Utkina, T. G., 1970, State of the automicroflora of skin tissues and certain natural immunity indices in the astronauts A. G. Nikolaev and V. I. Serast'ianov before and after flight, Kosm. Biol. i Med., 4:54-59.
Zaloguyev, S. N., Utkina, T. G., Shinkareva, M. M., 1971, The microflora of the human integument during prolonged confinement, Life Sci. Space Res., 9:55-59.
Zhukov-Verezhnikov, N. N., Mayskiy, I. N., Yazdovskiy, V. I., Pekhov, A. P., Rybakov, N. I., Klemparskaya, N. N., Gyurdzhian, A. A., Tribulev, G. P., Nefed'yeva, N. P., Kapichnikov, M. M., Podoplelov, I. I., Antipov, V. V., Novikova, I. S., and Kop'yev,

V. Ya., 1962, Problem of Space Microbiology and Cytology, Probl. Space Biol.,1:133-48.

Zhukov-Verezhnikov, N. N., Mayskiy, I. N., Yazdovskiy, V. I., Pekhov, A. P., Rybakov, N. I., Tribulev, G. P., Saksonov, P. P., Dobrov, N. N., Antipov, V. V., Kozlov, V. A., Vysotskiy, V. G., Mishchenko, B. A., Rybakova, K. D., Parfenov, G. P., Pantyukhova, V. V., Yudin, Ye. N., and Aniskin, Ye. D., 1963, Evaluating the biological effectiveness of spaceflight factors by means of the lysogenic bacterial E. coli K-12 lambda, Aviation & Space Med., pp. 158-160.

Zhukov-Verezhnikov, N. N., Rybakov, N. I., Kozlov, V. A., Saksonov, P. P., Dobrov, N. N., Antipov., V. v., Podoplelov, I. I., and Parfenov, G. P., 1965, Results of microbiological and cytological investigation conducted during the flights of "Vostok" type vehicles, Probl. Space Biol., 4:252-59.

HUMAN MONONUCLEAR CELL IN VITRO ACTIVATION IN MICROGRAVITY AND POST-SPACEFLIGHT

Richard Meehan

Department of Internal Medicine
University of Texas Medical Branch
Galveston Texas 77550

ABSTRACT

The results of postflight and inflight human in vitro lymphocyte experiments have been reviewed. The cumulative data indicate that mitogen-stimulated T-cell proliferation is blunted following short-duration missions. Since similar responses may also be obtained following exposure to non-spaceflight stressors (hypoxia and academic stress), it is unclear if microgravity per se aggravates this response. Our studies indicate that stress-induced impaired PHA- and PWM-stimulated activation can be detected within the first 24 hours in culture at the level of protein synthesis. While the mechanism for neuroendocrine-mediated blunted mitogen stimulated T cell proliferation has not been elucidated, it is not aggravated by autologous plasma and does not require changes in mononuclear cell subpopulations. While prior studies indicate lymphocyte activation is influenced by altering G forces on in vitro cultures, impaired cellular interactions or suboptimal microenvironments related to reduced cell densities in microgravity may contribute to the greatly impaired mitogen stimulated proliferation responses observed on Spacelab flights. It will be necessary to perform lymphocyte functional assays on crewmembers during spaceflight to determine the contribution of microgravity per se on altered human immune competence.

INTRODUCTION

The exotic environment of spaceflight contains a variety of novel hazards which would threaten crew health if immune homeostasis were impaired. Orbital flight is associated with exposure to unique sources of ionizing radiation (solar, galactic and geomagnetically trapped particles). The spacecraft air or water supply may become contaminated by pathogenic organisms, and numerous toxic chemical substances could be released into the cabin. Furthermore, since particles will remain airborne in the absence of gravity, the intercrew transfer of infectious agents may be facilitated. Since emergency evacuation may be difficult or impossible, the Soviet and American space programs have primarily focused upon medical issues which could compromise crew health. Because only one serious inflight infectious illness has occurred requiring an aborted mission (Canby, 1986), this may indicate the effectiveness of preflight quarantine procedures and the careful selection of flight crew.

Microgravity also induces a variety of physiologic responses which vary in severity, including cephalad fluid shifts, cardiovascular deconditioning, bone demineralization, muscle atrophy and temporary postural illusions or cerebral dysfunction which may progress to "space adaptation syndrome" among susceptible individuals. During the past 25 years of manned spaceflight, multiple immunology experiments have been conducted postflight and inflight to investigate the immune system's response to microgravity. Numerous investigators have performed in vitro mononuclear cell activation assays from crewmembers to assess cellular immune competence postflight. These assays were performed following Apollo (n=21), Skylab (n=9), Apollo-Soyuz Test Project (n=3) and Shuttle missions (n=36) as summarized in Table I. The results of other immunological studies are summarized by Dr. Taylor in the preceding paper. In reviewing these prior studies, it is important to appreciate that the in vitro mitogen-induced activation assays preceding the Shuttle program were performed over a decade ago, and lymphocytes were obtained and cultured under very difficult "field conditions" associated with mission operational constraints.

Table I Results of U.S. Astronauts' Peripheral Blood Mononuclear Cell In Vitro Mitogen-Stimulated Activation Following Space Flight

Program	Date	# Flights	# Crew	Flight Duration (days)	Reported Results
Apollo	1968-1970	7	21	6 to 11	Normal PHA-stimulated RNA and DNA synthesis (Fisher et al, 1972)
Skylab	1973-1974	3	7	28, 59, 84	Reduced PHA-stimulated RNA and DNA synthesis (Kimzey, 1977)
Apollo-Soyuz Test Project	1975	1	3	9	Reduced PHA-stimulated thymidine uptake and variable responses to Con A and PWM (Criswell, 1977)
Shuttle	1981-1984	10	36	2 to 6	Reduced PHA-stimulated thymidine uptake (Taylor et al, 1986)
TOTALS		21	69	294	

During the Apollo program, PHA-stimulated DNA and RNA synthesis were estimated by measuring 1-hour ^{3}H-thymidine and ^{3}H-uridine lymphocyte uptake at 72 and 24 hours in culture, respectively. The authors found that postflight results were within the normal range of values; therefore they concluded that short-duration spaceflights were not associated with immune suppression (Fisher et al., 1972).

The PHA-stimulated thymidine and uridine uptake results following the 28-, 59- and 84-day missions of the Skylab program, however, were reported in sufficient detail so that it is possible to evaluate the assay variability, and sensitivity and to critique the results (Kimsey 1977). Table II summarizes the results of the PHA-stimulated thymidine uptake from the crew and three control subjects. A range of 8,000 to 60,000 DPM obtained from 1 normal subject on 2 occasions (Skylab 2) indicates intra-subject variability with this assay, making detection of spaceflight-induced alterations of cellular immune function difficult. The uniformly low DPMS of Skylab 3 crew and pre- and postflight controls indicate mitogenic proliferation was very poor the day preceding launch. In contrast, more stable preflight responses from Skylab 4 suggest that blunted postflight proliferative responses occurred among all three crewmembers compared with controls. The low responses the day preceding launch (Skylab 3 and 4) may have indicated in vitro immune suppression associated with anticipation of launch (stress-induced).

Table II Skylab Astonauts and Control Subjects' PBNMC PHA-Stimulated ^{3}H-Thymidine Uptake

	Crew					Controls				
	Pre-flight					Pre-flight				
Skylab 2 (28 days)	F-29	F-11		Pre-$\bar{X}$	Post	F-29	F-11		Pre-$\bar{X}$	Post
1	3	10		7	6	60	8		34	22
2	13	32		23	8	38	38		38	24
3	3	32		18	21	42	37		39	15
Skylab 3 (59 days)	F-1				Post	F-1				Post
1	3				2.5	10				16
2	1.5				1.0	14				15
3	0.8				.7	13				14
Skylab 4 (84 days)	F-30	F-7	F-1	Pre $\bar{X}$	Post	F-30	F-7	F-1	Pre $\bar{X}$	Post
1	15	30	8	18	8	21	36	9	22	17
2	17	24	9	9	6	50	22	8	27	35
3	12	24	13	13	4	45	22	13	27	12

Data represent cpm (10^{-3}) per 10^6 MNC cultured (Kimsey, 1977)
PBMNC = peripheral blood mononuclear cells

The wide variation in results observed among subjects in the Apollo and Skylab missions was probably related to the methodology employed 10 to 15 years ago. Possible sources of variation which could influence assay sensitivity include the following: depleting adherent cells (monocytes and B cells) via a nylon wool column used for isolation of lymphocytes; variations in the mitogenic potency of nonpurified PHA; non-uniform lots of FCS (Apollo) or human AB serum (Skylab); diurnal variations and delay in culturing cells following collection (Apollo); measuring radiolabeled thymidine uptake in intact cells; and the inability to accurately determine the exact number of cells cultured or any combination of the above factors.

The mitogenic responses of mononuclear cells obtained from the Apollo-Soyuz crew have been reported to indicate a reduced postflight PHA-stimulated ^{3}H-thymidine uptake (Criswell 1977). The variability of preflight responses reported as stimulation indexes was so great for the Con A and PWM-stimulated responses that the author correctly chose not to comment on the significance of those postflight responses. This mission was unique, however, since the crew inhaled N_2O_4 during reentry. This toxic exposure resulted in radiographic evidence of pneumonitis and arterial O_2 desaturation within 24 hours (Nicogossian et al., 1977). Despite receiving high dose glucocorticoid therapy, 2 of the 3 crew had normal PHA-stimulated thymidine uptake responses 8 days after splashdown. Therefore, this assay was insensitive for detecting drug- induced immune depression. As a result it is not surprising that earlier studies failed to detect significant postflight immune suppression. These confounding variables make interpretation difficult despite some improved changes in the assay including ficoll-hypaque gradient separation and using an automatic harvester following a 2-hour pulse.

PHA-stimulated tritiated thymidine uptake was determined by a more sensitive assay from 36 crewmembers following the first 11 flights of the Space Shuttle (Taylor et al., 1986). Using optimum incubation times (72, 84 or 96 hours) and mitogenic concentrations of PHA, Taylor reported a decrease of 33+3% (mean +S.E.M.) from 29 crewmembers who exhibited a reduced maximal proliferative response compared to 3 preflight baseline values. Only 5 crewmembers had an increase response postflight (1%, 9%, 13%, 24%, and 44%). Cell surface phenotype analysis was also performed on mononuclear cells from 11 crewmembers prior to culture. An association between the postflight decrease in the percentage of M_3 positive cells (r=.697) and the change in postflight tritiated thymidine uptake was noted; whereas, no significant changes or correlations were detected between B_1, T_4 or T_8 populations of lymphocytes.

The Soviet postflight immunology studies have been reviewed and summarized by Cogoli (1980 and 1984). While the Soviet investigators have also reported impaired mitogenic responses following most missions (Konstantinov et al, 1978; Vorob'yev et al., 1984), the lack of published details regarding their immunologic methods prevents a critical analysis of their data or conclusions.

Cogoli and colleagues have been the pioneers of gravitational immunobiology and this area has been reviewed by Barone and Caren (1984). The effects of gravity per se on mitogen-induced in vitro lymphocyte proliferation has been studied by Cogoli for the past 10 years. Cogoli's group first reported that maximum Con A-stimulated thymidine incorporation in mouse spleen cells occurred 24 hours earlier during 2-G culture conditions compared with 1-G control cells (Cogoli et al., 1979). Con A-stimulated human lymphocytes exhibited a 50% reduction in thymidine uptake compared with 1-G controls when cultured in a rapidly rotating clinostat device simulating "functional weightlessness" (Cogoli et al., 1980). They also reported increased Con A-stimulated thymidine incorporation into human lymphocytes during 10-G, which exceeded the 20-30% increase observed in 4 different cell lines: HeLa, chicken fibroblasts, sarcoma cells and Friend leukemia virus transformed cells (Tschopp and Cogoli, 1983). In addition, Tschopp and Cogoli also demonstrated that this effect was independent of the increased hydrostatic pressure associated with centrifugation (Tschopp and Cogoli, 1983). During Spacelab 1 Cogoli and colleagues reported that cultured human mononuclear cells stimulated with Con A in flight had a 97% reduction in thymidine incorporation compared with ground 1-G controls, despite good glucose utilization and viability in 8 ml culture tubes containing 2 x 10^6 cells/ml (Cogoli et al., 1984). This finding was reproduced in an expanded protocol during the D-1 Spacelab mission which also included an in-flight 1-G control reference centrifuge in addition to ground controls (Bechler and Cogoli, 1986). Furthermore, they confirmed a postflight decrease in Con A-stimulated lymphocyte responsiveness which returned to preflight values in one astronaut by day 7 and another by day 13. The 50% blunted response observed in the 1-G flight control centrifuge is especially interesting because the effects of intermittently stopping the centrifuge in microgravity, with subsequent disruption of sedimented cells or biophysical changes in cells secondary to microgravity (more spheroid shape or alteration in cell morphology) during activation, may have prevented an optimum response. This landmark experiment provides the strongest evidence that microgravity per se may blunt T cell activation.

Therefore, in summarizing the U.S.post-spaceflight in vitro cellular immunology studies, the methods used before Shuttle were probably only sensitive enough to detect dramatically impaired in vitro activation responses. Nevertheless, the blunted responses following the 84-day mission of Skylab 4 suggest that long-duration flights induce responses similar to those observed post-Shuttle flights. The return of responses to preflight values within 1 to 2 weeks post-landing (Skylab and Shuttle) indicate that spaceflight induced altered immune function is quickly reversed upon return to Earth. This prompt recovery, the lack of association between mission duration and in vitro responses (Skylab or Shuttle), the low preflight responses the day before liftoff on Skylab 3 and 4 missions, and lower responses during the test phase of the Shuttle (first 4 flights) suggest that blunted post-spaceflight responses could be stress-induced and do not necessarily reflect microgravity-impaired responses.

We have performed a number of in vitro immunology studies on subjects' PBMNC following exposure to various environmental stressors to determine the following:

1) If physiological responses which accompany stress could induce similar responses to those observed post-space flight;

2) Which in vitro immune assays are most sensitive to stress or neuroendocrine-mediated influences; and

3) Possible mechanisms for stress-induced impaired in vitro mononuclear cell activation.

MATERIALS AND METHODS

SAMPLE PREPARATION

Peripheral blood mononuclear cells were obtained from volunteers participating in the following separate studies:

1) A decompression chamber exposure simulating extravehicular activity of U.S. Astronauts at NASA-Johnson Space Center (Meehan et al., 1985)

2) An altitude chamber study simulating a 6-week ascent from sea level to 29,000 ft, resulting in progressive hypobaric hypoxia (Operation Everest II, U.S. Army Research Institute of Environmental Medicine, Natick MA.)

3) A psychological stress study associated with major academic examinations by first-year UTMB medical students.

All subjects were healthy, denied using any drugs and freely gave informed consent. Approval was granted by Institutional Human Subject Review Committees (NASA, U.S.Army and UTMB). Peripheral blood was collected into sterile vacutainer tubes containing heparin (Becton-Dickinson) and within 1-hour after collection, mononuclear cells were isolated over ficoll-Hypaque (Sigma) density gradients as previously described (Taylor and Dardano, 1983). Activation assays were performed in triplicate 200ul wells using round bottom microtiter plates (Linbro) at 1.0 $x10^6$ mononuclear cells/ml in RPMI 1640 (Gibco) containing 5% 200mM glutamine (Gibco), 20% HIFCS (Gibco), or in some cultures, 20% autologous plasma and 1% v/v antibiotic (PCN, amphotericin and streptomycin-Gibco). Multiple concentrations of PHA (.1,.5, 1, 3, and 5 ug/ml Burroughs-Wellcome) and PWM (1:100, 1:200 and 1:400 Gibco) were used to determine the optimum mitogenic dose for each subject. Activation assay results were expressed as cpm per 1.0 $x10^6$ cells cultured. Protein synthesis was determined after 24 hours in culture following a 3-hour pulse with ^{35}S-methionine (2 uCi/well-sp. act. 1mCi/mM) as previously described (Meehan and Ashman, 1984). ^{3}H-Thymidine uptake was determined at 72 hours in culture following a 2-hour pulse with 1uCi/well as previously described (Taylor and Dardano, 1983), to allow comparison with data obtained post spaceflight.

Peripheral blood was collected in EDTA and mononuclear cells were stained by indirect immunoflourescence using monoclonal antibodies. Phenotype positive cells were analyzed by flow cytometry for the simulated EVA study as previously described (Taylor et al., 1986; Meehan et al., 1986). Direct immunoflourescence using phycoerythrin-conjugated MoAb (Becton-Dickinson) was used for the Academic stress and Hypoxia studies (anti-leu3a, anti-leu2a, anti-leuM_3, anti-leu11c, anti-leu_{12}, and anti-HLe1).

Statistical data analysis was performed with the UTMB-CRC Clinfo^R data management system. Data are reported as mean $\pm$ standard error of the mean. The results from multiple control and test days were analyzed by ANOVA with repeated measures-BMDP and significant differences were identified with the University of Rochester Weighted Multivariate ANOVA system. A paired t test was used on data from only 2 test periods. Linear regression analysis was performed on data to identify significant correlations.

RESULTS

Association Between Monocytes and T Helper/Suppressor Subsets on PHA- and PWM-Stimulated Thymidine Uptake

The combined data from the Academic stress and Hypoxia studies are displayed in Figures 1,2,4 and 5. The control data are from 9 male students, 3 weeks prior to their first major, medical school exam (stress) and from 7 male subjects during sea level in the

Hypoxia study. Stress data corresponded to samples obtained between 7 and 8 a.m. on the exam morning and after a 4-week ascent to 25,000 ft. A significant depression of PHA-stimulated thymidine uptake was observed in both studies during exposure to stressful environments (108+7 vs 85+5 cpm x 10^3 for academic stress $p<.01$ and 129+7 vs 106+12 cpm x 10^3 for hypoxic stress $p<.001$, control vs stress respectively). The unstimulated culture thymidine uptake values were similar between stress and nonstress periods (4+1 vs 4+1 cpm x 10^3 academic and 6+1 vs 8+1 cpm x 10^3 hypoxia). A significant correlation ($r=-.841$, $p<.005$) between the percentage of cultured monocytes (M_3 cells) and PHA-stimulated thymidine uptake was only observed in the medical students during the control period as shown in Figure 1. Despite reduced thymidine uptake at 72 hours in both separate studies during stress, no significant correlations were apparent between monocytes and proliferation responses during the stress periods.

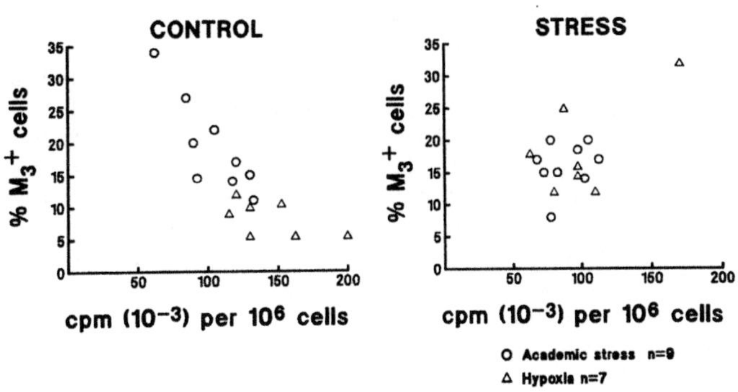

Figure 1. The relationship between the percentage of M_3+ cultured peripheral blood mononuclear cells and PHA-stimulated thymidine uptake by subjects participating in 2 different stress studies.

As noted in Figure 2, there were also no significant correlations between the percentages of cultured mononuclear cells expressing the T-cell surface phenotype subset markers (as ratios of Helper to Suppressor cells) and PHA-stimulated thymidine uptake. There were also no significant differences observed between control and stress periods in the percentage of cultured B-cells (leu12+), T Helper (leu3a+), T Suppressor (leu2a+) or NK cells (leu11c+ cells were only identified in the academic study). A stress-induced increase in monocytes (leu M_3+) was observed during hypoxia (9+1% vs 19+3% sea level vs 25,000ft $p<.05$), but not academic stress (19+2% vs 16+1% control vs stress). Therefore, the blunted PHA-stimulated thymidine uptake responses following 2 different stressors (academic and hypoxic) cannot be accounted for exclusively by culturing different proportions of monocytes, T Helper or T Suppressor subsets.

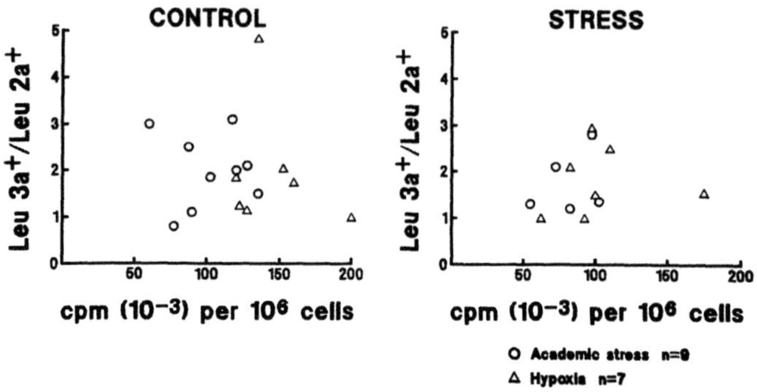

Figure 2. The relationship between cultured cells positive for leu3a+/leu2a+ antigens and PHA-stimulated thymidine uptake from subjects participating in 2 stress studies.

The results from 15 men and 13 women participating in the simulated EVA study were also analyzed to identify any associations between stress and changes in mononuclear cell subsets. Blood was obtained twice from each subject at 3 p.m. (pre chamber) and 24 hours later after completing the chamber exposure which included a 6-hour 100% O_2 prebreathe (14.7 psi) followed by 6 hours of simulated EVA activity at 4.3 psi. Despite this intervention, which also included loss of normal sleep patterns and venous bubbles detected by precordial doppler in 1/3 of the subjects, no changes were detected in any cell phenotypes before or after chamber exposure (M_3+, T_4+, T_8+ or leu12+). We were also unable to detect any differences in PHA-stimulated thymidine uptake following this acute stress episode (Meehan et al., 1986). There were no significant correlations between the percentage of M_3+ or T_4+/T_8+ cultured cells and mitogen stimulated activation (Figure 3) either before or after chamber exposure.

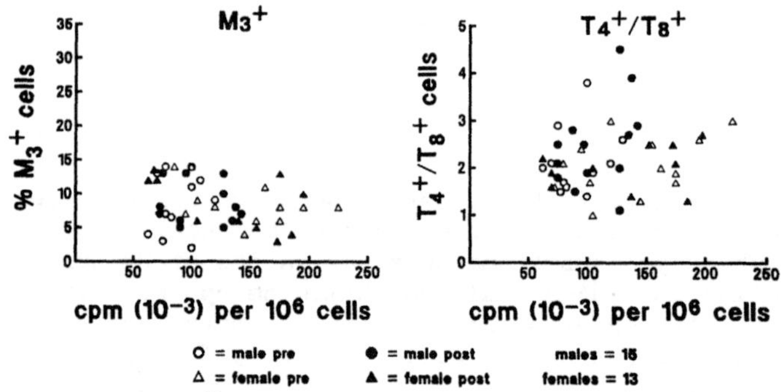

Figure 3. The association between cultured M_3+ and T_4+/T_8+ mononuclear cells and PHA-stimulated thymidine uptake from subjects before and after exposure to a decompression chamber simulating EVA conditions.

The combined data from the Academic and Hypoxia studies during PWM-stimulated thymidine uptake are displayed in Figure 4. There were no significant associations between thymidine uptake and the percentage of cultured monocytes during stress or control days. This lack of association was also true for leu3a+/leu2a+ cells (data not shown). Therefore, a reduced PWM-stimulated thymidine uptake during stress was similar to the PHA responses (Figure 1) since reduced proliferation occurred unassociated with culturing different percentages of monocytes or T-cell subsets. The combined data from all subjects participating in these various studies also suggest that inter-subject variations in mitogen-stimulated proliferative responses are not exclusively due to culturing different percentages of various mononuclear cell phenotypes.

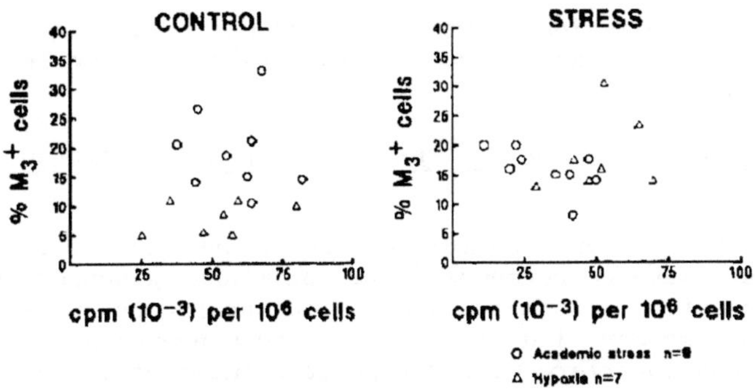

Figure 4. The association between cultured M_3+ cells and PWM-stimulated thymidine uptake using mononuclear cells from subjects participating in 2 stress studies.

Association Between Monocytes and T Helper/Suppressor Subsets on Mitogen-Induced Protein Synthesis

We had previously analyzed PWM-stimulated human mononuclear cell protein synthesis to investigate the contribution of cellular interactions on biochemical events which influence early B-cell activation signals (Meehan and Ashman, 1984). Therefore, we measured PWM-stimulated ^{35}S-methionine incorporation to determine if stress-induced immunoregulatory influences could be detected within the first 24 hours of activation in culture. Since monocytes contribute greatest to this PWM-stimulated protein synthetic response (compared with equal numbers of B-cells or T-cells) in a serum-free system, the demonstration of a slight positive trend ($r=.63$, $p=.07$) between the percentage of cultured monocytes and PWM-stimulated protein synthesis noted in Figure 5 was not surprising. A reduced PHA and PWM-stimulated protein synthetic response (36+1 vs 21+1 cpm x10^3 control vs stress for PHA $p<.001$, and 14+1 vs 10+1 cpm x10^3 control vs stress for PWM $p<.001$) was observed after the first 24 hours in culture during academic stress. As a result, reduced PHA and PWM-stimulated proliferation responses are preceded by reduced mitogen stimulated protein synthesis following stress.

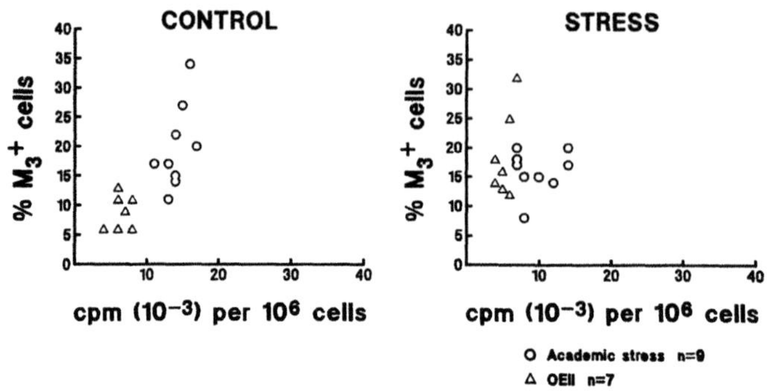

Figure 5. The association between cultured M_3+ cells and PWM-stimulated protein synthesis from subjects participating in 2 different stress studies.

Effect of Autologous Plasma on Impaired Mitogenic Activation following Stress

One possible explanation for impaired blastogenesis following stress is that elevated hormones (catecholamines, glucocorticoids, brain peptides etc.) or other unidentified substances present at the time of phlebotomy may bind or adhere to the mononuclear cell surfaces or receptors and interfere with mitogenic-stimulated activation signals. To investigate this possible mechanism, we simultaneously cultured each subject's cells in 20% autologous plasma in addition to 20% fetal calf serum during stress and nonstress periods. The results of this strategy are summarized in Table III. There was no difference between autologous plasma before or after stress in the EVA study. There were also no differences in thymidine uptake measured at the same times with 20% FCS (Meehan et al, 1986). In contrast, mononuclear cells obtained during academic stress had a 30% reduction in PHA-stimulated (1ug/ml) thymidine uptake with autologous plasma, which was less than the 40% reduction noted with fetal calf serum. A failure of autologous plasma to aggravate stress-induced blunted mitogen responses was also observed following another academic stress exposure (Meehan et al., 1985). A 48% reduction in maximum PHA-stimulated thymidine uptake occurred during an academic examination compared with 10 days later (control). No reduction was observed, however, in cultures with 20% autologous plasma collected and stored at -20°C from stress vs nonstress periods and in PHA-stimulated thymidine uptake from cells obtained during a nonstress period.

Table III Effect of Autologous Plasma on PHA Stimulated ^{3}H-Thymidine Uptake Stress vs Non-Stress

	20% FCS			20% AD		
EVA	CONTROL	STRESS		CONTROL	STRESS	
N=35	103±7	110±7		105±5	107±5	
ACADEMIC STRESS						
N=8	100±6	61±4	(↓40%)	141±14	98±10	(↓30%)

ALL DATA ARE $\bar{x}$ ± S.E.M. (10^{-3}) OF PHA (1μG/ML) STIMUALTED CULTURES HARVESTED AT 72 HOURS AFTER A TWO HOUR PULSE WITH ^{3}H-THYMIDINE.

We have performed PHA and PWM-stimulated in vitro lymphocyte activation studies on PBMNC from 60 subjects following exposure to various stressors including an altitude of 25,000 ft which is incompatible with successful adaptation,(Meehan and Zavala, 1982). We have not, however, observed the dramatic reductions in mitogen-stimulated thymidine uptake which were reported from in flight experiments performed on the Shuttle Spacelab missions (Cogoli et al., 1984 and Bechler and Cogoli, 1986). Therefore, we investigated the hypothesis that reduced cell densities per se (occurring during culture in microgravity ($2x\ 10^6$ cells/ml in 8 ml tubes) could impair mitogen-stimulated proliferation. The results in Table IV are from 3 separate subjects using round and flat bottom 200ul wells containing cells at various concentrations. Data are reported as cpm per million cells cultured. As noted, a ten fold reduction in final cell concentrations resulted in almost complete loss of PHA-stimulated thymidine uptake in flat bottom wells; whereas less reduction was noted in the round bottom wells. Therefore, while we used different culture conditions than those used during prior in flight experiments, this data supports the hypothesis that the profound loss of mitogen-induced DNA synthesis in PBMNC during 0-G culture reflect the loss of normal cellular interactions provided by higher cell densities which are necessary for optimum in vitro activation and proliferation.

Table IV Effect of Cell Density on PHA-Stimulated ^{3}H-Thymidine Uptake

	Round Bottom			Flat Bottom		
Cultured Cell Concentrations	Unstimulated	PHA	% of Max PHA	Unstimulated	PHA	% of Max PHA
2.0×10^6	8±2	83±8	(100%)	7±1	127±10	(100%)
1.0×10^6	4±1	84±5	(100%)	4±1	123±9	(97%)
$.5 \times 10^6$	4±1	56±14	(68%)	4±1	74±12	(59%)
$.1 \times 10^6$	4±2	18±2	(22%)	8±2	11±4	(9%)

Data are $\bar{x}$ ± S.E.M. cpm (10^{-3}) per 10^6 cells cultured from 3 subjects

DISCUSSION

The result of postflight PBMNC mitogen-induced in vitro thymidine uptake responses have been reviewed. While the results from more sensitive assays indicate blunted responsiveness, the magnitude of this reduction is certainly less than in-flight Con A-stimulated thymidine uptake observed during microgravity conditions on Spacelab 1 and D1. The most likely explanation for these disparate results is that postflight responses reflect stress-induced neuroendocrine mediated-alterations in immune regulation; whereas in-flight impaired mitogenesis is due primarily to unique 0-G related cell culture conditions. Since Con A-stimulated lymphocytes flown on Spacelab 1 had microscopic evidence of agglutination, as well as increased glucose utilization (compared with non-mitogen cultures), the cells probably underwent some early activation events. The failure to undergo mitogenesis in 0-G, as reflected by virtually no Con A-stimulated thymidine uptake, is probably due to insufficient cell contact with accessory cells and/or the subsequent generation of immunoregulatory cytokines (IL_1 and IL_2) in sufficient concentration in the microenvironment for biochemical amplification responses (example, up regulation of IL_2 receptors) to proceed. The importance of cellular interactions and accessory cells in mitogen-stimulated T-cell mitogenesis has been reviewed by Unanue (1981) and clarified by the report of Davis and Lipsky (1985). We have used various cell concentrations and well bottom geometries in this paper to demonstrate that greatly reduced PHA-stimulated thymidine uptake similar to the responses obtained by Con A in microgravity could occur by reducing in vitro cell densities.

Lectin stimulated mitogenesis involves a complex series of biochemical processes including: cross linking of surface molecules, cation and Ca++ influx, increased synthesis of phospholipids, proteins, cyclic nucleotides, and increased glucose utilization (Ashman, 1984). For the reasons listed above and/or due to biophysical cellular properties altered in reduced gravity, activation by Con A was probably not followed by normal DNA synthesis in microgravity.

No apparent positive correlations were observed between mission duration and reduction of mitogen-stimulated responses following the Soviet or American flights. Responses usually returned to preflight values within 2 weeks after landing. We have obtained similar reduced responses in normal subjects following exposure to various stressors. Therefore, blunted post-spaceflight mitogenic activation responses are probably due to stress per se.

Our studies indicate that while stress-induced blunted thymidine uptake can be associated with an increase in monocytes (hypoxia stress), it can also occur without changes in monocytes and does not depend upon changes in T Helper or Suppressor subsets. Furthermore, alterations in PHA- and PWM-induced activation can be detected as early as 24 hours in culture at the level of mitogen-increased protein synthesis. One possible mechanism for impaired mitogen-induced blastogenesis following stress could involve modulation of biochemical signals (via hormone-receptor interactions which blunt protein synthesis during the first 24 hours of mitogenic activation. Our studies with autologous plasma, however, suggest that the reduced in vitro responsiveness to mitogen following stress may involve more complex regulatory signals rather than simply reflect depressed in vitro T cell function due to the presence of various stress hormones.

Neuroendocrine modulation of human T-cell function following stressful events (including spaceflight) could be investigated by using lymphocyte activation strategies which have been useful in elucidating mechanisms of altered immune regulation in diseases (Fauci et al., 1983). Since the CNS and immune system interact as a regulatory circuit complete with feedback mechanisms and share common peptide hormones and receptors (Blalock and Smith, 1985), future studies may need to focus on the role of endogenous brain peptides and other hormones in modulating human T cell function following exposure to various stressful events.

Acknowledgements

The contributions of multiple collaborators in these studies were essential including; G. Taylor, U. Duncan, and L. Neale. The Principal Investigators for OE II, C. Houston, J. Sutton and A. Cymerman, and J. Waligora for the EVA study, were generous for allowing us to study their subjects. Secretarial assistance from Elaine Singleton and editorial support from Lynn Buguo were also greatly appreciated. Support was provided to R.Meehan by a 1984 and 1985 NASA/ASEE summer faculty fellow at the Johnson Space Center and NASA contract NAG -170 for the Academic Stress study. The UTMB CRC is supported by NIH grant MOI RR00073 .

BIBLIOGRAPHY

Ashman, R. F., 1984, Lymphocyte activation, in: "Fundamental Immunology," W. E. Paul ed., Raven Press, New York.

Barone, R. P., and Caren, L. D., 1984, The immune system: effects of hypergravity and hypogravity, Aviat. Space Environ Med. 55:1063.

Bechler, B., and Cogoli, A., 1986, Lymphozyten sind schwerkraftempfindlich, Naturwissenschaften 73:400.

Blalock, J.E., and Smith, E. M., 1985, A complete regulatory loop between the immune and neuroendocrine system, Am. Soc. Exp. Biol. 44:108.

Canby, T. Y., 1986, Are the soviets ahead in space?, Natl Geographic 170:420.

Cogoli, A., Valluchi-Morf, M., Bohringer, H. R., Vanni M.R., and Muller, M., 1979, Effect of gravity on lymphocyte proliferation, Life Sci. Space Res. 17:219.

Cogoli, A., Valluchi-Morf, M., Mueller, M., and Briegleb, W., 1980, Effect of hypogravity on Human lymphocyte Activation, Aviat. Space Environ. Med. 51:29.

Cogoli, A., 1981, Hematological and immunological changes during space flight, Acta/Astronatica 8:995.

Cogoli, A., Tschopp, A., and Fuchs-Bislin, P., 1984, Cell sensitivity to gravity, Science 225:228.

Cogoli, A., and Tschopp, A., 1985, Lymphocyte reactivity during spaceflight, Immunology today, 6:1.

Criswell, B. S., 1986, Cellular immune response experiment MA-031, in: Apollo-Soyuz test project Preliminary Science Report, TM X 581783 U.S. Govt. Printing office Washington D.C.

Davis, L., and Lipsky, P. E., 1985, Signals involved in T cell activation, J Immunol. 135:2946.

Fauci, A. S., Lane, H. C., and Volkman, D. J., 1983, Activation and regulation of human immune responses: implications in normal and disease states. Ann. Int. Med. 99:61.

Fischer, C.L., Daniels, J. C., Levin, W.E., Kimzey, S.L., Cobb, E. K., and Ritzmann, S.E., 1972, Effects of the space flight environment on Man's immune system: II. Lymphocyte counts and reactivity, Aerospace Med. 43:1122.

Kimzey, S.L., 1977, Hematology and Immunology Studies, in: "Biomedical Results From Skylab" NASA SP-377, U.S. Govt. Printing Office, Washington D.C.

Konstantinova, I.V., Nefedov, Y. G., Yeremin, A. V., Drozdova, V.I., Skryabin, A. S., Guseva, D. A., and Mukhina, N.N., 1978, Immunological reactivity and prediction of allergic complications in the crew of the second expedition of Salyut-4, Space Biol Med 12:16 [translation of Kosmicheskaya Biologiya i Aviakosmicheskaya Meditsina 12:15.]

Meehan, R.T., Dardano, J.R., Neale, L., Yokoyama W., and Taylor, G.R., 1985, Effect of Stress on human lymphocyte activation, Clin. Res. 33:509A.

Meehan, R. T., and Ashman, R.F., 1985, Early protein synthesis in activated human peripheral blood mononuclear cells, Mol. Immunol. 22:1893.

Meehan, R. T., Duncan, U., Neale, L., Waligora, J., and Taylor, G.R., 1985, The use of decompression to simulate the effect of extravehicular activity on human lymphocyte activation, in: "Proceedings of the 2nd International Conf. on Space Physiology." ESA SP-237

Meehan, R.T., and Zavala, D. C., 1982, The pathophysiology of acute high altitude illness. Am. J Med.73:393.

Nicogossian, A. E., LaPinta, C. K.,Burchard, E. C., Hoffler, G.W., and Bartelloni, P. J., 1986, Crew health, in: "The Apollo-Soyuz Test Project Medical Report," NASA SP- 411, U.S. Govt. Printing Office Washington D.C.

Taylor, G. R., and Dardano, J. R., 1983, Human cellular immune responsiveness following space flight, Aviat. Space Environ. Med. 54:S55

Taylor, G. R., Neale, L.S., and Dardano, J. R., 1986, Immunological analysis of U.S. Space Shuttle crewmembers, Aviat. Space. Environ. Med. 57:213.

Tschopp, A., and Cogoli, A., 1983, Hypergravity promotes cell proliferation, Experientia 39:1323.

Unanue, E.R.,1981 The regulatory role of macrophages in antigenic stimulation, II: symbiotic relationship between lymphocytes and macrophages, Advances in Immunology 31:1.

Vorob'yev, Y.I., Gazenko, O.G., Genin, A. M., Gurovskiy, N.N., Yegorov,A.D., and Nefedov, Y. G., 1984, Main results of medical studies on Salyut-6-Soyuz program. Space Biol. Med. 18:27, [Translation of Kosmicheskaya Biologiya i Aviakosmicheskaya Meditsina 18:22].

THE MAMMALIAN HEAT SHOCK (OR STRESS) RESPONSE:
A CELLULAR DEFENSE MECHANISM

William J. Welch

Cold Spring Harbor Laboratory
Cold Spring Harbor, New York 11724

All organisms display homeostatic-like responses to adverse changes in their local growth environment. These responses can include temporary modifications of protein function or more long-term changes including altered patterns of gene expression which allow for adaption to the new environmental circumstance. In addition, organisms have also developed what appears to be a pre-planned strategy to confront abrupt changes in their environment such as that experienced during exposure to slightly elevated growth temperatures. This latter response, termed the heat shock response, entails the rapid and preferential synthesis of a group of proteins, the heat shock proteins, whose collective function appears to afford the cell protection until a return of the cell to its normal growth temperature (for reviews, see Ashburner and Bonner, 1979; Schlesinger et al., 1982; Craig, 1985; Subjeck and Shyy, 1986; Lindquist, 1986).

Since the initial discovery of the heat shock response in isolated salivary glands of the fruit fly, Drosophila melanogaster (Ritossa, 1962), work from many laboratories has demonstrated that all organisms, be they prokaryotes, yeast, plants, on up to all higher eukaryotes, respond in a remarkably similar fashion to elevated growth temperatures. Moreover, a heat shock like response can also occur when the cell is exposed to a wide variety of other environmental insults including amino acid analogs, various heavy metals, ethanol, certain ionophores, and agents which perturb mitochondrial function (Ashburner and Bonner, 1979; Thomas et al., 1982). Consequently, this evolutionary conserved response to environmental traumas is now more commonly referred to as the "stress" response and the proteins induced as the stress proteins. Therefore, any circumstance that results in the increased synthesis of the stress proteins constitutes a stress response with the extent of the response depending upon the particular agent used and the amount of the stress proteins produced.

Collectively, the stress proteins appear to serve a function in the protection and enhanced survival of the cell experiencing stress. For example, it has been demonstrated that cells given a mild sublethal heat shock treatment, then returned to their normal growth temperature and subsequently exposed to a second more lethal heat shock challenge, display significantly higher survival rates than do cells which are immediately brought to the lethal temperature (Gerner et al., 1976; Henle and Leeper, 1976). This phenomenon, referred to as acquired thermotolerance, appears dependent upon the production of the stress proteins. Drugs which inhibit their production or agents which result in production of non-functional stress proteins (e.g., amino acid analogs) prevent the acquisition of thermotolerance. As will be discussed later, the key to thermotolerance appears to reside in the ability of the cell to function normally when presented with conditions which are typically toxic and/or which inhibit basic cellular functions like transcription and translation.

For a considerable period of time after the discovery of heat-induced changes in Drosophila transcription patterns, the heat shock response largely remained in the hands of molecular biologists interested in the regulation and mechanisms of gene transcription. Hence, a large part of what we know regarding the response concerns those genes which encode the stress proteins and the regulatory regions which govern their expression. Only in the past ten years or so has interest been paid to the biological changes occurring in the stressed cell and the properties of the individual stress proteins. Hence, work in our laboratory has centered around defining pertinent morphological changes which occur following stress, identifying and purifying the individual stress proteins, and determining the biochemical function of the stress proteins. In what follows, I will discuss much of our present knowledge concerning the biology of the stressed cell, placing an emphasis on the properties and possible functions of the stress proteins and the work done in our laboratory.

RESULTS AND DISCUSSION

Morphological Changes Which Occur Following Stress

Using a combination of light and electron microscopy, as well as immunological methods, we have defined some of the major morphological lesions which occur in mammmalian cells when subjected to stress. We have observed that in rat embryo fibroblasts exposed to a 42.5^{o}C heat shock treatment there occurs a number of significant changes with respect to the organization of components present in both the cytoplasm and nucleus. In the case of the former, physiological stress results in a rapid collapse of the vimentin-containing intermediate filaments in and around the nucleus (Thomas et al., 1982; Welch et al., 1985; Welch and Suhan, 1985). Concomitant with this collapse we find that both the mitochondria and ribosomes similarly relocalize within this tight network of collapsed filaments. During recovery from the heat stress, the cells slowly regain normal intermediate filament morphology and both the mitochondria and ribosomes regain their normal cytoplasmic distribution. Moreover, high voltage electron microscopy reveals that the structure and integrity of the mitochondria are visibly altered following the heat shock treatment (Welch and Suhan, 1985). Specifically, the mitochondria appear enlarged and show a corresponding change in the appearance of the individual cristae. These latter changes appear analogous to those described for the mitochondrion of cells treated with various agents which interfere with either electron transport or oxidative phosphorylation (Buffa et al., 1970) and therefore are indicative of there being a perturbation in mitochondrial function following heat shock. Indeed, others have described a rapid reduction in overall ATP levels following heat shock in Tetrahymena (Findly et al., 1985). In addition, we now have preliminary evidence which indicates there to be a depolarization of the mitochondria after induction of the stress response

(Welch, in preparation). These observations, in sum, may turn out to be very significant owing to suggestions that changes in mitochondrial function may play a role in triggering the stress response and/or be integral to the ability of the cells to recover from stress.

Striking alterations also occur within the nucleus of mammalian cells after stress. We and others have observed: i) increases in the accumulation of perichromatin granules, a result perhaps consistent with the observations of Yost and Lindquist (1986) demonstrating an inhibition of hnRNA processing in heat treated Drosophila cells; ii) the appearance of rod-shaped intranuclear bodies which consist of finely packed and parallel actin microfilaments; and iii) considerable alterations in the integrity of the nucleolus, specifically a relaxation in their condensation state and changes in both the number and size of the

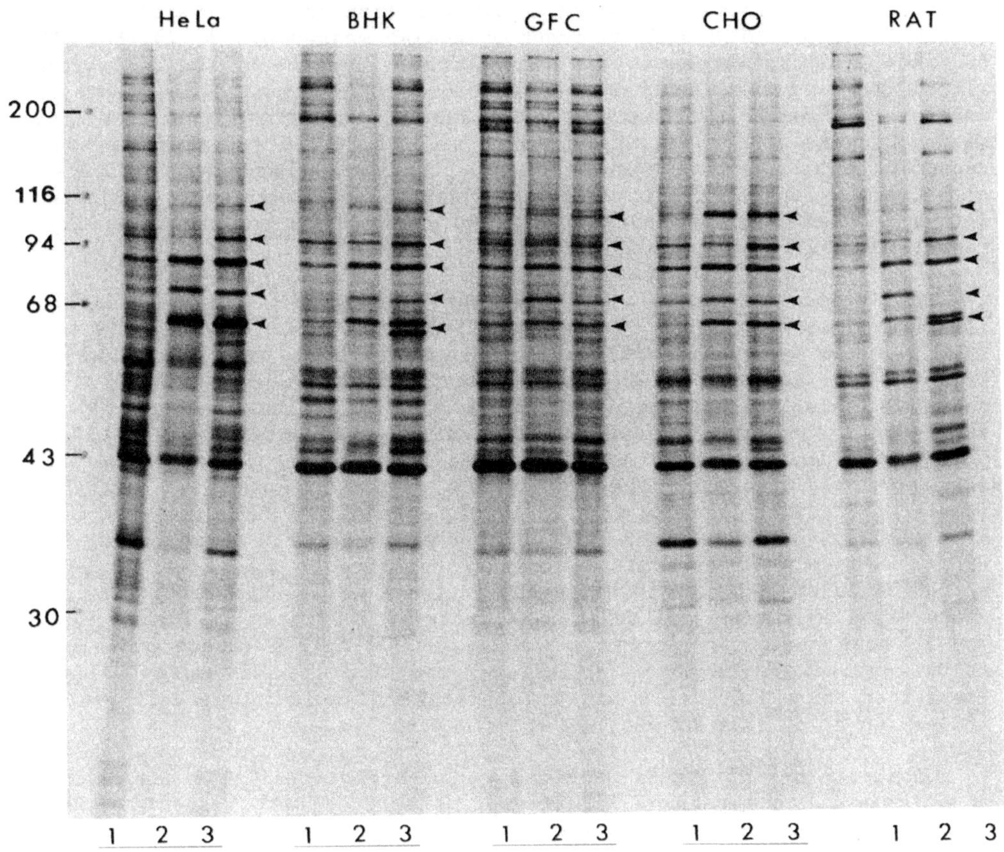

Fig. 1. Patterns of stress protein synthesis in five different mammalian cell lines. Hela, baby hamster kidney (BHK) cells, gerbil fibroma (GFC) cells, Chinese hamster ovary (CHO) cells, and rat-1 (RAT) cells were pulse-labeled with [^{35}S]-methionine after a 5 hour incubation at 37°C (lanes 1), at 37°C in the presence of 5mM Azc, an amino acid analog of proline (lanes 2) or at 42°C (lanes 3). The cells were solubilized and the labeled proteins analyzed on a 10% polyacrylamide gel. Shown is an autoradiograph of the gel. Molecular mass markers are indicated at the left and the stress proteins indicated at the right (in descending order: 110, 100, 90, 80, 73/72 kDa proteins).

pre-ribosomal granular components (Welch and Suhan, 1985). These latter changes in the structure of the nucleolus may be correlated with the observed repression of ribosomal RNA synthesis and ribosomal assembly following heat shock (Rubin and Hogness, 1975). As will be outlined below, one function of the major stress-induced protein, 72kDa, appears to be involved in the repair of such nucleolar abnormalities during recovery from heat shock treatment.

The Mammalian Stress Proteins

In Figure 1 is presented an example of the changes which occur in protein expression following induction of the stress response in five different mammalian cell lines. The cells were metabolically labeled with [^{35}S]-methionine after incubation at either the normal temperature, 37°C (lanes 1); exposure to the amino acid analog of proline, Azc (lanes 2); or after a 2 hour, 42.5^{o}C heat shock treatment (lanes 3). All of the different cell lines respond in a similar fashion by elevating the synthesis of proteins with apparent molecular masses of 72, 73, 80, 90, 100, and 110 kilodaltons (kDa). In addition, in some of the cell lines placed under stress, synthesis of most other polypeptides is somewhat reduced. Increased synthesis of the stress proteins continues even after the particular stress agent is removed with the extent of such synthesis dependent upon the stress agent itself, its amount, and the particular cell type (Welch and Suhan, 1986). In general, by 6-12 hours following return to normal growth conditions, the cells begin to regain their normal translation patterns.

The proteins synthesized in response to stress are more clearly illustrated when analyzed by two-dimensional gel electrophoresis (Figure 2). Here rat embryo fibroblasts or human Hela cells were radiolabeled with [^{3}H]-leucine at either 37°C or following exposure to a 42.5^{o}C, 2 hour heat shock treatment, and the labeled proteins analyzed by isoelectric focusing followed by SDS-gel electrophoresis on a 15% polyacrylamide gel. Such analysis reveals that: 1) all of the major stress-induced proteins are relatively acidic polypeptides with isoelectric points between pH 5.0-7.0; 2) most all of the stress proteins are synthesized at modest to even high levels in cells incubated at the normal 37°C growth temperature; and 3) synthesis of some, but not all, normal cellular proteins is decreased in those cells experiencing stress. Along with the higher molecular mass proteins indicated in Figure 1, it can be seen that there occurs a small, 28,000 dalton stress protein. 28kDa contains few methionine residues and therefore is more easily visualized when the cells are metabolically labeled with different [^{3}H]-amino acids (Kim et al., 1984; Welch, 1985).

Analysis of the stress proteins by two-dimensional gels has revealed an interesting and perhaps significant difference with respect to the 70kDa stress proteins synthesized in human cells as opposed to those synthesized in rodent cells. Both species, when cultured at 37°C, synthesize rather abundant levels of the 73kDa protein, or what is referred to as the constitutive or cognate member of the 70kDa stress protein family. After heat shock treatment, there occurs an increase in 73kDa as well as a dramatic induction of a related member, the 72kDa stress protein, in both cell types. What is different, however, is that this highly inducible 72kDa species is also constitutively synthesized in the human cells incubated at 37°C while in rodent cells little or no 72kDa can be detected at the normal growth temperature. Moreover, three other points have emerged concerning this unusual constitutive synthesis of the major stress-induced 72kDa protein in human cells: i) its expression appears cell-cycle regulated with such expression occurring at the G_1/S boundary (Milarski and Morimoto, Proc. Natl. Acad. Sci., in press); ii) 72kDa expression generally appears to increase in human cells following transformation (Welch, submitted); and iii) the expression of 72kDa increases in human cells, but not rodent cells, following transfection (or infection) with either of two cooperating oncogenes, E1A or myc (Nevins, 1982; Kingston et al., 1984).

Owing to the brevity of this report, I have compiled a table summarizing much of what we know concerning the structure and properties of the individual mammalian stress proteins. This data, presented in Table 1, consists of a composite of studies performed in our and many other laboratories and represents the current status of our understanding of the biology of the individual stress proteins. Examining each stress protein:

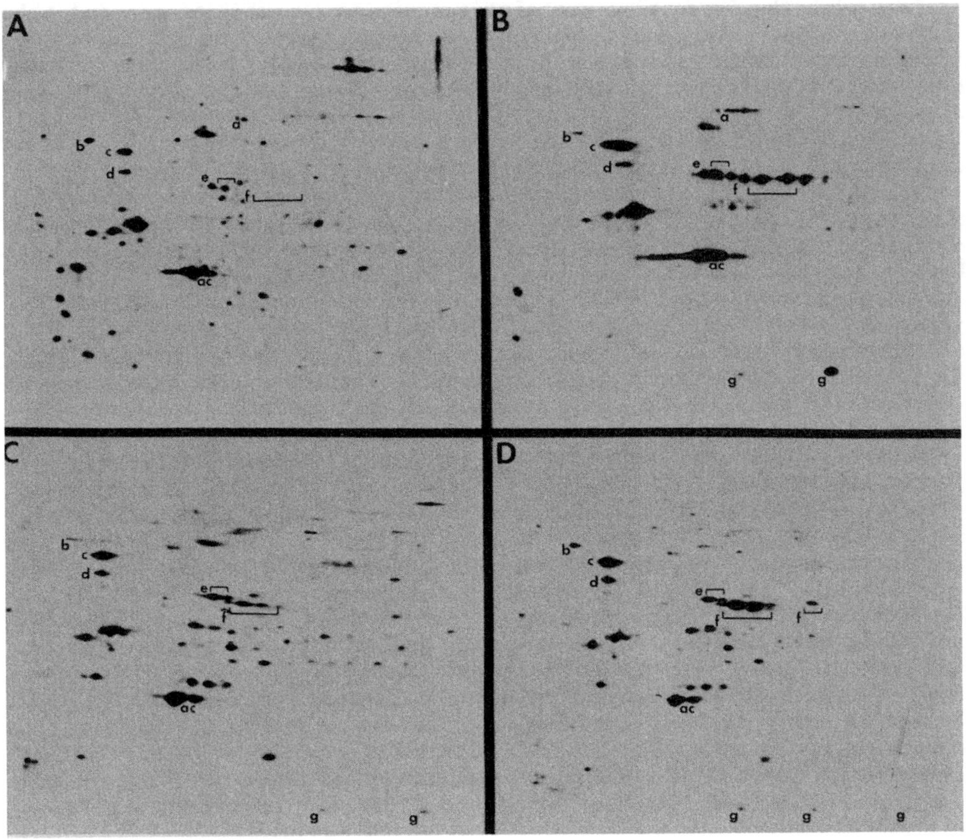

Fig. 2. Analysis of the stress proteins by two-dimensional gel electrophoresis. Rat embryo fibroblasts (REF-52) and Hela cells were incubated at either 37°C or at 42.5°C for 2 hours, were labeled with $[^3H]$-leucine and the labeled proteins analyzed by isoelectric focusing (pH 5-7) followed by SDS-gel electrophoresis on 15% polyacrylamide gels. (Acidic end of the gel is to the left.) Panel A, 37°C REF cells; panel B, 42°C REF cells; panel C, 37°C Hela cells; panel D, 42°C Hela cells. Stress proteins designation: a, 110kDa; b, 100kDa; c, 90kDa; d, 80kDa; e, 73kDa; f, isoforms of 72kDa; g, isoforms of 28kDa; ac, actin.

28kDa. Does not label efficiently with $[^{35}S]$-methionine and therefore is most commonly detected using a mixture of $[^{3}H]$-amino acids. In cells grown at 37°C, synthesis of 28kDa is quite low and is generally difficult to detect. In contrast, the protein is easily visualized in the 37°C cell following labeling with $[^{32}P]$-H_3PO_4 (Kim et al., 1983; Welch, 1985). The protein consists of at least four isoforms, three of which contain phosphate (Welch, 1985). More interesting is the fact that 28kDa phosphorylation, but not synthesis, increases dramatically in cells exposed to a variety of different mitogens or tumor promoters (Welch, 1985). Hence, it will be interesting to see if the mammalian 28kDa, like the Drosophila small molecular weight heat shock proteins, shows differential expression and/or changes in phosphorylation during early development and/or differentiation (Sirotkin and Davidson, 1982; Cheney and Shearn, 1983; Ireland and Burger, 1982; Zimmerman et al., 1983). This is suggested since the mammalian 28kDa protein exhibits sequence homology with the Drosophila proteins and similarly exhibits an unusually high native molecular mass (≥400,000 daltons) (Arrigo et al., 1985; Hickey et al., 1986; Arrigo and Welch, submitted to J. Biol. Chem. 1986). To date, the precise intracellular locale of mammalian 28kDa has not been determined.

90kDa. The mammalian 90kDa stress protein, homologous to the Drosophila 83kDa stress protein, is a very abundant protein in cells grown under normal conditions and whose synthesis increases approximately 3-5 fold after induction of stress. 90kDa is heavily phosphorylated with there being at least 12 isoforms, half of which appear to contain phosphate (Welch et al., 1983). The protein has been purified from the cytosolic fraction of cells, exists as a dimer (and perhaps higher molecular mass forms), and co-purifies with a small amount of the 100kDa stress protein (Welch and Feramisco, 1982). 90kDa has also been shown to interact with a number of other interesting intracellular proteins. For example, the protein displays a transient interaction with a number of tyrosine kinases (see review by Brugge, 1985). Specifically, newly synthesized kinases, such as $pp60^{src}$, associate with 90kDa and another cellular protein of 50kDa. While present in this complex, the src protein shows neither tyrosine kinase activity nor phosphorylated tyrosine residues. As the complex containing $pp60^{src}$ reaches its final destination at the plasma membrane, the complex dissociates with src being deposited at the inner side of the membrane and the protein now exhibiting both tyrosine kinase activity and autophosphorylated tyrosine. In a somewhat analogous situation, 90kDa is found associated with the 8S form of various steroid hormone receptor complexes (Catelli et al., 1985; Sanchez et al., 1985). Upon binding of the steroid, there is a conversion of the receptor to the biologically active 4S form with an accompanying loss of the 90kDa stress protein. These studies, then, point toward a role for the 90kDa stress protein in regulating the activity of other biologically important macromolecules.

110kDa. Of all of the members of the stress protein family, we know the least regarding the properties of this protein. 110kDa is a constitutively expressed protein whose synthesis increases approximately five-fold after stress. The protein is present within the nucleolus in what appears to be the fibrillar region, i.e., that site within the nucleolus involved in rRNA transcription (Subjeck et al., 1983).

80kDa and 100kDa. In cells placed under stress by exposure to the amino acid analog of proline, Azc, increased synthesis of the classical heat shock proteins (28, 72, 73, 90, and 110kDa) occurs along with two other proteins designated 80kDa and 100kDa. Synthesis of these latter two proteins, for the most part, does not increase very dramatically in

Table 1. Properties of Mammalian Stress Proteins

Stress Protein ($x10^{-3}$ dalton)	Modification	Location 37	Location 42	Remarks
Major				
28	phosphorylation	N.D.	N.D.	increased phosphorylation to growth factors, tumor promoters or calcium perturbations; partial homology to lens alpha crystallins; native molecular mass $\geq$400,000 daltons
72	methylation	----	cytoplasmic nuclear nucleolar	most highly induced stress protein; binds nucleotides (ATP) and perhaps RNA; portion colocalizes with ribosomes; expression in primates at 37°C and cell cycle regulated; elevated expression in human cells after transformation
73	methylation	cytoplasmic	cytoplasmic nuclear (nucleolar?)	homology with 72kDa; portion present with cycled microtubules/intermediate filaments; homology to clathrin coated vesicle uncoating ATPase
90	phosphorylation methylation	cytoplasmic	cytoplasmic (nuclear?)	abundant cellular phosphoprotein with multiple isoelectric forms; increased phosphorylation in response to ds DNA; transient association with tyrosine kinases; present in steroid hormone receptor complex; synthesis repressed following glucose/calcium deprivation
110		nucleolar	nucleolar cytoplasmic	
Minor				
80	phosphorylation ADP-ribosylation	endoplasmic reticulum	endoplasmic reticulum	increased synthesis following glucose/calcium deprivation; homology to immunoglobulin heavy chain binding protein; binds ATP and immunologically related to 72kDa/73kDa stress proteins
100	phosphorylation glycosylation	Golgi plasma membrane	Golgi plasma membrane nuclear	increased synthesis during glucose/calcium deprivation; portion associated with 90kDa stress protein

cells placed under stress by other agents such as heat shock or exposure to heavy metals. Hence, we classify 80kDa and 100kDa as special members of the stress protein family. We and others have shown that 80kDa and 100kDa are identical to the previously described "glucose regulated proteins" (Hightower, 1980; Welch et al., 1983). These are the proteins whose synthesis increases in cells grown in the absence of extracellular glucose or calcium (Shiu et al., 1977; Wu et al., 1981). Interestingly, these latter treatments, while resulting in an increased synthesis of 80kDa and 100kDa, also cause a rather significant repression in the synthesis of the 90kDa stress protein (Welch et al., 1983).

Both 80kDa and 100kDa are relatively abundant proteins in cells grown under normal conditions. Both contain phosphate and in the case of 100kDa also carbohydrate. Cell fractionation and immunological studies have shown 80kDa to be present within the endoplasmic reticulum and 100kDa to be present within the Golgi and perhaps present in the plasma membrane (Welch et al., 1983). Similarly, we now know that the 80kDa stress protein is structurally similar to the 70kDa stress protein family, and as discussed further below, 80kDa displays ATP binding properties in vitro (Welch and Feramisco, 1985). As will be discussed later, this observed relationship of the glucose regulated proteins with the major members of the heat shock protein family indicates that the stress proteins, in general, are a structurally related family of proteins who may have diverged from a small number of gene(s) and which serve similar functions in the cell, albeit within different subcellular locales.

72kDa and 73kDa. Of all of the stress proteins, we know the most concerning the so-called "70kDa" stress protein members. As was mentioned earlier, there appear to be two major members of this family: the rather abundant 73kDa protein whose synthesis is readily apparent in all cells grown under normal conditions. Consequently, 73kDa is referred to as the "cognate" or "constitutive" 70kDa stress protein. In contrast, the second member, what we refer to as 72kDa, is not obvious in most cells grown at 37°C. Rather synthesis of 72kDa, in general, occurs only after induction of the stress response and in most cases represents the major translational activity of the stressed cell. An exception to this rule occurs in primate cells, as was discussed earlier. For example, in most human and monkey cells, synthesis of 72kDa can be detected in the cells grown under normal conditions, although generally at much lower levels than that observed for 73kDa. Moreover, it appears that the levels of constitutive expression of 72kDa may be influenced by the "transformation" state of the cells. Specifically, evidence is accumulating that a number of highly transformed human cell lines (many established from isolated human tumors) express rather high levels of 72kDa (Welch and Morimoto, in preparation). In concert with this observation is the fact that certain cooperating oncogenes, including E1A and myc, when transfected into human lines, result in an increased constitutive expression of 72kDa (Nevins, 1982; Kingston et al., 1984). Indeed, human 293 cells (developed many years ago from Adenovirus infected Hela cells) express high levels of both E1A and of the 72kDa stress protein.

Immunological, biochemical, and DNA sequence analysis has demonstrated that while the 72kDa and 73kDa proteins are related, they are in fact distinct gene products (Hightower, 1980; Welch and Feramisco, 1982; Hunt and Morimoto, 1985; Lowe and Moran, 1986; O'Malley et al., 1985; Voellmy et al., 1985). In addition, both proteins show very similar biochemical properties including their stoichiometric co-purification during either gel filtration or ion exchange chromatography (Welch and Feramisco, 1982). Finally, both proteins are found to display an affinity for various nucleotides, with the highest affinity being observed for ATP (Welch and Feramisco, 1985). This property of the proteins provided the impetus by which one possible function of these proteins was recently described. Specifically, Jim Rothman's laboratory had described and purified a 70,000 dalton protein from bovine brain which, in vitro, facilitated the uncoating or release of clathrin triskelions from clathrin coated vesicles in an ATP dependent manner (Schlossman et al., 1984). The reported properties described for this uncoating ATPase appeared very similar to the properties we had observed for the human 70kDa stress protein members. Under a collaborative effort using biochemical and immunological methods, we demonstrated that the bovine uncoating ATPase was indeed similar, if not identical, to the constitutively abundant 73kDa stress protein (Chappell et al., 1986). Work from Ungewickel's laboratory (Ungewickel, 1985) served to corroborate this finding. The question then arises as to why the cell would require increased levels of a protein (e.g., 73kDa) whose function is involved with membrane biogenesis events (i.e., the shuttling of membranes via clathrin coated vesicles). A possible answer to this question follows from observations in our laboratory demonstrating that both the endoplasmic reticulum and Golgi complex fragment and vesicularize following severe heat shock treatment (Welch and Suhan, 1985). Hence, to rebuild these structures, cells recovering from heat shock might require increased amounts of a protein involved in the repair and/or rebuilding of these intracellular membranous organelles. Indeed, preliminary studies indicate a considerable increase in the amount of clathrin coated vesicles in the perinuclear region of cells recovering from heat shock treatment (Welch, unpublished observations). Such an increase in clathrin staining may represent the reformation of the endoplasmic reticulum and Golgi in the recovering cell.

Considerable efforts in our laboratory have and will continue to focus on the biology of the 72kDa stress protein. This follows from the aforementioned observations that 72kDa: i) represents the most highly induced protein in cells experiencing physiological stress; ii) appears highly conserved amongst different organisms; and iii) is integral in the protection of the cell and the acquisition of thermotolerance (discussed in more detail below). Consequently we believe that the key to understanding how cells defend against physiological stress will ultimately lie in our dissecting the function of 72kDa.

After stress, synthesis of 72kDa represents the major translation product of the cells. 72kDa consists of multiple related members, the exact number depending upon the cell type, the agent used to induce the response, and finally the severity of the stress treatment (Welch et al., 1983; Buzin and Petersen, 1982; Welch, 1985). Biochemical fractionation and immunological studies have shown that the majority of 72kDa localizes within the nucleus shortly after its synthesis (Welch and Feramisco, 1984). Here the protein appears present within the nucleoplasm, the nuclear matrix, and large amounts within the nucleoli. This nucleolar deposition of the protein always appears correlated with marked alterations in the integrity of the nucleoli. As was discussed earlier, such alterations in the nucleoli appear to coincide with a diminishment of nucleolar function, most notably the shutdown of rRNA synthesis and ribosomal assembly. Using immunoelectron microscopy, we have shown that most of the nucleolar distributed 72kDa is present within the so-called granular region--that area of the nucleolus involved in the assembly of small ribonucleoproteins and pre-ribosomes. As the nucleoli slowly regain their normal morphology during recovery from the stress treatment, there occurs a corresponding exit of 72kDa (Welch and Suhan, 1985).

During the later periods of recovery from physiological stress, the majority of 72kDa begins to accumulate within the cytoplasm. Three distinct cytoplasmic locales are observed: a strong perinuclear distribution; a portion present within unusually large and phase dense structures; and finally a portion present directly underneath the plasma membrane, again in association with phase dense material. Using electron microscopy and double-label indirect immunofluorescence analysis, we have found that much of the cytoplasmic 72kDa is in very close association with ribosomes and polysomes (Welch and Suhan, 1986) (Figure 3). This co-localization of 72kDa with the translational machinery, we think, is integral to the functioning of the protein synthesis during and after recovery from heat shock treatment (discussed further below).

A Family of ATP Binding Proteins

In the course of studies examining possible biochemical properties of the stress proteins, we discovered that the 72kDa/73kDa stress proteins displayed an affinity for various nucleotides with the highest affinity being for ATP. This property was then exploited to develop a rapid two-step purification of the proteins utilizing ion exchange chromatography followed by affinity chromatography on agarose columns containing covalently linked ATP (Welch and Feramisco, 1985). Using the cytosolic fraction from Hela spinner cells (e.g., 12,000xg supernatant from hypotonically lysed cells), it is possible to purify 3-5mg of these proteins from approximately 20-30 liters of cells using this procedure.

Because a significant fraction of both 72kDa and 73kDa is also present in the particulate fraction (12,000xg pellet from hypotonically lysed cells), we also examined whether one could purify the proteins using ATP-agarose affinity chromatography. The proteins in the particulate fraction were extracted with nonionic detergent and the proteins then applied and eluted from a DEAE-52 ion exchange chromatography. The peak fractions containing 72kDa/73kDa were then applied to and eluted off the ATP-agarose column. In addition to the 72kDa/73kDa proteins, we were somewhat surprised to find two other proteins which co-purified with the 72kDa/73kDa proteins. One of these proteins has an approximate apparent molecular mass of 75kDa and the other 80kDa. Using biochemical and immunological methods, we have determined that both of these proteins are in fact related to the 72kDa/73kDa stress proteins. Moreover, we have determined that the 80kDa ATP binding protein is identical to the above-described 80kDa glucose regulated protein, a member of the stress protein family (Welch and Feramisco, 1985). The 75kDa ATP binding protein does not appear to be a

Fig. 3. Colocalization of the 72kDa stress protein with ribosomes in cells recovering from physiological stress. REF-52 cells growing on glass coverslips were placed under stress by heat shock treatment (42.5°C for 3 hours), exposure to Azc (5mM for 10 hours), or exposure to sodium arsenite (80uM for 1.5 hours). The cells were then returned to normal culture conditions for either 4 hours (heat shock) or 8 hours (Azc and arsenite) at which time the cells were fixed and permeabilized. The cells were then incubated with a mixture of the mouse monoclonal anti-72kDa serum and the human autoimmune anti-ribosomal antibody. The primary antibodies were visualized with a mixture of rhodamine-conjugated goat anti-mouse and fluorescein-conjugated rabbit anti-human antibodies. A, D, and G are phase contrast micrographs; B, E, and H show the anti-72kDa staining; C, F, and I show the anti-ribosomal staining. (A-C) Cells heat shock treated and recovered for 4 hours. (D-F) Cells treated with Azc and recovered for 8 hours. (G-I) Cells treated with sodium arsenite and recovered for 8 hours. Bar, 20um.

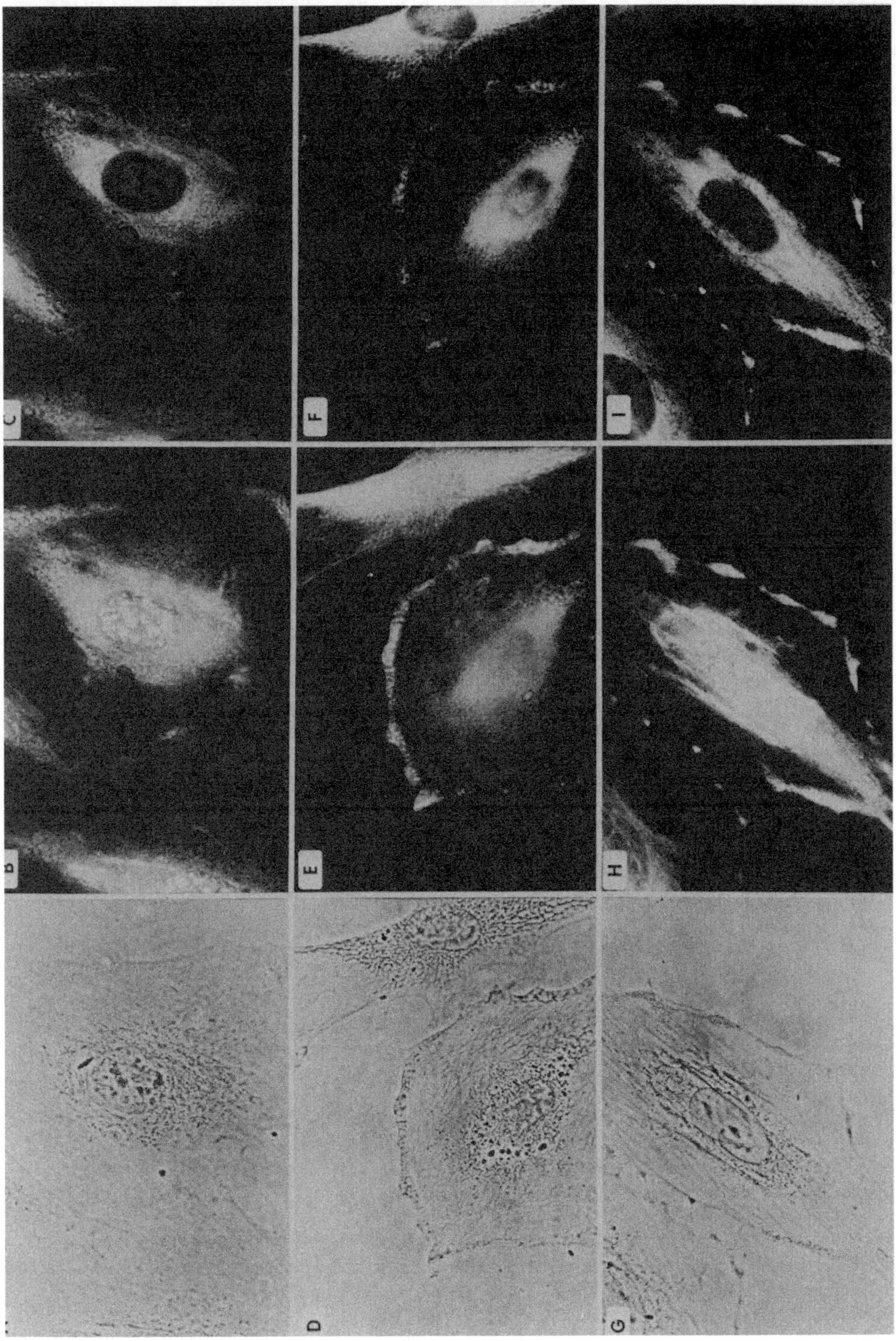
B
C
D
E
F
G
H
I

major member of the stress protein family. We do not observe any increases in its synthesis following heat shock or other forms of physiological stress. Preliminary studies, utilizing subcellular fractionation techniques, indicate that 75kDa is present within the mitochondria (Welch, unpublished results).

These studies, in sum, then indicate that a number of proteins whose synthesis increases in response to stress (e.g., 72kDa, 73kDa, and 80kDa) are structurally related proteins who also share a common property of binding ATP in vitro (summarized in Table 2). Moreover, each of these proteins appear to reside in different compartments within the cell. Specifically, 73kDa appears to reside primarily within the cytoplasm; 72kDa within the nucleus, nucleolus and cytoplasm (a portion in association with ribosomes as discussed above); and the 80kDa protein present exclusively in the endoplasmic reticulum. In the case of the non-stress-induced, ATP binding 75kDa protein, we find it present within the mitochondria. Hence the cell appears to produce a family of related ATP binding proteins, all with different intracellular locales, and which appear to function in the response of cells to environmental stress.

Possible Function of the Stress Proteins

Having described the properties, location in the cell, and biochemical interrelationships of the stress proteins, the obvious question arises as to what function these proteins serve in the cell. Because most of what we know concerns the 70kDa family, let us focus first on their possible biological role. Most workers in the field have begun to lean toward the idea that the 70kDa stress proteins serve a rather promiscuous function involved with the assembly/disassembly of proteins and/or protein-containing macromolecular complexes. More specifically, the 70kDa stress proteins appear to function in the repair of denatured proteins and/or prevent further denaturation events. Although there is no definitive data to prove this hypothesis, there does exist considerable corroborative data. First, it must be remembered that the only obvious common denominator amongst the various agents of the stress response is their ability to perturb protein structure (e.g., heat, amino acid analogs, heavy metals which bind free sulfhydryls, etc.) (see Ashburner and Bonner, 1979; Thomas et al., 1982). Hence, when

Table 2. A Family of Immunologically Related Stress Proteins Which Bind ATP

1) 73kDa: Abundant, constitutive protein whose synthesis increases modestly after stress; present in cytoplasm and nucleus; homology to clathrin coated vesicle uncoating ATPase.

2) 72kDa: Present in low or negligible levels in cells grown at 37°C; most highly induced protein after stress; highly related to 73kDa; co-localization with pre-ribosomes/RNP's in nucleolus and with cytoplasmic ribosomes; binds fatty acids.

3) 80kDa: Abundant constitutive protein whose synthesis increases modestly after stress; increased synthesis following glucose, calcium or O_2 deprivation; present in endoplasmic reticulum; homology with immunoglobulin heavy chain binding protein.

4) 75kDa: Constitutive protein whose synthesis remains the same or decreased after stress; increased synthesis following glucose/calcium deprivation; present in mitochondria.

thinking about the function of the stress proteins, one must always keep in mind that a major problem of the stressed cell is to somehow cope with an accumulation of polypeptides which may become denatured and/or aggregated. Along these lines then, it is of considerable interest that in the case of the 70kDa stress proteins one finds these proteins accumulating to rather high levels and localized throughout the stressed cell. Consequently, I would argue that the proteins are not "classical" enzymes with high catalytic activity but rather have a somewhat more promiscuous or mass action role in the stressed cell. Considering these two points in sum, most workers in the field would argue that the 70kDa stress proteins serve a general role in the assembly/disassembly of proteins or proteins containing macromolecular complexes whose structure has been perturbed by the stress treatment. Moreover, the presumed ability of the proteins to bind and hydrolyze ATP (mentioned above) may prove integral to the function of the 70kDa proteins in either refolding proteins after partial denaturation and/or protecting proteins from further denaturation.

Two recent lines of evidence point toward a role for the 70kDa stress proteins in protecting and/or restoring the function of protein-containing macromolecular complexes. First, Petersen and Mitchell (1981) have demonstrated that translation is sharply curtailed in Drosophila larvae given a rather severe heat shock treatment. If, however, the cells are first given a mild heat shock treatment, allowed to recover at the normal growth temperature and then subsequently given the more severe heat shock challenge, the cells now display a marked increased ability to translate protein. That is, similar to increased survivability, cells made thermotolerant (e.g., mild heat shock, recovery, and a second more severe heat shock), also display tolerance with respect to their translational capacity. How might the translational machinery acquire such tolerance? I suggest that one or more of the stress proteins, made during the initial heat shock treatment, becomes associated with the translational machinery during the recovery period and upon the subsequent heat shock challenge now results in protection of the translational machinery. Indeed we have now observed that the major stress-induced 72kDa protein does show a co-localization with cytoplasmic ribosomes in rat embryo fibroblasts recovering from heat shock treatment (Welch and Suhan, 1986). Moreover, we find that maximal translation in these recovering cells correlates with maximal co-localization of 72kDa with the cytoplasmic ribosomes. Finally, we find that we can also make rat embryo fibroblasts translationally thermotolerant by prior incubation of the cells under mild heat shock conditions and that such tolerance is maximal only when the cells have finished synthesizing the 72kDa stress protein (Mizzen and Welch, manuscript submitted). Similarly, tolerance can be achieved by other agents, such as sodium arsenite, which also elicit production of the heat shock proteins. Finally, we observe no tolerance if we elicit production of the heat shock proteins with amino acid analogs. However, the lack of tolerance appears to be due to the fact that the analogs, while resulting in an elevation of 72kDa, render the protein "nonfunctional" as assayed by its failure to localize within the nucleolus and/or co-localize with the cytoplasmic ribosomes. In summary then, we think it highly plausible that 72kDa, by virtue of its association with the translation machinery, serves to protect the ability of the machinery to translate proteins even under conditions (e.g., severe heat shock) which normally result in translational inhibition.

As was stated above, I think that 72kDa serves a rather general role in the stabilization of macromolecular complexes, not just the translation machinery. Consistent with this idea is the recent results of Yost and Lindquist (1986) who have shown that a brief but severe heat shock treatment in Drosophila cells results in a diminishment of hnRNA processing. However, a mild heat shock treatment followed by a recovery period before the more severe treatment rescues the ability of the cells to correctly process new mRNA transcripts. Hence, similar to the rescue of translation, the thermotolerant cell has now also regained the ability to process hnRNA.

The last piece of evidence consistent with the idea of the stress proteins being involved with the recognition and/or stabilization of altered proteins concerns the 80kDa glucose regulated stress protein. As was discussed earlier, 80kDa shows sequence homology and immunological cross-reactivity with the 70kDa stress protein family and like the 70kDa proteins binds ATP *in vitro*. However, unlike 70kDa, 80kDa is a compartmentalized protein present within the endoplasmic reticulum (Welch et al., 1983; Welch, in preparation). A clue to the function of 80kDa has come from studies demonstrating its homology to a previously described polypeptide termed the BiP protein (Munro and Pelham, 1986). This protein was first shown to show a tight association with immunoglobulin heavy chains in various myeloma cells (Morrison and Scharff, 1975; Haas and Wabl, 1983; Bole et al., 1986). Here it was found that in the absence of light chains, the heavy chains of the IgG were not transported into the Golgi but rather remained and accumulated within the endoplasmic reticulum in association with BiP. BiP has now been observed in a wide variety of different mammalian cells and has been shown to bind to a number of different mutated nascent secretory and/or transmembrane proteins which for one reason or another are not transported out of the endoplasmic reticulum. Pelham's laboratory has found that BiP (equivalent to the 80kDa stress protein) can be released from the heavy chains by incubation with ATP but not nonhydrolyzable ATP analogues (Munro and Pelham, 1986. This then is reminiscent of the previously described situation in which the 72kDa stress protein can be released from isolated nuclei/nucleoli by addition of ATP (Lewis and Pelham, 1985).

SUMMARY

The response of mammalian cells to abrupt changes in their local environment entails a series of coordinated transcription and translation events leading to the accumulation of a group of proteins, the stress proteins. As evidenced by the high similarities in the structure of the stress proteins amongst different organisms, the stress response appears to be a well-conserved, pre-planned strategy by which cells protect themselves against changes in their environmental circumstance. In addition to their presumed protective role, most of the stress proteins are expressed at significant levels in cells grown under normal conditions and participate in a number of biological phenomenon apparently distinct from their role during stress. For example, we have described here the role of some of the stress proteins in clathrin coated vesicle assembly/disassembly, tyrosine kinase and steroid hormone receptor function, and cell proliferation. In this regard it seems likely that we have only touched the surface regarding the many different biological processes which occur normally in cells and which involve the participation of the individual stress proteins.

Of particular importance, as well, is to understand the role of the stress proteins, both individually and collectively, in protecting the cell during and after recovery from physiological stress. A breakthrough in this endeavor has come from the recent observation demonstrating the structural and biochemical similarities of many of the stress proteins and notably their ability to bind ATP. In this regard, I have described the immunological and biochemical similarities of the 70kDa heat shock proteins with that of the 80kDa glucose regulated protein and suggest that this family of proteins serves basically similar functions but within different intracellular compartments: the 70kDa proteins being cytosolic and nuclear and 80kDa being present within the endoplasmic reticulum. That a general rule is emerging here comes from the recent observation of Sorger and Pelham (in press) describing a significant sequence homology of the 90kDa heat shock protein with that of the other glucose-regulated protein, 100kDa. Here again, however, the proteins are distributed differently: 90kDa is a soluble cytoplasmic protein and 100kDa is present within the Golgi and perhaps the plasma membrane (Welch et al., 1984). Might all of the stress proteins have evolved from only a few genes with selection having resulted in different compartmentalization of the stress proteins?

Finally, a picture is slowly emerging concerning the role of the major stress induced 72kDa protein (and perhaps the related 73kDa and 80kDa proteins) in protecting macromolecular complexes such as the transcription and translation machinery. This idea seems rather common sensical owing to the fact that most all of the stress inducing agents are rather potent protein denaturants. With the availability of the purified proteins (and corresponding antibodies), this idea seems readily amenable to experimental confirmation. In the next few years I feel confident that we will experience a rapid and successful furthering of our understanding of how such protection may occur at both the biochemical and cellular levels.

REFERENCES

Arrigo, A.P., Darlix, J.L., Khandijan, E.W., Simon, M., and Spahr, P.F., 1985, Characterization of the prosome from Drosophila and its similarities with the cytoplasmic structures formed by the low molecular weight heat shock proteins, EMBO J., 4:399.

Ashburner, M., and Bonner, J.J., 1979, The induction of gene activity in Drosophila using heat shock (review), Cell, 17:241.

Bole, D.G., Hendershot, L.M., and Kearney, J.F., 1986, Posttranslational association of immunoglobulin heavy chain binding protein with nascent heavy chains in secreting and nonsecreting hybridomas, J. Cell Biol., 102:1558.

Brugge, J.S., 1985, Interaction of the Rous sarcoma virus protein, pp60src, with the cellular proteins pp50 and pp90, in: "Current Topics in Microbiology and Immunology," P.D. Vogt, ed., Springer Press, Heidelberg, Germany, vol. 122.

Buffa, P., Guarriera-Bobyleva, V., Muscatello, V., and Pasquali-Ronchetti, I., 1970, Conformational changes of mitochondria associated with uncoupling of oxidative phosphorylation in vivo and in vitro, Nature (Lond.), 226:272.

Buzin, C.H., and Petersen, N.S., 1982, A comparison of the multiple Drosophila heat shock proteins in cell lines and larval salivary glands by two-dimensional gel electrophoresis, J. Mol. Biol., 158:181.

Catelli, M.G., Binart, N., Jung-Testas, I., Renoir, J.M., Baulieu, E.E., Feramisco, J.R., and Welch, W.J., 1985, The common 90kd protein component of non-transformed "8S" steroid receptors is a heat shock protein, EMBO J., 4:3131.

Chappell, T.G., Welch, W.J., Schlossman, D.M., Palter, K.B., Schlesinger, M.J., and Rothman, J.E., 1986, Uncoating ATPase is a member of the 70kDa family of stress proteins, Cell, 45:3.

Cheney, C.M., and Shearn, A., 1983, Developmental regulation of Drosophila imaginal disc proteins: synthesis of a heat shock protein under non-heat-shock conditions, Dev. Biol., 95:325.
Craig, E.A., 1985, The heat shock response, CRC Crit. Rev. Biochem., 18:239.
Findly, R.C., Gillies, R.J., and Shulman, R.G., 1983, In vivo phosphorous-31 nuclear magnetic resonance reveals lowered ATP during heat shock of tetrahymena, Science, 219:1223.
Gerner, E.W., Boone, R., Connor, W.G., Hicks, J.A., and Boone, M.L.M., 1976, A transient thermotolerant survival response produced by single thermal doses in Hela cells, Cancer Res., 36:1035.
Haas, I.G., and Wabl, M., 1983, Immunoglobulin heavy-chain binding protein, Nature, 306:387.
Henle, K.J., and Leeper, D.B., 1976, Interaction of hyperthermia and radiation in CHO cells: recovery kinetics, Radiat. Res., 66:505.
Hickey, E., Brandon, S.E., Potter, R., Stein, G., and Weber, L.A., 1986, Sequence and organization of genes encoding the human 27kDa heat shock protein, Nucleic Acids Res., 14:4127.
Hightower, L.E., 1980, Cultured animal cells exposed to amino acid analogues or puromycin rapidly synthesize several polypeptides, J. Cell. Physiol., 102:407.
Hunt, C., and Morimoto, R.I., 1985, Conserved features of eukaryotic hsp 70 genes revealed by comparison with the nucleotide sequence of human hsp 70, Proc. Natl. Acad. Sci. USA, 82:6455.
Ireland, R., and Burger, E., 1982, Synthesis of low molecular weight heat shock proteins stimulated by ecdysterone in a cultured Drosophila cell line, Proc. Natl. Acad. Sci. USA, 79:855.
Kim, Y.J., Shuman, T., Sette, M., and Przybyla, A., 1984, Nuclear localization and phosphorylation of three 25-kilodalton rat stress proteins, Mol. Cell. Biol., 4:468.
Kingston, R.E., Baldwin, A.S., Jr., and Sharp, P.A., 1984, Regulation of heat shock protein 70 gene expression by c-myc, Nature, 312:280.
Lewis, M.J., and Pelham, H.R., 1985, Involvement of ATP in the nuclear and nucleolar functions of the 70 kd heat shock protein, EMBO J., 4:3137.
Lindquist, S., 1986, The heat shock response, Ann. Rev. Biochem., 55:1151.
Lowe, D.G., and Moran, L.A., 1986, Molecular cloning and analysis of DNA complementary to three mouse M_r=68,000 heat shock protein mRNA's, J. Biol. Chem., 261:2102.
Morrison, S.L., and Scharff, M.D., 1975, Heavy chain-producing variants of a mouse myeloma cell line, J. Immunol., 114:655.
Munro, S., and Pelham, H.R.B., 1986, An HSP70-like protein in the ER: identity with the 78 kd glucose regulated protein and immunoglobulin heavy chain binding protein, Cell, 46:291.
Nevins, J.R., 1982, Induction of the synthesis of a 70,000 dalton mammalian heat shock protein by the adenovirus ElA gene product, Cell, 29:913.
O'Malley, K., Mauron, A., Barchas, J.D., and Kedes, L., 1985, Constitutively expressed rat mRNA encoding a 70-kilodalton heat shock-like protein, Mol. Cell. Biol., 5:3476.
Pelham, H.K.B., 1986, Speculations on the functions of the major heat shock glucose-regulated proteins, Cell, 46:959.
Peterson, N.S., and Mitchell, H.K., 1981, Recovery of protein synthesis after heat shock: prior heat treatment affects the ability of cells to translate mRNA, Proc. Natl. Acad. Sci. USA, 78:1708.
Ritossa, F., 1962, A new puffing pattern induced by heat shock and DNP in Drosophila, Experientia, 18:571.

Rubin, G.M., and Hogness, D.S., 1975, Effect of heat shock on the synthesis of low molecular weight RNAs in Drosophila accumulation of a novel form of 5S RNA, Cell, 6:207.
Sanchez, E.R., Toft, D.O., Schlesinger, M.J., and Pratt, W.B., 1985, Evidence that the 90kDa phosphoprotein associated with the untransformed L-cell glucocortoid receptor is a murine heat shock protein, J. Biol. Chem., 260:12398.
Schlesinger, M.J., Ashburner, M., and Tissieres, A., 1982, "Heat Shock: From Bacteria to Man," Cold Spring Harbor Laboratory, New York.
Schlossman, D.M., Schmid, S.L., Bruell, W.A., and Rothman, J.E., 1984, An enzyme that removes clathrin coats: purification of an uncoating ATPase, J. Cell Biol., 99:723.
Shiu, R.P.C., Pouyssegur, J., and Pastan, I., 1977, Glucose depletion accounts for the induction of two transformation-sensitive membrane proteins in Rous sarcoma virus-transformed chick embryo fibroblasts, Proc. Natl. Acad. Sci. USA, 74:3840.
Sirotkin, K., and Davidson, N., 1982, Developmentally regulated transcription from Drosophila melanogaster chromosomal site 67B, Dev. Biol., 89:196.
Subjeck, J., and Shyy, J., 1986, Stress protein systems of mammalian cells, Am. J. Physiol., 250:C1.
Subjeck, J.R., Shyy, T., Shen, J., and Johnson, R.J., 1983, Association between the mammalian 110,000-dalton heat-shock protein and nucleoli, J. Cell Biol., 97:1389.
Thomas, G.P., Welch, W.J., Mathews, M.B., and Feramisco, J.R., 1982, Molecular and cellular effects of heat shock and related treatments of mammalian tissue culture cells, Cold Spring Harbor Symp. Quant. Biol., 46:985.
Ungewickel, E., 1985, The 70-kd mammalian heat shock proteins are structurally and functionally related to the uncoating protein that releases clathrin triskelia from coated vesicles, EMBO J., 4:3385.
Voellmy, R., Ahmed, A., Schiller, P., Bromley, P., and Rungger, D., 1985, Isolation and functional analysis of a human 70,000 dalton heat shock protein gene segment, Proc. Natl. Acad. Sci. USA, 82:4949.
Welch, W.J., 1985, Phorbol ester, calcium ionophore, or serum added to quiescent rat embryo fibroblast cells all result in the elevated phosphorylation of two 28,000-dalton mammalian stress proteins, J. Biol. Chem., 260:3058.
Welch, W.J., and Feramisco, J.R., 1982, Purification of the major mammalian heat shock proteins, J. Biol. Chem., 257:14949.
Welch, W.J., and Feramisco, J.R., 1984, Nuclear and nucleolar localization of the 72,000-dalton heat shock protein in heat-shocked mammalian cells, J. Biol. Chem., 259:4501.
Welch, W.J., and Feramisco, J.R., 1985, Rapid purification of mammalian 70,000-dalton stress proteins: affinity of the proteins for nucleotides, Mol. Cell. Biol., 5:1229.
Welch, W.J., Garrels, J., Thomas, G.P., Lin, J.J.C., and Feramisco, J.R., 1983, Biochemical characterization of the mammalian stress proteins and identification of two stress proteins as glucose and Ca^{++}-ionophore-regulated proteins, J. Biol. Chem., 258:7102.
Welch, W.J., Feramisco, J.R., and Blose, S.H., 1985, The mammalian stress response and the cytoskeleton: alterations in intermediate filaments, Ann. N.Y. Acad. Sci., 455:57.
Welch, W.J., and Suhan, J.P., 1985, Morphological study of the mammalian stress response: characterization of changes in cytoplasmic organelles, cytoskeleton and nucleoli, and appearance of intranuclear actin filaments in rat fibroblasts after heat shock treatment, J. Cell Biol., 101:1198.
Welch, W.J., and Suhan, J.P., 1986, Cellular and biochemical events in mammalian cells during and after recovery from physiological stress, J. Cell Biol., 106; in press.

Wu, F.S., Park, Y.C., Roufa, D., and Martonosi, A., 1981, Selective stimulation of the synthesis of an 80,000-dalton protein by calcium ionophores, J. Biol. Chem., 256:5309.
Yost, H.J., and Lindquist, S., 1986, RNA splicing is interrupted by heat shock and is rescued by heat shock protein synthesis, Cell, 45:185.
Zimmerman, J.L., Petri, W., and Meselson, M., 1983, Accumulation of a specific subset of D. melanogaster heat shock mRNA's in normal development without heat shock, Cell, 32:1161.

Acknowledgements

The author greatly acknowledges the staff of the McClintock laboratory, including J.Feramisco, P. Arrigo, L. Mizzen, and J. Lamb for many helpful discussions and participation in these studies. Technical assistance of M Mulcahy, N. Kronenberg, M. Szadkowski, and P. Renna is greatly appreciated. This work was supported by National Institutes of Health grants GM 33551 and HL 23848.

PHASE PARTITIONING IN SPACE AND ON EARTH

James M. Van Alstine[1,2], Laurel J. Karr[1], J. Milton Harris[3], Robert S. Snyder[1], Stephan B. Bamberger[4], Helen C. Matsos[1], Peter A. Curreri[1], John Boyce[5], and Donald E. Brooks[4,5]

[1]Biophysics Branch, ES76, Space Science Laboratory, NASA/Marshall Space Flight Center, Huntsville, AL 35812
[2]Universities Space Research Association
[3]Department of Chemistry, University of Alabama at Huntsville, Huntsville, AL 35899
[4]Department of Neurology, Oregon Health Sciences University, Portland, OR 97201
[5]Departments of Pathology and Chemistry, University of British Columbia, Vancouver, Canada V6T 1W5

ABSTRACT

In aqueous solution at low concentrations, the neutral polymers dextran and poly(ethylene glycol) (PEG) rapidly form a two-phase system consisting of a PEG-rich phase floating on top of a dextran-rich phase. Biological particles and macromolecules tend to partition differentially between the phases and the liquid-liquid phase interface in these systems. Bioparticle partitioning has been shown to be related to physiologically important surface properties such as membrane charge or lipid composition.

Affinity partitioning into the PEG-rich phase can be accomplished by coupling PEG to a ligand having affinity for specific cells or macromolecules. Subpopulations can be identified or separated using multi-step countercurrent distribution (CCD).

Incomplete understanding of the influence of gravity on the efficiency and quality of the impressive separations achievable by partitioning, and appreciation for the versatility of this efficient technique, have led to its study for low-gravity biomaterials processing. On Earth, two-phase systems rapidly demix because of density differences between the phases. In low-gravity, demixing has been shown to occur primarily by coalescence. Polymer surface coatings, developed to control localization of demixed phases in low-g, have been found to control electroosmosis which adversely affects electrophoretic separation processes on Earth and in space. In addition PEG-derivatized antibodies have been synthesized for use in immunoaffinity cell partitioning.

Correspondence: James M. Van Alstine at the above address.

When polymers such as the poly(glucose) dextran and poly(ethylene glycol)(PEG) are mixed in low concentrations (i.e., approx. 5% w/w) in water they typically form a two-phase system consisting of a PEG-rich phase floating on top of a dextran-rich phase (Fig. 1). On Earth an emulsion formed by mixing the phases rapidly demixes, primarily because of phase density differences. Aqueous polymer two-phase systems can be rendered physiological by adding salts or other low molecular weight solutes, and have proven to be very useful for preparative and analytical separation of a wide range of biological particles and macromolecules (for reviews see Albertsson, 1986; and Walter, Brooks, and Fisher, 1985). This is possible since biological materials tend to partition differentially, in a stochastic manner, between both phases and the liquid-liquid phase interface.

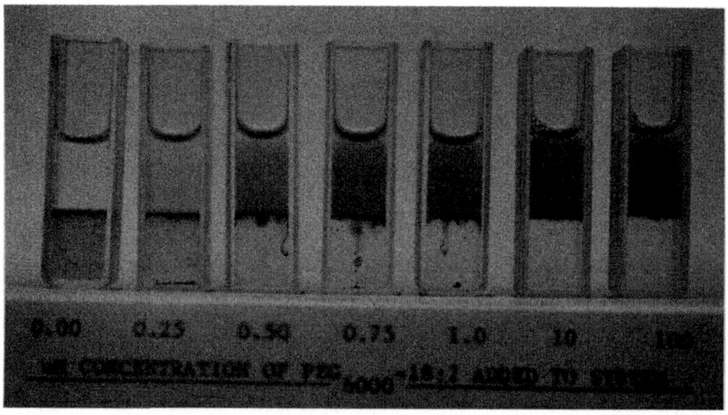

Fig. 1. Hydrophobic affinity partition of human erythrocytes in an NaCl-enriched two-phase system containing the indicated micromolar amounts of PEG 6000-18:2 linoleate fatty acid ester.

A typical single-step partition is illustrated in Figure 2. The phase system is allowed to demix in a separatory funnel. The phases, which are in equilibrium, are separated and recombined in equal volumes in a test tube. Cells or macromolecules are added to the system, frequently dissolved or suspended in the sample of PEG-rich phase. The system is emulsified by gentle agitation and allowed to demix until a definite planar interface is formed. The PEG-rich phase is sampled, and the partition is expressed as the percentage of added material partitioning back into the upper phase, or in terms of a partition coefficient K which reflects the ratio of material in the two phases. In the case of particles, which typically partition between one phase and the interface (Fig. 1), K is taken to be the ratio of cells in one phase compared to cells not in that phase.

Certain ions (i.e., phosphate and sulfate) tend to partition asymmetrically between the phases creating electrostatic millivolt bulk-phase potentials, while other ions (e.g., sodium and chloride) show little preference for either phase (Brooks et al., 1984b; Reitherman et al., 1973; Walter et al., 1976a). In systems possessing electrostatic potentials, cell partition into the PEG-rich phase appears to be related to particle surface charge, detected electrophoretically (Albertsson, 1986; Brooks et al., 1971; Walter et al., 1973; Walter et al., 1976). Similarly, protein partition has been shown to be related directly to protein isoelectric pH (Albertsson, 1970; Albertsson, 1986; Walter et al., 1972).

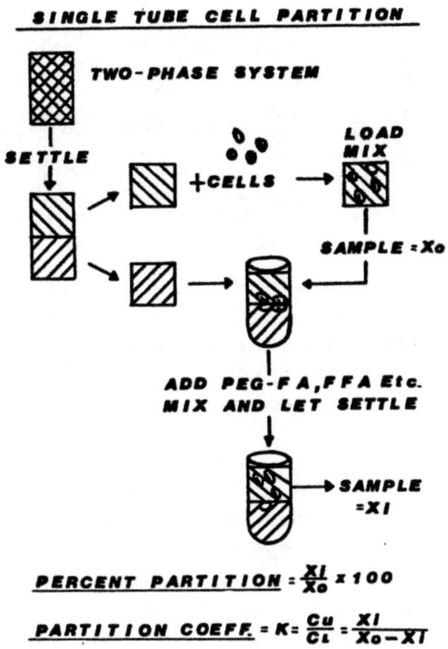

Fig. 2. Typical single chamber partition procedure illustrated for cells.

Cell-polymer interactions (i.e., PEG and dextran adsorption) are also important partition determinants and appear to be influenced by non-charge-related cell surface properties. For instance, the differential partition of various mammalian erythrocytes in two-phase systems containing predominantly NaCl has been correlated with the degree of membrane lipid unsaturation and/or phospholipid head group structure (Eriksson and Albertsson, 1978; Walter et al., 1976a; 1976b). Other membrane properties affect partition, which in a number of two-phase systems has been shown to vary with cell surface carbohydrate (Kessel et al., 1983; Van Alstine et al., 1986b, 1986c; Walter, 1985; Walter et al., 1976a, 1976b, 1986).

Polymer-particle surface interaction can be increased by covalently coupling affinity ligands onto one of the polymers, typically PEG (Flanagan et al., 1976; Flanagan, 1984; Harris, 1986). PEG-fatty acid esters hydrophobically adsorb to particle surfaces or interact with macromolecules, and at low concentration dramatically increase partition into the PEG-rich phase (Fig. 1). Hydrophobic affinity partition has been shown to be sensitive to surface differences among a wide range of bioparticles (see below) (Eriksson and Albertsson, 1978; Eriksson et al., 1976; Kihlström and Magnusson, 1980; Van Alstine and Brooks, 1984; Van Alstine et al., 1986a, 1986b, 1986c; Walter et al., 1976b). PEG-fatty acid esters and other PEG associated affinity ligands (e.g., Cibacron dyes) have also been used to partition specific proteins, enzymes and nucleic acids (Flanagan, 1984; Kopperschläger et al., 1983; Matiasson, 1984; Müller, 1985; Müller and Kütemeier, 1983; Shanbhag and Johansson, 1974).

Multi-step sequential partitions can be performed using thin-layer countercurrent distribution (CCD) (Figure 3). The shallow chamber depth allows rapid phase demixing so that many partitions can be performed in a few hours (Albertsson, 1986; Van Alstine et al., 1985). CCD provides increased resolution of partition differences and indicates the degree of heterogeneity present in the sample, in direct analogy to the behavior of molecular mixtures subjected to column chromatography (Brooks et al.,

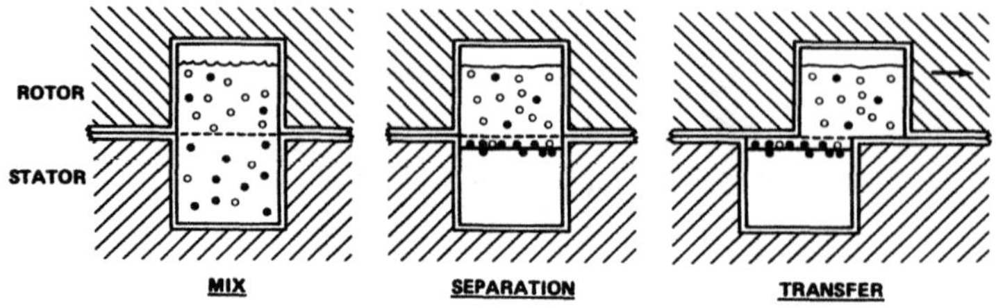

Fig. 3. Thin-layer countercurrent distribution (CCD). The phases are mixed, allowed to demix and material partitioned between both phases is separated by transferring the upper cavity onto a new lower cavity. The process is then repeated.

1971; Walter, 1985; Walter et al., 1976a, 1976b, 1976c.). For example, Figure 4 (taken from Van Alstine et al., 1985) depicts the separation of an equal mixture of human and mouse erythrocytes over thirty transfer steps in a phosphate-containing system. The separation required approximately four hours and, despite the large number of cells processed, the CCD profiles obtained closely resemble their theoretical (binomial) counterparts.

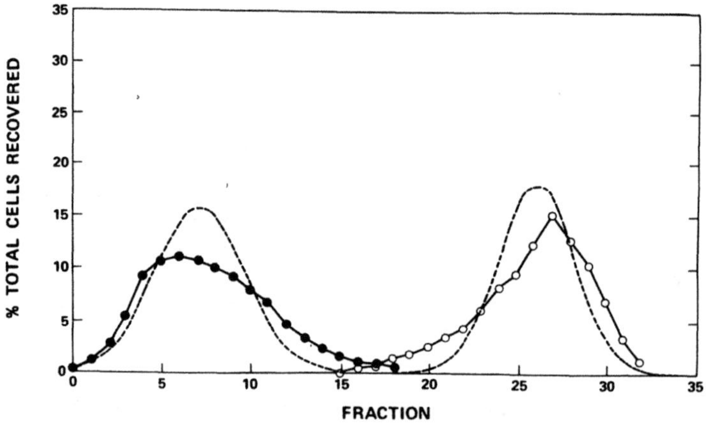

Fig. 4. Thirty transfer CCD of an equal mixture of 2.7×10^8 human (O) and mouse (O) erythrocytes (see text); observed (——) and predicted (---) distributions.

Hydrophobic-affinity CCD of a single culture sample of B16-F10 mouse melanoma cells is shown in Figure 5 (Van Alstine et al., 1986b). In comparison with the B16-F1 parental line, cells from this subline, exhibit high lung-colonizing (metastatic) capability when injected intravenously into mice (Fidler, 1973; Poste et al., 1981). Comparison of the CCD profiles in Figure 4 and 5 indicates considerable cell surface F10 sample heterogeneity which has been shown to be related to ^{125}I-iododeoxyuridine (^{125}I-UdR) specific activity and hence DNA synthesis. F1 cells also exhibit a wide, symmetric distribution peak (not shown) centered at cavity 32. The ^{125}I-UdR specific cell activity of F1 cells subjected to CCD mimicked that of the F10 distribution, although maximal F1 specific activity reached only 40 cpm per cell. These results, in keeping with those of other investigators (Kessel et al., 1982; Miner et al., 1981) suggest a relationship between cell metastatic capability and surface properties reflected by partition. They also indicate the ability of CCD to isolate subpopulations of cells.

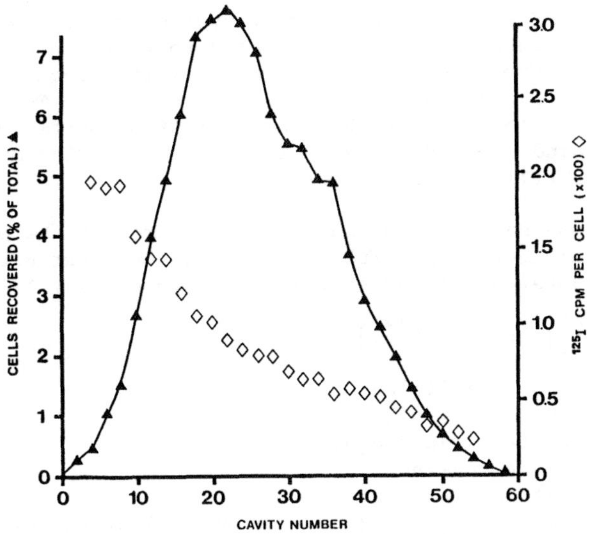

Fig. 5. Countercurrent distribution of B16-F10 (▲) mouse melanoma cell sample exhibiting high metastatic capability, and the ^{125}I-UdR specific activity (◇) of cells along the distribution. Buffered saline system containing 1 μm PEG 8000-18:2 linoleate ester.

Many interesting and useful partitions involving cells, bacteria, viruses, cell particles, and liposomes have been carried out. Cells have been separated according to type, age, developmental stage, and response to surface modifying agents (Albertsson, 1986; Brooks et al., 1971; Eriksson and Albertsson, 1978; Eriksson et al., 1976; Van Alstine and Brooks, 1984; Van Alstine et al., 1986b, 1986c; Walter et al., 1976a; 1976b; Walter, Fisher, and Brooks, 1985). Lymphocytes have been separated into subpopulations (i.e., B,T,N and NK as evaluated by rosetting techniques) (Malstrom et al., 1978, 1980; Michalski et al., 1983; Walter et al., 1979; 1980). Human peripheral blood monocytes have been separated into fractions differing in their phagocytic activity (Walter et al., 1980).

Given the above it is not surprising that many types of proteins, including isozymes, have been differentially partitioned. The separation of DNA and RNA molecules of different base pair composition, molecular weight, origin and helicity has also been accomplished (Albertsson, 1965, 1970, 1986; Müller and Kütemeier, 1982; Müller, 1985; Pettijohn, 1967; Walter et al., 1972).

Partitioning is very gentle, due in part to the ease with which the phases, whose interfacial tensions are very low (i.e., 1 to 20 μN/m, Bamberger et al., 1984), can be mixed. Cells can be cultured in a normal fashion following CCD. Cancer cells retain their ability to live in a host and to metastasize (Miner et al., 1981; Van Alstine et al., 1986b). Reticulocytes isolated via CCD mature normally when injected into autologous hosts (Walter et al., 1971). Macromolecules retain their native structure and function (Albertsson, 1986; Johansson, 1985). In addition to being powerful, versatile, and sensitive to physiologically important macromolecular and particle surface properties, partitioning is also relatively inexpensive and easily scaled up. As a result the technique enjoys growing interest for both biotechnical and biomedical applications (Albertsson, 1986; Brooks, 1983; Brooks et al., 1986; Hustedt et al., 1985; Kula et al., 1982; Matiasson, 1983).

The strength of partitioning is that system properties which determine K (e.g., interfacial tension, electrostatic interfacial potential, polymer type and concentration, affinity ligand type and concentration) are largely under experimental control. The effectiveness of partition is due to the fact that the partition coefficient, K, has been shown to depend exponentially on the relevant system as well as macromolecular or cell surface properties.

From a thermodynamic standpoint one would predict the above observations given that (for a full discussion see Albertsson, 1986; Brooks et al., 1984a, Brooks et al., 1985; Sharp et al., 1987):

$$K \;\alpha\; \exp\left(\frac{\Delta G}{kT}\right) \;\alpha\; \exp\left(\frac{\Delta\gamma A}{kT}\right) \tag{1}$$

where: K = partition coefficient
α = proportionality sign
ΔG = interfacial free energy
k = Boltzman's constant
T = temperature, K
A = particle surface area or, for molecules, macromolecular area (which is proportional to MW)
Δγ = net interfacial free energy per unit area in the two phases

In the case of particles, interfacial tension (γ_{tb}) between the two liquid phases (which increases dramatically with slight increases in polymer concentration (Bamberger et al., 1984)) is an important partition determinant. This is because particle adsorption at the interface lowers the free energy of the system by an amount proportional to the area occupied, times the interfacial tension. Hence, the larger the particle, or the higher the interfacial tension, the greater the expected particle interfacial localization. Consideration of this factor and the role of particle surface charge and system phase potential in determining particle partition leads to the following thermodynamic description for particle partition between the interface and a bulk phase.

$$K = \text{const} \times \exp\left(-\gamma_{tb}A[1-(\Delta\gamma + \sigma\Delta\psi)/\gamma_{tb}]^2/4kT\right) \tag{2}$$

where: K = no. particles in bulk phase/no. particles at interface
A = surface area of particle
σ = surface charge density of particles
Δψ = electrostatic potential difference between bottom and top phase
$\Delta\gamma = \gamma_{pb} - \gamma_{pt}$
γ_{pb}, γ_{pt} = interfacial free energy per unit area of particle in bottom (γ_{pb}) or top (γ_{pt}) phase
γ_{tb} = interfacial tension between top and bottom phases

The σΔψ term in the exponential in equation (2) describes the electrostatic dependence of the partition coefficient. Clearly, the larger the value of Δψ, the greater will be the dependence on cell surface charge density. Δψ is determined by the equilibrium distribution of ions between the two phases, any concentration difference producing a type of Donnan potential across the boundary (Brooks et al., 1984a). Conditions which maximize ionic partition should therefore produce the optimal conditions for charge-dependent cell separations.

The remaining terms embody the effects of interfacial tension, γ_{tb}, and of particle-polymer interaction, (e.g., affinity partitioning) through the Δγ term. The greater the preferential binding of one of the two phase polymers to the particle surface, the lower will be the interfacial free energy of the particle in the phase in which that polymer predominates and the larger will be $\Delta\gamma$ in the other phase. It is also seen that K decreases exponentially with increasing γ_{tb} provided other properties of the system do not change.

The above expression accounts very well for the qualitative features of cell partition. Moreover, in a number of systems the exponential dependence of K on $\Delta\gamma$, γ_{tb}, and $\Delta\psi$ has been observed (Brooks et al., 1984a; Brooks et al., 1985; Sharp, 1985; Sharp et al., 1987). However, eqn. 2 assumes that the particles are randomly distributed by thermal forces and ignore mechanistic (e.g., fluid dynamic) aspects of particle partition. Biological cells exhibit very limited Brownian motion and have extremely small diffusion coefficients (i.e., 10^{-10} cm^2 s^{-1}). Even at the low interfacial tensions present in these systems, cell size should allow for strong interfacial adsorption.

The graph of log K versus interfacial tension for the partition of particles between the PEG-rich phase and the interface approximates linearity for a variety of particles of different sizes in systems devoid of electrostatic potentials ($\Delta\psi = 0$). The slopes of such graphs (e.g., Figure 6, taken from Brooks et al., 1984a), which approximate -A/4kT, suggest that the cell partitions observed should occur at much higher temperatures (i.e., 10^4 to 10^5 °K) (Brooks et al., 1984a; Sharp et al., 1987). Thermodynamic factors therefore appear to be important in determining particle partition, but nonthermodynamic, randomizing forces are also present. These forces, which appear to vary with particle size, are believed to be associated with rapid fluid movement during phase emulsion demixing at unit gravity (see below). Such forces could dislodge particles from the surfaces of phase droplets and "streaming structures" (see below) present during the early stages of phase demixing (Clark and Wilson, 1983; Sharp et al., 1987) (Fig. 7). As a result it may be impossible to achieve theoretically predictable separations, such as of two sets of particles differing only in size, on Earth.

If the source(s) of the randomization could be identified, it should be possible to design a separation process that minimizes this influence. Much higher resolution separations would result, with attendant benefits to biomedical investigation and biotechnology. It is towards this goal that our microgravity experiments are directed.

DEMIXING OF POLYMER PHASE SYSTEMS IN MICROGRAVITY

NASA's interest in phase partitioning began in the late 1970's with a proposal from D. E. Brooks to evaluate the role of gravity in the partitioning of biological cells and to develop alternate methods to demix the phases in low-g. A small instrument was built by Beckman Instruments to fly on a sounding rocket. Although this instrument was not flown before sounding rocket experiments were phased out in favor of space shuttle experiments, developmental research showed the feasibility and advantages of using electrophoretic methods to demix the phases in low-g (Brooks and Bamberger, 1982; Brooks et al., 1984). Research presently encompasses:

1. Theoretical and practical studies directed towards gaining a greater understanding of phase partitioning in unit-g and low-g.
2. Development of novel methods, both passive (e.g., polymeric wall coatings) and active, to localize demixed phases in low-g.
3. Development of novel applications of two-phase systems and new polymer phase systems with unique properties.

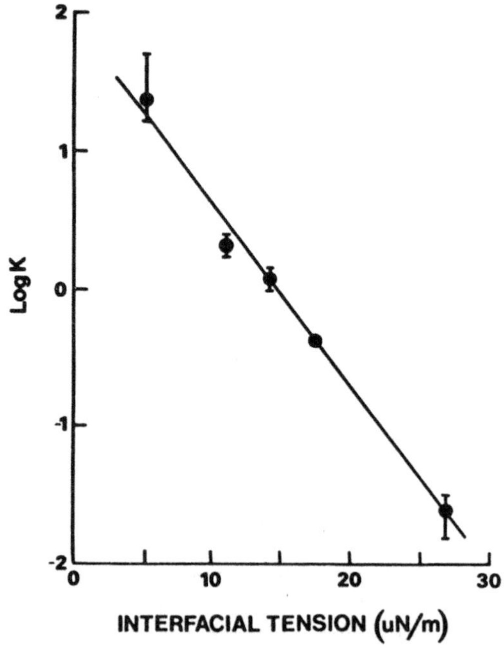

Fig. 6. Logarithm of the partition coefficient of spherical A. laidlawii B cells vs interfacial tension for a series of buffered saline two-phase systems.

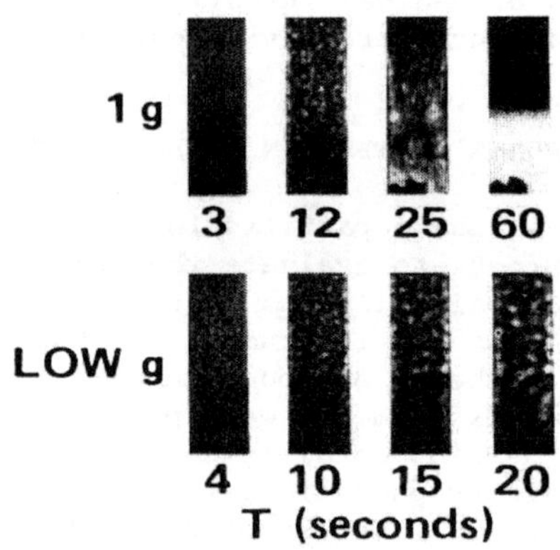

Fig. 7. Effect of gravity on the demixing of an NaCl-enriched two-phase system containing 7% (w/w) dextran T40 and 5% PEG 8000. The PEG-enriched phase was dyed with Trypan blue (0.05 mg/ml).

These interests are supported by the advantages of carrying out phase system demixing and partition studies under low gravity conditions:

1. Elimination of particle sedimentation effects so that large particles (e.g., cells cultured on carrier beads, or megakaryocytes) can be partitioned, and systems can completely demix before sampling.
2. Control of the rate and mechanism of demixing and its effect on particle partition (see below).

In addition, the energy-efficient, versatile, safe, inexpensive nature of the technique recommends its possible use as a preparative step in Space Bioprocessing protocols involving other purification procedures.

Initial low-gravity demixing studies were performed aboard KC-135 aircraft (Van Alstine et al., 1984). As shown in Figures 8 and 9, the KC-135 flies a series of parabolic trajectories providing up to 30 seconds of low-g and up to one and one-half minutes of pull out and climb (high-g). The acceleration experienced by the partition module was monitored by three accelerometers (model 300 Al, Sunstrad Data Controls) mounted to the same assembly in orthogonal axes, one of which was parallel to the sample vertical axis (aircraft yaw axis). For a typical maneuver, the low-g acceleration on all axes averaged less than 10^{-2} g with a maxima of 3 x 10^{-2}g (Fig. 8).

Unit-gravity and low-g phase separation experiments were undertaken using an apparatus consisting of a Nikon FM2 camera, equipped with Kodacolor ASA 400 film, a 55 mm 1:2.8 macrolens and shutter release cable, anchored to a platform holding a removable plexiglass phase-partition module backlit by a fluorescent light box. The phase partition module contained four rectangular partition chambers 30 mm high, 8 mm wide, and 6 mm thick and a digital clock. One steel ballbearing (5 mm dia.) was added to each chamber to facilitate complete mixing of the phases. A typical experiment involved mixing the phases by inverting the module 30 times, starting the timer, attaching the module to the platform and taking pictures as the phases separated.

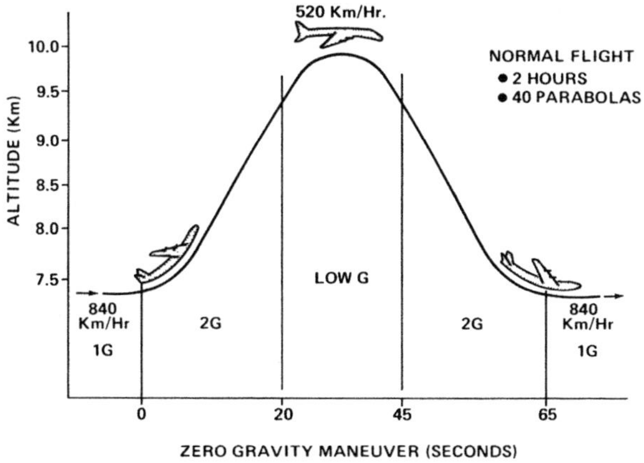

Fig. 8. KC-135 aircraft parabolic flight trajectory.

Figure 7 illustrates phase demixing for a polymer two-phase system at unit-gravity and aboard the KC-135. The PEG-rich phase was dyed with 0.05 mg/ml Trypan blue. At this low concentration the dye does not alter system physical properties (Bamberger et al., 1987). On Earth, gentle mixing is sufficient to create an emulsion of micrometer-sized droplets and solutes (or particles) are evenly distributed throughout the chamber. After a brief period (5-10 s) during which the phase droplets coalesce to form larger droplets, approximately one minute of rapid phase streaming can be seen in the system. This streaming is characterized by the presence of columnar regions of both phases in the central region of the chamber. Clear regions of upper and lower phase rapidly appear at the top and bottom of the chamber. As demixing progresses the middle emulsion region slowly contracts to form a planar interface. This last stage lasts approximately 60 seconds. Phase systems containing greater concentrations of polymers of equal molecular weight, and therefore possessing larger interfacial tensions and phase density differences, tend to demix faster, despite increased phase viscosity. Varying the phase volume ratio decreases the demixing rate. Utilizing polymers of lower MW can decrease phase viscosity and increase the demixing rate, all other factors being equal.

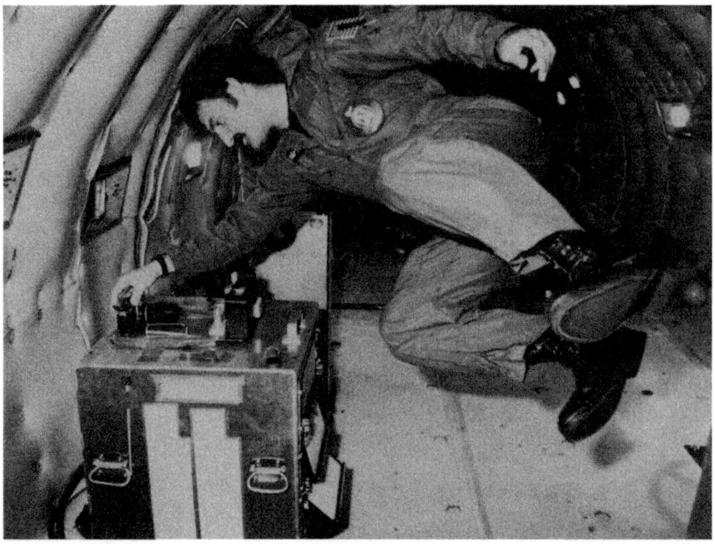

Fig. 9. KC-135 low-g (10^{-2} g) phase system demixing experiment. Operator initiating photo sequence.

Demixing of systems possessing phases of equal volume in low-gravity appears to progress primarily by a coalescence mechanism. The columnar structures indicative of phase streaming are absent and demixing involves fusion of phase droplets into larger and larger regions. To quantitatively analyze these results slides of demixing phase systems, taken at defined time intervals, were projected and the outlines of connected domains traced on paper. The area of each domain was estimated using an IBM-PC computer equipped with a Microsoft mouse mechanically fixed to a single orientation. A program was developed to digitize and store the pictures of the domain areas as polygons. Domain area was calculated by adding the areas of the trapezoids formed from the individual sides of the polygon and the projection of each side onto the horizontal axis. Drop area distributions were analyzed and for each interval the mean and standard deviation drop size was found, the radius (r) of a circle of area equal to the mean area determined, and results expressed as a function of time (t) on a log-log plot. These plots (not shown) were subjected to linear regression analysis. Correlation coefficients between 0.9 and 1.0 were found and as well as positive line slopes between 0.6 and 0.8 (Bamberger et al., 1987).

The above analysis indicates that the slow, mechanism of Ostwald ripening which involves the growth of large phase droplet regions by diffusive transport of material from smaller droplets culminating in a single large region of radius, r, growing asymptotically with time ($t^{1/3}$), is not responsible for demixing of these systems in low-g. The most probable mechanism is droplet coalescence, self-driven by coalescence initiated at the end of mixing when micrometer sized droplets of each phase are in close proximity and possess some residual fluid movement (Bamberger et al., 1987). These results are somewhat analogous to those of other researchers investigating the structures of immiscible metal alloys and liquid-liquid two-phase systems solidified via cooling under microgravity (Curreri et al., 1985; Feuerbacher, Hamacher, and Naumann, 1986; Van Alstine et al., 1984). In agreement with unit-g modeling studies conducted with various isopycnic polymer two-phase systems (to which a third polymer, Ficoll, was added to achieve equal phase density) our KC-135 results indicated:

1. Spontaneous phase demixing of dextran-PEG two-phase systems is mechanistically different at low-gravity than at unit-gravity, proceeding at a slower, but still useful rate.
2. The equilibrium configuration of a demixed phase system is expected to be one phase in the shape of a sphere, to minimize surface area of contact, completely surrounded by the phase which prefers to "wet" the container walls.
3. Given the above, it should be possible to influence the rate of spontaneous demixing and final disposition of the phases by varying phase volume ratio, phase viscosity, liquid-liquid interfacial tension, chamber geometry, chamber wall material or wall coatings.

In April 1985 a small hand-held Phase Partition Experiment (PPE) module (Fig. 10) was flown aboard STS-51D. The experiment, performed by Senator E. J. "Jake" Garn (R-Utah), consisted of shaking the module to mix the phases, placing the module in front of a fluorescent light source, and photographing demixing of the systems with a Nikon camera equipped with an hour-min.-sec. data back. The module contained fifteen chambers, each fitted with a 5 millimeter diameter stainless steel ball bearing to facilitate complete emulsification of the phases.

The systems flown (Fig. 11) were chosen to provide initial insight into the effects of several factors (phase viscosity, interfacial tension, phase volume ratio, etc.) on demixing in the 10^{-3} to 10^{-4} g environment provided by the Shuttle. Fixed erythrocytes were included in the right-hand side, bottom and middle row chambers as an initial test of low-g polymer phase cell partition. In addition the middle chamber in the middle row contained a control "isopycnic" phase system having phases of approximately equal density (Bamberger et al., 1987).

Figure 12 indicates the equilibrium appearance of the PPE module in low-g aboard the Shuttle. It can be seen that in all cases the metal mixing balls become isolated in the center of the chamber inside the clear dextran-rich phase which, itself, is surrounded by the dyed PEG-rich phase. The PEG-rich phase prefers to wet the glass (top row) and plexiglass (bottom two rows) chambers' walls.

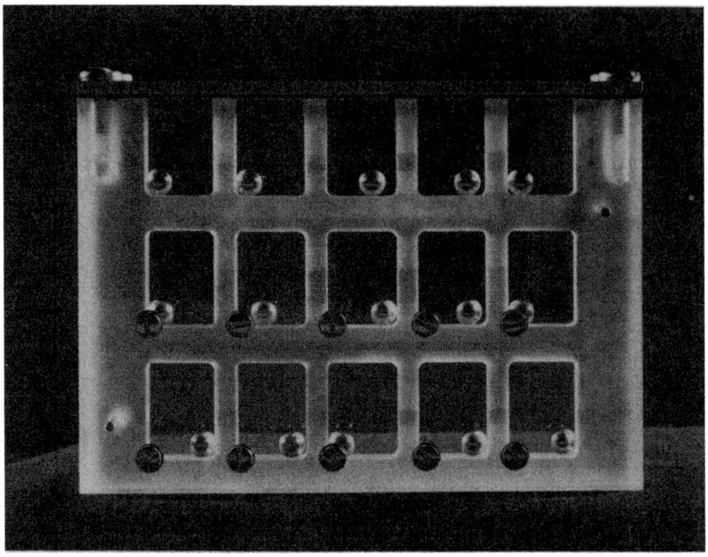

Fig. 10. STS-51D, Phase Partition Experiment (PPE) hand-held module.

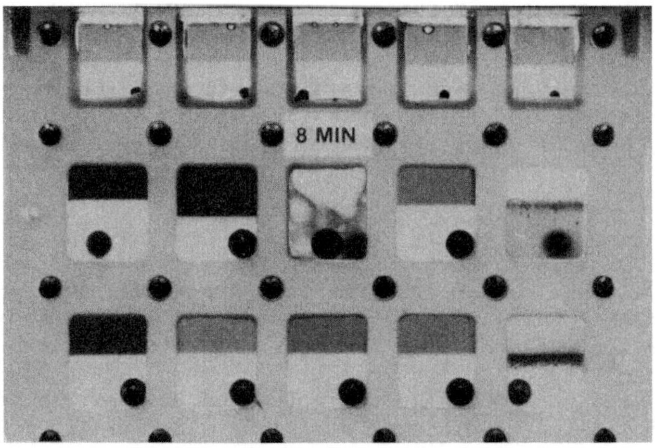

Fig. 11. STS-51D, PPE appearance after demixing in unit-gravity.

Phase systems typically useful for cell partitioning on Earth were shown to demix fairly rapidly in low-g. Phase systems compounded with larger differences in polymer concentration between the phases, and hence larger differences in viscosity, interfacial tension, and density differences, demixed at a much slower rate. In all cases the time necessary to appreciably demix the phase systems was greater than on the ground. Figure 13 provides more detail of the low-g demixing for four systems whose physical properties are given in Table 1 (Bamberger et al., 1986). Although the relative importance of interfacial tension and viscosity is not clear it appears that, in keeping with theoretical work by other investigators (Allan and Mason, 1962; Chappelear, 1961; McKay and Mason, 1963), increased interfacial tension may impart increased stability to the polymer emulsion by mechanically hindering droplet-droplet coalescence (Bamberger et al., 1987; Curreri et al., 1985).

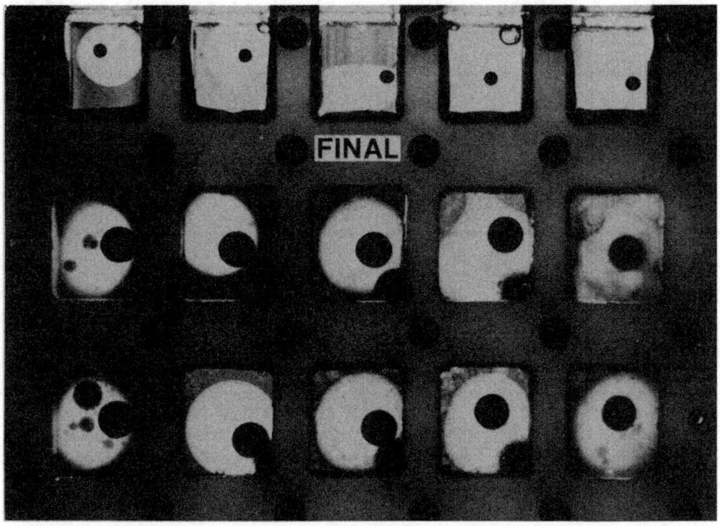

Fig. 12. STS-51D, PPE appearance after demixing in low-gravity.

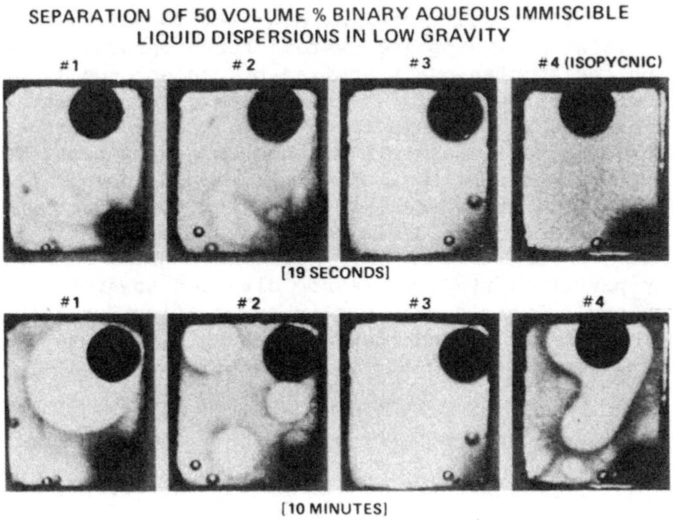

Fig. 13. STS-51D, PPE detail of four chambers demixing in low-gravity (see text).

The other parameter that had a large effect on the demixing rate was the phase volume ratio. When the PEG-rich phase, which prefered to wet the container wall, was mixed at a ratio of 2:3 (vol:vol) with dextran-rich phase, demixing occurred more rapidly than when the phases were at a 1:1 ratio. Similarly a 1:1 system demixed much more rapidly than a 3:2 system (not shown).

The presence of cell particles in the phase systems was seen to noticeably but not drastically alter system demixing kinetics. Effects of chamber geometry (not shown) were also noted.

Table 1. Composition and Physical Properties of Polymer Phase Systems in Figure 13.

[a]System	Interfacial Tension (μN/m)	[b]Phase Viscosity (cP) D	[b]Phase Viscosity (cP) PEG-F	[b]Phase Density (g/cm^3) D	[b]Phase Density (g/cm^3) PEG-F
1 (5,3.5,0)	1.9	20	3.4	1.052	1.015
2 (5,4.0,0)	8.3	30	3.3	1.057	1.016
3 (6,4.0,0)	20.0	50	3.8	1.065	1.016
4 (7,0.5,11)	5.0	50	30.0	1.080	1.080

[a]Systems designated by chamber number (Figure 13) followed by composition (%w/w) of Dextran T500, PEG 8000 and Ficoll 400.
[b]Phases are designated Dextran-rich (D) or PEG/Ficoll-rich (PEG-F).

Time sequence pictures from the 51-D PPE experiment are currently undergoing quantitative analysis using the method described above. A more sophisticated Baush and Lomb Omicon computer-enhanced analysis system is being employed. Initial results mimic those reported for systems demixed on board the KC-135 (Bamberger et al., 1987).

In general this first shuttle experiment reinforced belief in the potential of utilizing polymer phase systems for bioprocessing experiments in space. The phases spontaneously demixed by coalescence (Fig. 13) at a rate compatible with cell separation experiments. The rate at which demixing occurs and the final disposition of the demixed phases evidently depends on system composition as well as chamber shape, coatings and materials; all of which can be controlled. It would appear that the low gravity shuttle environment is ideal for studying the effect of varying the rate and mechanism of phase demixing on particle partition.

Low gravity partition studies are now directed towards improving apparatus design and polymeric coatings in preparation for future shuttle flight. At the same time, ground-based research is progressing in a number of exciting areas related to cell separation technology.

RELATED GROUND-BASED RESEARCH

Polymeric wall coatings have been developed utilizing PEG and dextran. A simplified presentation of the chemistry is given in Figure 14. (For more details refer to Harris, 1986; Harris and Yalpani, 1986; Harris et al., 1984; Herren et al., 1986). Glass surfaces were activated with a silating reagent which was reacted with PEG (monomethyl ether) activated by conversion to the cyanuric chloride derivative (PEG-CC) in the presence of butyl-lithium (Abuchowski et al., 1984; above references). PEG-CC was then reacted (typically) with aminosilane activated glass to yield PEG-amino-glass and HCl. Dextran was attached to amino-glass using sodium cyanoborohydride reduction (Harris and Yalpani, 1986; Harris et al., 1984). Approximately 1.4 aminopropylsilane molecules were bound per 100 $Å^2$ of glass surface and one polymer molecule was bound per 10 aminopropyl groups.

The effect of surface alteration on phase wetting behavior was evaluated by contact angle measurements after the method of Schurch et al., 1981. This involved measuring the angle of contact between a 5 µl droplet of the more dense dextran-rich phase resting on an appropriate glass or plexiglass slide immersed in PEG-rich phase. Contact angles of 0°, 90° and 180° represent, respectively, complete wetting of the surface by the dextran-rich phase, equal wetting of the surface by both phases, and complete wetting of the surface by the PEG-rich phase.

Typical results are shown in Figure 15. As expected, contact angle measurements support shuttle results, regarding the preference of PEG-rich phases to wet plexiglass and uncoated glass container walls, as well as dextran-rich phases to prefer metal surfaces (not shown). They also indicate the ability of polymeric coatings to control phase wall wetting in a manner somewhat analogous to polymer affinity ligands ability to alter particle phase interactions.

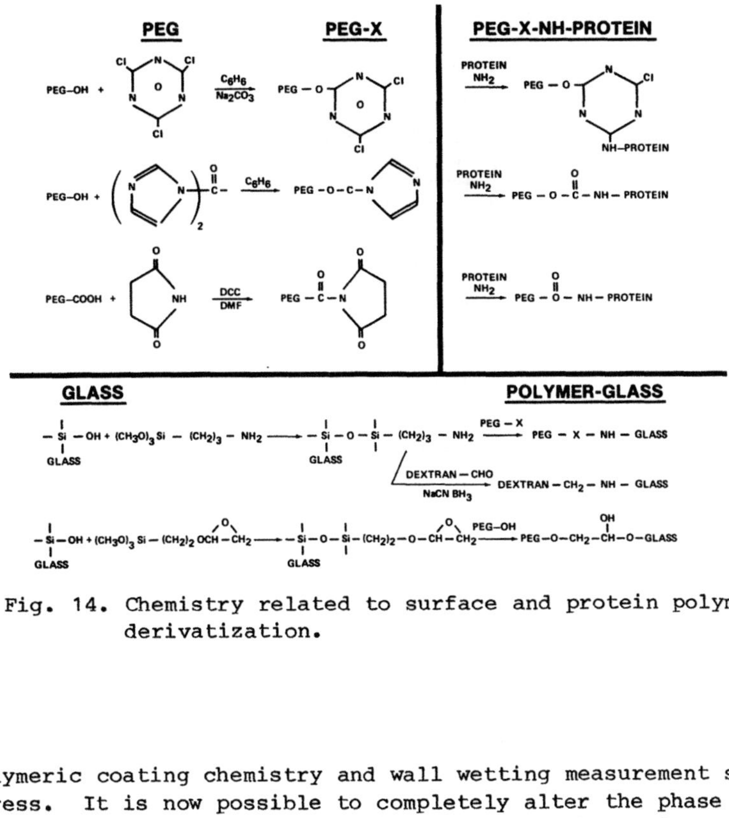

Fig. 14. Chemistry related to surface and protein polymer derivatization.

Polymeric coating chemistry and wall wetting measurement studies are in progress. It is now possible to completely alter the phase preferring to wet the container wall (not shown) and we hope that polymer coatings will prove useful in a number of low-g materials processing applications. These coatings have already shown promise in a number of Earth-bound applications (Harris et al., 1986). For example, PEG coatings have been demonstrated to control the electroosmosis which hinders the resolution of electrophoretic separations both on Earth and in space (Herren et al., 1986). The reduction in electroosmosis is related to PEG coating molecular weight. PEG coatings are stable for at least 1 year and are more effective than dextran, methylcellulose or silane coatings. In addition the coatings are expected to render chamber surfaces less susceptable to protein absorption (Hlady et al., 1985).

The same chemistry used to covalently couple PEG to amino groups on glass surfaces can be employed to covalently link PEG molecules to protein gamma amino groups (Figure 14) (Abuchowski et al., 1984; Harris, 1986; Harris and Yalpani, 1986; Karr et al., 1986; Sharp et al., 1986). This chemistry has been utilized to covalently link PEG molecules to antibody molecules in order to create affinity ligands with which to carry out immunoaffinity cell partition (Karr et al., 1986; Sharp et al., 1986).

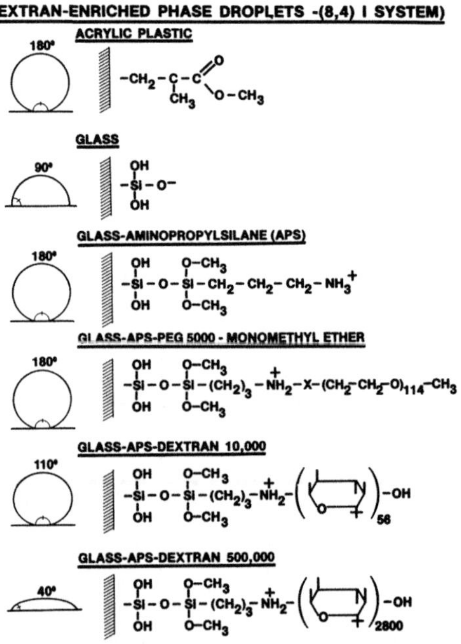

Fig. 15. Variation in partition chamber surface wetting with surface coating.

Figures 16 to 18 are taken from Karr et al. (1986). Figure 16, the graph of log K versus PEG-IgG (rabbit anti-human erythrocyte) incubation concentration, for human erythrocytes in an NaCl enriched, dextran T500, PEG 8000, containing two-phase system is in keeping with equation 2. Approximately half of the 90 IgG lysine groups were derivatized by monomethyl PEG 5000. Cells were incubated with PEG-IgG in upper phase for 15 min at 37 °C, washed and partitioned in a normal manner. PEG derivatization did not appear to alter IgG specificity although, fortuitously, it did significantly decrease, in a manner dependent on the degree of derivatization, antibody induced cell aggregation (Karr et al., 1986).

Figures 17 and 18 indicate the ability of immunoaffinity CCD to separate cell mixtures. Following a single incubation with PEG-IgG a mixture of sheep and human erythrocytes (distinguishable on the basis of size) was completely separated in 100 minutes using 30 transfer CCD and a two-phase system which normally offers little resolution.

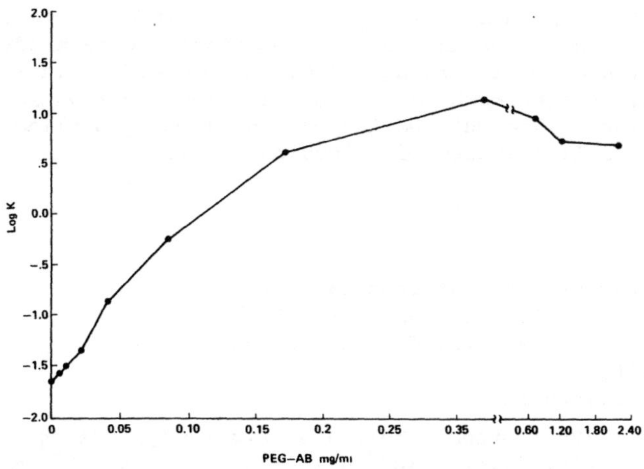

Fig. 16. Effect of PEG 5000 derivatized rabbit anti-erythrocyte IgG on the partition (log K) of 2×10^7 human erythrocytes in a buffered saline system containing 4.9% (w/w) dextran T500 and 3.6% (w/w) PEG 8000.

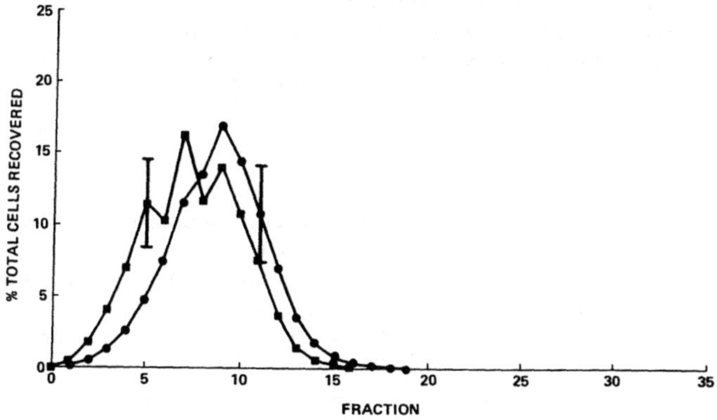

Fig. 17. Countercurrent distribution of 3×10^7 human (●) and sheep (■) erythrocytes for 30 transfers in the same system used in Figure 16.

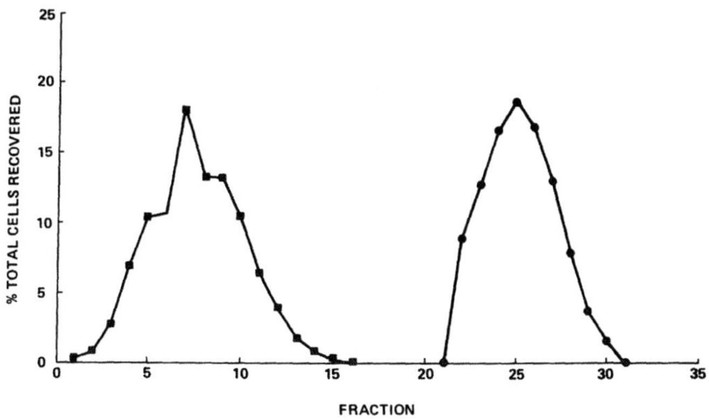

Fig. 18. Countercurrent distribution of 3×10^7 human (●) and sheep (■) erythrocytes, in the same system used in Fig. 16, following incubation with 1.3 mg/ml PEG 5000-IgG.

Development of immunoaffinity partitioning, which in terms of simplicity, resolving power and capacity possesses certain advantages over fluorescent activated cell sorting, (FACS) is proceeding in a number of different areas. Better methods of protein polymer derivatization and analysis are being worked out and the method is being applied to the fractionation of cell mixtures of biomedical interest.

ABBREVIATIONS

CCD	countercurrent distribution
51D	Designated STS Mission, April 1985
FACS	fluorescent activated cell sorting
g	gravity
IgG	immunoglobulin G
^{125}I-UdR	Iodine 125 isotope labelled deoxyuridine, DNA precursor
low-g	low gravity (i.e., $<10^{-2}$ g KC 135; $<10^{-3}$ to 10^{-4} g STS)
MC	methylcellulose
MSFC	Marshall Space Flight Center
MW	molecular weight
NASA	National Aeronautics and Space Administration
PEG	poly(ethylene glycol)
PEG-CC	PEG-cyanuric chloride derivative
PPE	Phase Partitioning Experimental (Program)
SSL	Space Science Laboratory
STS	Space Transportation System (Shuttle)

ACKNOWLEDGEMENTS

This research was supported by the National Aeronautics and Space Administration - Microgravity Science and Applications Office via contracts NAS8-35333, NAS8-35334, NAS8-35362, and NAS8-36045 and the Medical Research Council of Canada. J.V.A. is supported by a Universities Space Research Association, Visiting Scientist Fellowship and J.B. is supported by a Canadian Heart Foundation Fellowship. The authors wish to thank Susan Burrer for typing and editorial assistance.

REFERENCES

Albertsson, P. Å., 1965, Partition studies on nucleic acids I. Influence of electrolytes, polymer concentration and nucleic acid conformation on partition in the dextran-polyethylene glycol system, Biochim. Biophys. Acta, 103:1.

Albertsson, P. Å., 1970, Partition of cell particles and macromolecules, Adv. Prot. Chem., 24:309.

Albertsson, P. Å., 1986, "Partition of Cell Particles and Macromolecules," 3rd Edn., John Wiley and Sons, New York.

Abuchowski, A., Kazo, G. M., Verhoest, Jr., C. R., van Es, D., Nucci, M. L., Kafkewitz, T., Viau, A. T., and Davis, F. F., 1984, Cancer therapy with chemically modified enzymes. I. Antitumor properties of polyethylene glycol-asparaginase conjugates, Cancer Biochm. Biophys., 7:175-186.

Allan, R. S., and Mason, S. G., 1962, Particle motions in sheared suspensions XIV. Coalescence of liquid drops in electric and shear fields, J. Colloid Sci., 17:382.

Bamberger, S., Seaman, G. V. F., Sharp, K. A., and Brooks, D. E., 1984, The effects of salts on the interfacial tension of aqueous dextran poly(ethylene glycol) phase systems, J. Colloid and Interf. Sci., 99: 194.

Bamberger, S., Brooks, D. E., Sharp, K. A., Van Alstine, J. M., and Webber, T. J., 1985, Preparation of phase systems and measurement of their physicochemical properties, in: Walter, Brooks, and Fisher, 1985, p. 85.

Bamberger, S., Van Alstine, J. M., Harris, J. M., Baird, J. K., Snyder R. S., Boyce, J., and Brooks, D. E., 1987, Demixing of aqueous polymer two-phase systems in low gravity, Sepn. Sci. and Technol., submitted.

Brooks, D. E., 1984, Two-phase systems for biotechnical isolations, Biotechnology, 1:668.

Brooks, D. E., Seaman, G. V. F., and Walter, H., 1971, Detection of differences in surface charge associated properties of cells by partition in two polymer aqueous phase systems, Nature New Biology, 234:61.

Brooks, D. E., and Bamberger S., 1982, Studies on aqueous polymer two-phase systems useful for the partitioning of biological materials, in: "Materials Processing in the Reduced Gravity Environment of Space," G. E. Rindone, ed., Elsevier, Amsterdam, p. 233.

Brooks, D. E., Bamberger, S. B., Harris, J. M., and Van Alstine, J., 1984a, Rationale for two phase polymer system microgravity separation experiments, in: "Proceedings of the 5th European Symposium on Material Sciences Under Microgravity", European Space Agency Publication SP-222, p. 315.

Brooks, D. E., Sharp, K. A., Bamberger, S., Tamblyn, C. H., Seaman, G.V.F., and Walter, H., 1984b, Electrostatic and electrokinetic potentials in two polymer aqueous phase systems, J. Colloid Interf. Sci., 102:1.

Brooks, D. E., Sharp, K. A., and Fisher, D., 1985, Theoretical aspects of partitioning, in: Walter, H., Brooks, D. E., and Fisher D., 1985, p. 11.

Brooks, D. E., Boyce, J., Bamberger, S. B., Harris, J. M., and Van Alstine, J. M., 1986, Separation of biological materials in microgravity, Proceedings of National Research Council of Canada NRC Publications Meeting on Space Biomedicine and Biotechnology, Ottawa, May 29-30, 1986.

Chappelear, D. C., 1961, Models of a liquid drop approaching an interface, J. Colloid Sci., 16:186.

Clark, A. N., and Wilson, D. J., 1983, Foam Flotation Theory and Applications, Marcel Dekker Inc., New York, pp. 97-128.

Curreri, P. A., Van Alstine, J. M., Brooks, D. E., Bamberger, S., and Snyder, R. S., 1985, On the stability of high volume fraction immiscible dispersions in low gravity, NASA, Space Science Laboratory, Alabama, 35812, Preprint No. 85-156.

Eriksson, E., Albertsson, P. Å., and Johansson, G., 1976, Hydrophobic surface properties of erythrocytes studied by affinity partition in aqueous two-phase systems, Molec. Cell. Biochem., 10:123.

Eriksson, E., and Albertsson, P. Å., 1978, Partition of liposomes in aqueous two-phase systems, Biochim. Biophys. Acta, 507:425.

Feuerbacher, B., Hamacher, H., and Naumann, R. J., 1986, "Materials Sciences in Space", Springer Verlag, New York.

Fidler, I. J., 1973, Selection of successive tumor lines for metastasis, Nature New Biol., 97:597.

Flanagan, S. D., and Barondes, S. H., 1978, Affinity partitioning: A method for purification of proteins using specific polymer ligands in aqueous polymer two-phase systems, J. Biol. Chem., 251:858.

Flanagan, S. D., 1984, Affinity phase partitioning, in: "Receptor Purification Procedures", J. C. Venter and L. C. Harrison, eds., Alan R. Liss Inc., New York, p. 15.

Harris, J. M., 1985, Laboratory synthesis of polyethylene glycol derivatives, J. Macromol. Sci., Rev. Macromol, Chem. Phys., C25(3):325.

Harris, J. M., Struck, E. C., Case, M. G., Paley, M. S., Van Alstine, J. M., and Brooks, D. E., 1984, Synthesis and characterization of poly(ethylene glycol) derivatives, J. Polymer Sci., Polymer Chem. Edn., 22:341.

Harris, J. M., and Yalpani, M., 1985, Polymer-ligands used in affinity partitioning and their synthesis, in: Walter, Brooks, and Fisher, 1985, p. 590.

Harris, J. M., Brooks, D. E., Boyce, J. F., Snyder, R. S., and Van Alstine J. M., 1986, Hydrophillic polymer coatings for control of electroosmosis and wetting, in: "Dynamic Aspects of Polymer Surfaces: Proceedings of the 5th Rocky Mountain ACS Meeting", J. D. Andrade, ed., American Chemical Society, Washington, in press.

Hlady, V., Van Wagenen, R. A., and Andrade, J. D., 1985, Total internal reflection intrinsic fluorescence (TIRIF) spectroscopy applied to protein adsorption, in: "Surface and Interfacial Aspects of Biomedical Polymers," Vol. 2, Protein Adsorption, J. D. Andrade, ed., Plenum Press, New York, p. 81.

Hustedt, H., Kroner, K. H., and Kula, M. R., 1985, Applications of phase partitioning in biotechnology, in: Walter, Brooks, and Fisher 1985, p. 529.

Johansson, G., 1985, Partitioning of proteins, in: Walter, Brooks, Fisher, 1985, p. 161.

Karr, L. J., Shafer, S. G., Harris, J. M., Van Alstine, J. M., and Snyder, R. S., 1986, Immuno-affinity partition of cells in aqueous polymer two-phase systems, J. Chromatography, 354:269.

Kessel, D., Butler, W. B., Iyer, V. K., and Horwitz, J. P., 1982, Estrogen bridged purines: A new series of anti-tumor agents which alter cell membrane properties, Biochem. Biophys. Res. Commun., 109:45.

Kihlström, E., and Magnusson, K. E., 1980, Association of Hela cells of LPS mutants of "Salmonella typhimurium" and "Salmonella minnesota" in relation to their physiochemical surface properties, Cell Biophys., 2:177.

Kopperschläger, G., Lorenz, G., and Usbeck, E., 1983, Application of affinity partitioning in aqueous two-phase systems to the investigation of triazine dye-enzyme interactions, J. Chrom., 259:97.

Kula, M. R., Kroner, K. H., and Hustedt, H., 1982, Purification of enzymes by liquid-liquid extraction, in: "Advances in Biochemical Engineering," A. Fiechter ed., Springer-Verlag, Berlin, p. 73.

Matiasson, B., 1983, Applications of aqueous two-phase systems in biotechnology, Trends in Biotechnology, 1:16.

Malström, P., Nelson, K., Jönsson, A., Sjögren, H. O., Walter, H., and Albertsson, P. Å., 1978, Separation of rat leukocytes by countercurrent distribution in aqueous two-phase systems I. Characterization of subpopulations of cells, Cell. Immunol., 37:409.

Malström, P., Jönsson, A., Hallberg, T., and Sjögren, H. O., 1980, Countercurrent distribution of lymphocytes from human peripheral blood in aqueous two-phase systems. I. Separation into subsets of lymphocytes bearing distinctive markers, Cell Immunol., 53:39.

McKay, G. D. M., and Mason, S. G., 1963, The gravity approach and coalescence of fluid drops at liquid interfaces, Can. J. Chem. Eng., 41:203.

Michalski, J. P., Razandi, M., McCombs, C. C., and Walter, H., 1983, Surface properties of lymphocyte subpopulations in autoimmune NZB/NZW F1 hybrid mice: Alterations correlated with the immunodeficiency of aging, Clin. Immunol. Immunopathol., 29:15.

Miner, K. M., Walter, H., and Nicolson, G. L., 1981, Subfraction of malignant variants of metastatic murine lymphosarcoma cells by countercurrent distribution in two polymer aqueous phases, Biochemistry, 20:6244.

Müller, W., 1985, Partitioning of nucleic acids, in: Walter, Brooks, and Fisher, 1985, p.227.
Müller, W., and Kütemeier, G., 1982, Size fractionations of DNA fragments ranging from 20 to 30,000 base pairs by liquid/liquid chromatography, Eur. J. Biochem., 128:231.
Pettijohn, D. E., 1967, A study of partially devatured DNA, protein-DNA complexes in the polyethylene glycol-dextran phase system, Eur. J. Biochem., 3:25.
Poste, G., Doll, J., and Fidler, I. J., 1981, Interactions among clonal subpopulations affect stability of the metastatic phenotype in polyclonal populations of B16 melanoma cells, Proc. Nat. Acad. Sci., US, 78:6226.
Reitherman, R., Flanagan, S. D., and Barondes, S. H., 1973, Electromotive phenomena in the partition of erythrocytes in aqueous polymer two phase systems, Biochim. Biophys. Acta, 297:193.
Schürch, S., Gerson, D. F., and McIver, D. J. L., 1981, Determination of cell/medium interfacial tensions from contact angles in aqueous polymer systems. Biochim. Biophys. Acta, 640:557.
Shanbhag, V. P. and Johansson, G., 1974, Specific extraction of human serum albumin by partition in aqueous biphasic systems containing poly(ethylene glycol)-bound ligand, Biochem. Biophys. Res. Commun., 61:1141.
Sharp, K. A., 1985, Ph.D. Thesis, University of Britsh Columbia, Vancouver.
Sharp, K. A., Yalpani, M., Howard, S. J., and Brooks, D. E., 1986, Synthesis and application of a poly(ethylene glycol) antibody affinity ligand for cell separations in aqueous polymer two-phase systems, Anal. Biochem., 154:110.
Sharp, K. A., Brooks, D. E., Van Alstine, J. M., and Bamberger, S., 1987, Mechanisms of cell partition in aqueous polymer two-phase systems, Biophys. J., submitted.
Snyder, R. S., 1986, Separation techniques, in: B. Feuerbacher, R. Naumann, and H. Hamacher, p. 465.
Van Alstine, J. M., and Brooks, D. E., 1983, Cell membrane abnormality detected in erythrocytes from multiple sclerosis patients by partition in two-polymer aqueous-phase systems, Clin. Chem., 30:441.
Van Alstine, J. M., Harris, J. M., Snyder, S., Curreri, P. A., Bamberger, S., and Brooks, D. E., 1984, Separation of aqueous two-phase polymer systems in microgravity, in: Proceedings of the 5th European Symposium on Material Sciences Under Microgravity, European Space Agency Publication SP-222, p. 309.
Van Alstine, J. M., Karr, L. J., Snyder, R. S., and Harris, J. M., 1985, Cell separation with countercurrent chromatography and thin-layer countercurrent distribution in aqueous two-phase systems, J. Liq. Chrom., 8:2293.
Van Alstine, J. M., Sharp, K. A., and Brooks, D. E., 1986a, Critical micelle concentration dependence on head group size in polyoxyethylene nonionic surfactants, Colloids Surf., 17:115.
Van Alstine, J. M., Sorensen, P., Webber, T. J., Greig, R., Poste, G., and Brooks, D. E., 1986b, Heterogeneity in the surface properties of B16 melanoma cells from sublines with differing metastatic potential detected via two-polymer aqueous-phase partition, Exptl. Cell Res., 164:366.
Van Alstine, J. M., Trust, J., and Brooks, D. E., 1986c, Differential partition of virulent "Aeromonas salmonicida" and attenuated derivatives possessing specific cell surface alterations in polymer aqueous phase systems, Appl. Environ. Microbi., 51:1309.
Walter, H., 1985, Surface properties of cells reflected by partitioning: Red blood cells as a model, in: Walter, Brooks, and Fisher, 1985, p. 328.

Walter, H., Miller, A., Krob, E. S., and Ascher, G. S., 1971, Alterations in membrane surface properties of reticulocytes during maturation as determined by partition in two polymer aqueous phase systems, Exptl. Cell Res., 69:416.

Walter, H., Sasakawa, S., and Albertsson, P. A., 1972, Cross partition of proteins. Effect of ionic composition and concentration, Biochemistry, 11:3880.

Walter, H., Krob, E. J., and Brooks, D. E., 1976a, Membrane surface properties other than charge involved in cell separation by partition in polymer, aqueous two-phase systems, Biochemistry, 15:2959.

Walter, H., Krob, E. S., and Tung, R., 1976b, Hydrophobic affinity partition in aqueous two-phase systems of erythrocytes from different species. Systems containing polyethylene glycol-palmitate, Exptl. Cell Res., 102:14.

Walter, H., Moncla, B. J. Webber, T. J., and Nagaya, H., 1979, Membrane charge-associated heterogeneity of B-lymphocytes from human peripheral blood as reflected by cell partition in two-polymer aqueous phases, Exptl. Cell Res., 122:380.

Walter, H., Graham, L. L. Krob, E. G., and Hill, M., 1980, Correlation between phagocytic and membrane surface properties reflected by partitioning of human blood monocytes in two polmer aqueous phases, Biochim. Biophys. Acta., 602:309.

Walter, H., Brooks, D. E., and Fisher, D., 1985, "Partitioning in Aqueous Two-Phase Systems. Theory, Methods, Uses and Applications to Biotechnology," Academic Press, New York.

Walter, H., Krob, E. J., Pedram, A., Tamblyn, C. H., and Seaman, G.V.F., 1986, Effect of surface modification of rat erythrocytes of different ages on their partitioning behavior in charge-sensitive two-polymer aqueous phases, Biochim. Biophys. Acta, 860:650.

INDEX

GPSR Compliance

The European Union's (EU) General Product Safety Regulation (GPSR) is a set of rules that requires consumer products to be safe and our obligations to ensure this.

If you have any concerns about our products, you can contact us on ProductSafety@springernature.com

In case Publisher is established outside the EU, the EU authorized representative is:

Springer Nature Customer Service Center GmbH
Europaplatz 3
69115 Heidelberg, Germany

Batch number: 10684222

Printed by Printforce, the Netherlands